SNPBit Compe

Overviews, Culled Research, Pathway Drawings, and Our Two Cents

Featuring:
- Phase I and II Liver Detox SNPs
- Methylation SNPs
- Alcohol SNPs
- Histamine SNPs
- Neurotransmitter SNPs
- Mitochondrial SNPs

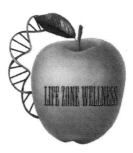

Compiled by Cynthia Smith, BSEE, JD
With contributions by Sterling Hill Erdei and Carolyn Ledowsky, ND
Life Zone Wellness, LLC.
Chicago, Illinois

SNPBit Compendium I

By Cynthia Smith, et. al.

Please credit use of graphics and flowcharts to this publication and/or to Life Zone Wellness, LLC. Any part of this document that is reproduced or transmitted in any form or by any means, electronic, mechanical, photocopying, recording, or otherwise, must be cited/referenced to the appropriate source as noted in this book.

First Printing, 2015

ISBN-10: 1517447275

ISBN-13: 978-1517447274

Life Zone Wellness, LLC.

116 W. Illinois St.

Suite 6W

Chicago, Illinois 60654

www.LifeZoneWellness.com

10 9 8 7 6 5 4 3 2

Contents

Introduction ix

Chapter 1 – Single Nucleotide Polymorphisms (SNPs) 1

- Section 1.1 - What is an SNP 1
  - Section 1.1.a - What is a Variant Report? 1
  - Section 1.1.b - Details about SNPs 2
  - Section 1.1.c - Why the interest in methylation SNPs? 4
  - Section 1.1.d – A few more details 5
    - Section 1.2 - The epigenome 6
    - FIGURE 1 – The epigenome 9

Chapter 2 – Liver Detoxification 10

- Section 2.1 - Review of liver detoxification basic 10
  - FIGURE 2 – Phase I & II liver detox 11
- Section 2.2 - Phase I detoxification (cytochrome P450 family) 12
  - Section 2.2.1 - The CYP1** Family 15
    - CYP1A1 16
    - CYP1A2 19
    - CYP1B1 21
      - FIGURE 3 – Hormone schematic 25
  - Section 2.2.2 - The CYP2** Family 26
    - CYP2A6 26
    - CYP2B6 28
    - CYP2C9 31
    - CYP2C19 34
    - CYP2D6 37
    - CYP2E1 44
  - Section 2.2.3 - The CYP3** Family 46
    - CYP3A4 46
    - CYP3A5 55
  - Section 2.2.4 - The CYP4** Family 58
    - CYP4A11 58
  - Section 2.2.5 – SNPs related to phase I detoxification 59
    - HFE 59

- PON1 62
- RAB6B related to HFE 64
- SOD3 65
- Section 2.3 - Phase II detoxification 67
  - Section 2.3.1 – Glutathione conjugation SNPs 68
    - GGT1 69
    - GPX3 72
    - GSR 74
    - GSS 76
    - GSTM1 78
    - GSTM3 80
    - GSTP1 81
  - Section 2.3.2 – Acetylation SNPs 84
    - NAT1 85
    - NAT2 86
  - Section 2.3.3 – Glucuronidation SNPs 89
    - UGT1A1 90
    - UGT2A1, UGT2A2 93
  - Section 2.3.4 – Peptide conjugation – glycine/ taurine 94
    - Section 2.3.4.1 – Glycine peptide conjugation 94
    - Section 2.3.4.2 – Taurine peptide conjugation 94
  - Section 2.3.5 - Sulfation SNPs 95
    - SULT1C3 96
    - SULT2A1 97
  - Section 2.3.6 – Methylation 98
  - Section 2.3.6.1 Methylation figures 99
    - FIGURE 4 – Folate & methionine/homocysteine pathway 99
    - FIGURE 5 – Trans-sulfuration pathway 100
    - FIGURE 6 – Neurotransmitter pathway 101
    - FIGURE 7 – Glutamate/GABA 102
    - FIGURE 8 – Mitochondria – electron transport chain 103
  - Section 2.3.6.2 – Methylation SNPs 103
    - ACAT1 103
    - ACE 106
    - ADA 109
    - ADD1 112

- ADK 113
- AGT 115
- AHCY 117
- AMT 118
- BHMT 119
- CBS 122
- CSAD 125
- CTH 126
- COMT 128
    - FIGURE 9 – COMT 134
- DHFR 134
- DMDGH 136
- FOLR1 137
- FOLR2 139
- FOLR3 140
- GAD1 141
- GAMT 144
- GCSH 146
- GGH 147
- MAT1A 149
- MAT2A 151
- MAT2B 152
- MAOA 154
- MAOB 156
- MMAB 158
- MTHFD1 159
- MTHFD1L 161
- MTHFD2 163
- MTHFR 164
- MTHFS 171
- MTR 172
- MTRR 173
- MUT 177
- NOS1 179
- NOS2 182
- NOS3 185

- PEMT 187
- SHMT1 189
- SLC19A1 191
- SPR 192
- SUOX 193
- TCN1 195
- TCN2 196
- TYMS 197
- VDR Bsm 199
- Section 2.3.6.3 – Other SNPs related to methylation 201
  - DAO 201
  - FUT2 205
  - HDC 209
  - HNMT 210
  - HRH1 212
  - HRH4 215
- Section 2.3.7 – Related to liver detox 217
- Section 2.3.7.1 – Figures related to liver detox 217
  - FIGURE 10 – Yeast/alcohol pathway 217
  - FIGURE 11 – Alcohol breakdown pathway 218
- Section 2.3.7.2 – SNPs related to liver detox 219
  - ADH1B 219
  - ALDH2 220
  - ALDH3A2 222
  - ADP1 224
  - ACAT1 226
  - APOC3 228
  - CAT 230
  - G6PD 233
  - MPO 238
  - NQO1 240

Chapter 3 – Neurotransmitters 242

- Section 3.1 – Neurotransmitter pathway 242
  - Figures related to neurotransmitter pathway 242
    - FIGURE 6 – Neurotransmitter pathway (repeated) 242

- FIGURE 9 – COMT (repeated) 243
- Section 3.2 – Neurotransmitter SNPs 244
    - AANAT 244
    - ADH1B 245
    - ALDH2 246
    - ALDH3A2 246
    - ANK3 247
    - ANKK1 250
    - CACNA1C 251
    - COMT 253
    - CSAD 254
    - DBH 255
    - DDC 257
    - DHFR 260
    - DISC1 260
    - DRD1 264
    - DRD2 268
    - DRD3 274
    - DRD4 276
    - GAD1 279
    - GCH1 279
    - HRT2A 282
    - MAOA 286
    - MAOB 287
    - NOS1 287
    - NOS2 288
    - NOS3 288
    - PAH 288
    - PEMT 291
    - PNMT 291
    - SLC6A2 292
    - SLC6A3 294
    - SLC6A4 297
    - TH 299
    - TPH1/TPH2 303

- Section 3.2.1 - Other SNPs related to neurotransmitters 304
    - DTNBP1 304
    - IDO1 308

Chapter 4 – Mitochondria – Electron Transport Chain (ETC) 311

- Section 4.1 – Review of mitochondria basics 311
    - FIGURE 8 – Mitochondria (repeated) 312
- Section 4.2 – Mitochondria SNPs 312
    - Section 4.2.1 – Mitochondria SNPs- complex I 313
        - NDUFS3 313
        - NDUFS7 314
        - NDUFS8 316
    - Section 4.2.2 – Mitochondria SNPs– complex III 316
        - UQCRC2 316
    - Section 4.2.3 – Mitochondria SNPs- complex IV 317
        - COX5A 317
        - COX6C 318
    - Section 4.2.4 – Mitochondria SNPs- complex V 319
        - ATP5c1 319
        - ATP5g3 320

Chapter 5 – My Favorite Books 322

Introduction

Over the past few years, Sterling and I have researched and compiled data that is the basis for Compendium I. In addition, much time was spent learning and drawing the included pathways. Carolyn, a Naturopathic Doctor (ND) with a large practice in Sydney, Australia assisted with some of the research and her clinical inputs. It has been a labor of love for all of us, prompted by our desire to provide information to those who are attempting to understand SNPs and their application, but without the hassle of researching each individual SNP. For those wishing to dig deeper without the guesswork of determining trustworthy sources, we have included relevant citations corresponding to the research we culled from various sources.

In a nutshell, this compilation includes phase I and II liver detoxification SNPs (detox SNPs), neurotransmitter SNPs, and mitochondrial SNPs (e.g., electron transport chain). Phase II detox SNPs are further broken down by their categories, including methylation. Alcohol metabolism SNPs and histamine metabolism SNPs are also included.

Most immune and other assorted SNPs will be included in SNPBit Compendium II, currently in the works. I intend to combine the best practices for GI health, in light of immune system SNPs and GI-related SNPs (e.g., FUT2). Like SNPBit Compendium I, SNPBit Compendium II will include logically grouped SNPs and will closely track to, "Sterling's App", found at http://www.MTHFRsupport.com. Sections will be broken down into SNPs associated with particular autoimmune conditions such as RA, Crohns, MS, and others. SNPBit Compendium II will also include GI repair protocols, clinical pearls, and 'Our Two Cents', as the GI and immune systems are intertwined.

For each SNP entry in Compendium 1, we have included a quick overview, a cited research section, and a data section which includes entries such as catalytic activity (e.g., 2 glutathione + H_2O_2 = glutathione disulfide + 2 H_2O), cofactors, molecular function, and biological processes. Where applicable, we have also included clinical pearls and what I call, 'Our Two Cents', which is based on our collective clinical experience, with the understanding that Sterling and I are NOT MDs. We have worked with hundreds of folks to interpret their variant reports in light of their health history and, in some cases, clinical data.

In this edition, the phase I detox section includes the CYP450 SNPs, plus a small group of SNPs that directly impacts phase I detox, but are not CYP450 enzymes. As an example, because heme is a center molecule of the CYP450 enzymes, HFE SNPs are included in the "OTHER" subsection under the phase I detox.

The phase II detox SNP section is extensive. Included are SNPs categorized by the six high-level pathways of phase II including; glutathione conjugation, acetylation, glucaronidation, amino acid (peptide) conjugation, sulfation, and methylation. As you can imagine, the methylation section alone is quite extensive, so it is further broken down into individual SNPs, including a category of methylation-related SNPs. In addition, some of the pathways associated with methylation are intimately tied to neurotransmitter production and breakdown, so some neurotransmitter SNP write-ups will be included in the methylation section, and listed again in the neurotransmitter section as a quick overview with a reference to the appropriate page number in the methylation section.

The pathway drawings were created by myself using an app called, "Pages", which is not very user friendly. Please forgive the crudeness of the drawings. It is my hope that SNPBits Compendium II will include professionally prepared drawings.

A few thoughts—

SNPs are an important tool for identifying the potential for, or the underpinnings of, chronic conditions. A combination of the variant report of SNPs, a comprehensive health history, and medical/health data is very powerful when determining and addressing (un)health issues. As such, this reference is not to be used as a solo diagnostic tool. Rather, its purpose is to assist in your understanding of enzyme, carrier protein, and receptor function - coded by your DNA. Lifestyle choices, food choices, and exposures (e.g., viruses, toxins, etc) are important as well.

It is also worth noting that enzymatic malfunction may not be due to SNPs, but may instead be due to lack of nutrient cofactors needed for optimal enzymatic function. Where possible, I have included nutrient cofactors for each of the SNPs. Besides vitamins and minerals, these nutrient cofactors also include enzymatic outputs such as those from intermediary steps of the Krebs cycle, phospholipid derivatives, and much more. A word of caution: It is important to address all enzymatic pathways, in the proper order, and not initially jump on the 5MTHF and methyl-B12 supplement bandwagons.

The three of us have collectively added our two cents, based on our clinical experience. 'Our Two Cents' does not override your physician's suggestions, but we wanted to share our clinical experience. Where you see, 'Our Two Cents', please understand that it is our anecdotal observation and NOT medical advice. We do understand liability and what is involved when going out on a limb and as such, we have chosen to share our experiences with the knowledge and understanding that it is our two cents and is not based on double-placebo testing.

In the past, I was an electrical engineer. For twelve years, I worked in aerospace and radio frequency (RF). After that, I was an Intellectual Property (IP) attorney for ten years, writing patents in the radio frequency and cellular technology fields at Motorola™ and law firms. Between the years in the RF and cell phone business and telecommunications law classes, I came to recognize that there may be health risks associated with constant exposure to high frequency electrical signals and their resulting perpendicular magnetic waves. Since the early 1990's we have been increasingly exposed to these signals in our daily lives; a grand experiment. As they can negatively impact some, please consider your exposures to transmitting devices as one aspect of health.

After leaving the corporate world, I went back to school to re-tool with a focus on health. My first stop was PCOM to study Chinese Medicine, then other classes followed in the health and nutritional area. Like many others who take this path, my original goal was to gain an understanding of my health issues and my family's health issue, particularly my mother who struggled life-long with depression. My interest shifted to genetics after I viewed a NOVA special called, "Ghosts in Your Genes". Subsequent to that viewing, I left PCOM after investing two years and began focusing on nutrition and genetics for the next 5 years, taking classes via the Institute of Functional Medicine, basics at the local community college, Poliquin, Nutraceutical companies, and many more. I also prepped for the Certified Clinical Nutritionist exam, including the Post Graduate Studies in Clinical Nutrition. I digress…

To get back to the contents of this book and how to use it, we suggest being mindful of the basics; GI/liver support, addressing HPATG axis issues, including insulin modulation, and addressing neurotransmitter imbalances. Once again, please do not simply focus on MTHFR/MTRR SNPs by first administering a 5MTHF/methyl-B12 combo supplement. In most cases, administering 5MTHF is often a last step AFTER the basics are addressed and other nutrients are repleted; for example, replete vitamins B-1, B-2, and B-3 for Krebs cycle function.

DO NOT TREAT SNPs in a vacuum. A comprehensive health history and testing from companies like, SpectraCell, Genova Diagnostics, DDI, Great Plains, Precision Analytical, and others, will provide additional data regarding biochemical pathway function. That data, plus health history and SNPs inform how enzymes, carrier proteins, and receptors are functioning in real time, given the environment in which they work.

Although enzyme function, carrier protein function, and receptor function <u>may</u> be adversely impacted by SNPs, their function <u>may also</u> be adversely impacted by lack of availability of nutrient cofactors, either due to poor diet and/or poor assimilation of food. As an example, poor gallbladder function and fat-soluble nutrient assimilation may be attributed to sludgy bile due to SNPs in BHMT, PEMT, MAT1, COMT and/ or SULT, or may be attributed to a less than robust gallbladder response due to hypochlorhydria from hypothyroidism or PPIs, etc. Similarly, high homocysteine from low levels of B-12 could be due to SNPs in TCN 1 and/or 2 required to transport B-12 in blood, low folate conversions via DHFR, MTHFD1 and/or MTHFR, or could be due to an ongoing autoimmune attack on intrinsic factor, required to carry B-12 through the intestine.

For a sound approach on combining SNP knowledge with functional medicine principles, please check out our two-day class that was held in Philadelphia in January 2015. Links to the class can be found at http://www.MABIM.org. You can also access our series of webinars at http://www.MTHFRsupport.com.au/product/snp-learning-masterclass/.

One last note; with pathways in mind, when looking at analytes from testing and/or SNP profiles, note their relationship to each other and their nutrient cofactors. Layer-in that knowledge with health history and a timeline of health issues, sibling health, and parent health. All of that data combined with SNPs can provide a powerful tool. Yes, draw an actual timeline with dates (birth through today's date) on a piece of paper and populate it with relevant data, including the last time wellness was experienced.

There is typically a relevant timeframe event(s) that precedes declining health. Sometimes it is as simple as identifying an increase, swing, or liver breakdown issue of steroid sex hormones (such as puberty, introduction of BCPs, post-partum, peri-menopause, etc.). Other times, it could follow a concussion, introduction of a food, exposure to a chemical, a move to a moldy house, a tick bite, a stressful situation such as a divorce, and more. It is best to figure out the environment and potential trigger(s) that came before a person's decline in health, in light of SNPs. Again, do not treat SNPs in a vacuum.

This SNPBit Compendium I will be updated and re-released with edits over the course of time, depending on research and new information.

We welcome any feedback to improve and/or update the contents. Please contact me at c.smith@lifezonewellness.com with research-supported additions, deletions, or updates.

Our intention is to build a community of folks who understand that knowledge of our individual genetics is our right to use, to empower our health and lifestyle choices. We also want to ensure that our individual genetics will not be corralled or controlled by big entities for a price, nor used against us if Big Whatever controls access to the data.

— Cynthia Smith 2015

The Internet addresses given in this compendium were accurate at the time it went to press.

The SNPs and their rs numbers given in this compendium were reflective of Sterling's App at the time it went to press. Over time, additional rs numbers may be added to Sterling's App.

Reference to specific organizations, companies and authorities in this compendium does not imply endorsement by the author, contributors, nor does mention of specific organizations, companies and authorities imply that they endorse this book, its author or contributors.

This compendium is intended as a reference for single nucleotide polymorphisms, and not as a medical book. The information herein is not intended as a substitute for testing suggested by, or treatment that may have been prescribed by, your physician. If you suspect that you have a medical problem, we urge you to seek competent medical assistance.

This Page Intentionally Left Blank

Chapter 1

Single Nucleotide Polymorphisms (SNPs)

Section 1.1 - What is an SNP?

The acronym "SNP" stands for, *single nucleotide polymorphism*. It is not a snip of DNA; rather it is a swap of a single nucleotide on one of the "rungs" of the DNA "ladder".

An SNP occurs when a single nucleotide differs from the majority (wild type is considered the "normal" expected nucleotide).

SNPs occurred during evolution; some granted protection at the time they occurred and were propagated to the subsequent generations. Now, they may be adversely impacting us in today's environment. Neanderthal HLA SNPs are one such example.

SNPs occur in coding regions, non-coding regions, or between genes (intergenic). We look at the coding regions.

SNPs vary in terms of severity and benefit due to location and redundancy. Our bodies typically have back-up pathways for redundancy, but they are not as good as the primary pathways. For example, estrogen breakdown via the phase II liver sulfation pathway is backed-up by the phase II liver glucuronidation pathway. The sulfation (SULT SNPs can affect) pathway can accept a larger variety of intermediate metabolites, but will defer to the glucuronidation pathway when it gets overwhelmed, so both need to be working optimally.

Although some are directly impactful (e.g., CBS C699T, COMT), mos SNPs do NOT govern genetic expression alone. Diet and lifestyle do.

SNPs may cause gene instability due to decreased cofactor affinity. A cofactor may be a vitamin, a mineral, or a byproduct of biochemical pathway processing (e.g., Krebs -> NADH).

SNPs may be by-passed by increasing cofactor concentration and/or providing end products directly. For instance, if you have an MTHFR C677T down-regulation, you can "bypass" the down-regulation via delivery of 5 MTHF (folate) as a supplement. Because the biochemical pathways interconnect, if one SNP is addressed in isolation, other pathways can destablize. For example, if a high dose of 5-MTHF (e.g., Deplin) is taken without considering neighboring SNPs/enzymes, 5MTHF supplementation may result in increased energy for a few days, then fatigue, and/or increased anxiety as, for example, epinephrine increases.

Section 1.1.a - What is a Variant Report?

A variant report is a listing of single nucleotide polymorphisms (SNPs), derived from the raw data results of "23andMe" saliva testing and generated via a software application (app). The most comprehensive and well-researched variant report can be obtained at, www.MTHFRsupport.com, using "Sterling's App". The variant report is organized into groups of SNPs, including phase I and phase II liver detoxification SNPs, IgE, IgA, and IgG SNPs, methylation SNPs, mitochondrial electron transport chain SNPs, and others. The variant report also includes biochemical pathway drawings and will be updated over time.

Section 1.1.b - Details about SNPs:

Each SNP is associated with an "rs" number (e.g., rs4880), which represents a particular location (rung) on the DNA genome (ladder). Using the ladder analogy, a consecutive series of rungs provides a blueprint, or code, for generating a particular polypeptide (e.g., protein or enzyme). For example, the well-known MTHFR enzyme, encoded using a length of the DNA genome equivalent to thousands of rungs of the ladder, is copied, and subsequently used as the blueprint for building the MTHFR enzyme outside of the nucleus.

There are coding and non-coding parts (possibly signaling the coding portions) of the DNA genome. The segments that code, versus the segments that do not, partially depend on the addition/deletion of a methyl group (think of the Great Oz, toggling segments of the DNA on and off with a CH3 molecule referred to as a methyl group) and histone winding (think garden hose wrapped/unwrapped around a portion of the DNA to "uncover or cover it up" for copying). Our diets, environment, and habits affect toggling on/off via methyl groups and histone winding/unwinding of our DNA via our "Epigenome".

The DNA is subsequently expressed as a "phenotype" after it is copied and is used to build enzymes, receptors, carrier proteins, and other polypeptides, which run our biochemical machinery.

The DNA genome is safely protected in the nucleus of each cell, where it remains as the blueprint for generating all polypeptides used in our body's biochemical pathways. DNA is a nucleic acid made up of nucleotides, where each nucleotide includes a nucleobase, deoxyribose (a pentose sugar) and a phosphate group. The nucleobases can be one of four possibilities; adenine "A", guanine "G", cytosine "C" or thymine "T". Going back to our ladder analogy, there are two nucleotides per ladder rung. Cytosine pairs with a guanine, while thymidine pairs with an adenine. It is a bit like a binary system of "I's" and "0's". Cytosine should pair with guanine, and thymidine should pair with adenine.

Day in and day out, messenger RNA moves into the nucleus, copies an "untwisted", unzipped segment (DNA unzips down the middle, lengthwise to produce two linear sequence of complementary nucleotides A, C, G, and T) of the ladder, and carries a copied portion out of the nucleus. The copied portion is then transported to its destination– a ribosome (part of assembly machinery) by mRNA. There are stop/start segments of DNA to signal where one enzyme blueprint starts and stops.

The ribosome assists in selecting amino acids (beads), where three linear sequential nucleotides translate/code into one amino acid. For example, if the three sequential nucleotides are G, G, T, then the resulting amino acid "bead" selected is glycine. If the next three sequential nucleotides are T, C, T, then the ribosomal machinery selects a serine amino acid (next bead). Recall that the amino acids are derived from protein foods we eat, which in turn, depend on our GI's ability to assimilated and digest them (GI health).

Through a series of complicated steps, the selected amino acids are strung together to form the polypeptide chain (necklace). If all goes well, a perfect polypeptide is formed, and that polypeptide does its thing as an enzyme (e.g., methylenetetrahydrofolate reductase or the MTHFR enzyme), carrier protein, or receptor (e.g., DRD - dopamine receptor). However, if an incorrect nucleotide (SNP) translates into an incorrect amino acid (bead) selection, then the resulting enzyme, receptor, or carrier protein function may not be optimal. The non-optimal function may be the result of an SNP in the DNA, which may change shape at a critical location on the enzyme. This could, in turn, result in an impaired cofactor affinity for a vitamin or mineral that is needed for its operation or could result in impairment of a docking site. If you google a particular enzyme, you will see that it looks like a ribbon (I analogized it to a beaded necklace) with curls and bends and docking sites for cofactors such as, magnesium, vitamin B-6, etc. Some of the curls and bends and docking sites are critical to its function, hence selection of researched SNP rs numbers.

As I mentioned earlier, the function of an "SNP-free generated" enzyme, receptor, or carrier protein function can be impaired by a simple lack of the nutrient cofactor. The co-factors are primarily B vitamins, minerals including lithium for vitamin B-12 transport, and output products from the Krebs cycle. The Krebs cycle is highly dependent on sufficient vitamin B-1, B-2, and B-3 and the ability to utilize fatty acids, amino acids and glucose. Similarly, the function of an "SNP-free generated" enzyme, receptor, or carrier protein function can be impaired by the presence of toxins, heavy metals, and chemicals, to name a few. Therefore, in addition to looking at SNPs, it is equally important to evaluate nutrient cofactors, toxins, heavy metals, and other things that influence enzymatic function.

Getting back to details about SNPs…Despite an incorrect amino acid selection due to an SNP in the DNA, the resulting polypeptide, with its alteration, is still utilized in its biochemical pathway to convert A into B. Due to the shape alteration, the conversion may be compromised; like a key that is not quite right for a particular lock, but with a bit of jiggling still works.

Returning to our MTHFR enzyme example where its job is to convert molecule A to molecule B, "A" would be *5,10 Methyl THF* and "B" would be *5- MTHF*. In the case of a C677T MTHFR SNP, the conversion of *5,10 Methyl THF* and "B" to *5- MTHF* would be slowed.

If the MTHFR SNP comes from one parent, it operates at a slower speed in its conversion of *5,10 Methyl THF* to *5- MTHF*, and is referred to as a heterozygous SNP (yellow). If the same SNP (nucleotide swap) comes from each parent, the resulting enzyme works even slower and is referred to as a homozygous SNP (red).

Expanding our MTHFR example, at location rs1801133 (rung) of the DNA genome, or position 677 of the MTHFR-encoding portion of DNA, one expects to find two cytosine (C) nucleotides. However, if one of the cytosine nucleotides has been replaced by a thymine (T), the SNP ("swap") is referred to as, a <u>MTHFR C677T</u> heterozygous SNP, and will reduce associated MTHFR enzymatic activity by twenty to thirty percent. If however, both of the cytosine nucleotides have been replaced by thymine, the SNP is referred to as, <u>MTHFR C677T</u> homozygous SNP, and will reduce associated MTHFR activity by as much as sixty percent. As a result, a person with an MTHFR C677T hetero- or homozygous SNP will have a decreased ability to convert 5,10-methylenetetrahydrofolate (substrate **A**) to 5-methyltetrahydrofolate (product **B**).

In layman's terms, a MTHFR SNP means that there may be poor conversion of dietary synthetic folic acid or folate to its usable form, 5-methyltetrahydrofolate. In that case, supplements that contain synthetic folic acid are not your friend. 5-methyltetrahydrofolate is one of the enzymes in methylation pathways required for serotonin and dopamine generation and conversion of homocysteine to methionine and subsequent SAMe generation, to name a few. DHFR and MTHFD1 are also in direct line between folic acid and MTHFR, so their function must also be considered with respect to ones ability to convert folic acid into 5-methyltetrahydrofolate.

Section 1.1.c - Why the interest in methylation SNPs?

There are many functions that require methylation:
1. Turn on and off genes (gene regulation via CH3).
2. Process chemicals, endogenous, and xenobiotic compounds (biotransformation via phase II liver clearing, especially estrogen and heavy metals).
3. Build neurotransmitters (dopamine-> norepinephrine à epinephrine, serotonin à melatonin). If one has neurotransmitter issues, then looking at methylation pathway genetics and lifestyle are key.
4. Metabolize/breakdown neurotransmitters (dopamine, epinephrine).
5. Build immune cells (T-cells, NK cells).
6. Build DNA "bits and pieces" and histone synthesis (thymine aka, 5-methyluracil).
7. Produce energy (CoQ10, carnitine, creatine, ATP via Krebs cycle).
8. Produce protective coating on nerves (myelination).

9. Build and maintain cell membranes (via utilization of phosphatidylcholine derived from phosphatidylethanolamine in the presence of estrogen and functioning PEMT enzyme).

Section 1.1.d – A few more details:

A note about SAMe...methionine adenosyltransferase (MAT) catalyzes the synthesis of S-adenosylmethionine (SAMe) from methionine. SAMe is the "prize" after many enzymatic steps, including DHFR, MTHFD1, MTHFR, MTR, MTRR and BHMT, as it is our major biological methyl donor. All enzymes that have names ending with methyl transferase, or "MT", require SAMe as a methyl donor in order to function. A methyl group is simply one carbon atom with three hydrogen atoms attached to it.

There are about 200 enzymes that require a donation of a methyl group from SAMe in order to function. **MT enzymes include those responsible for neurotransmitter production and breakdown (e.g., COMT, PNMT), those that contribute to building muscle (e.g., GAMT), those that contribute to generating cell membranes (e.g., PEMT), and those that toggle DNA expression. In the event of a shortage of SAMe, methyl groups can be culled from other sources such as cell membranes (not ideal). SAMe supplementation however, is not always the solution.

- A cautionary example of when SAMe supplementation is not a first step - SNPs in one SAMe dependant enzyme, catecholamine-O-methyltransferase (COMT), are particularly impactful. There has been much research on the affects of SNPs in COMT V158M and COMT H62H. It is often noted that folks with homozygous SNPs in COMT V158M and COMT H62H tend to be more productive and focused, hard charging, creative, and sensitive as compared to others without, as their dopamine levels tend to run higher. You can often find blood relatives in their family tree that were brilliant, and/or a bit crazy and/or lived outside of the mainstream expectations of their time. The downside is that those same folks may be less capable of breaking down fight/flight neurotransmitters (e.g., epinepherine) and they may have a difficult time relaxing and sleeping. Their adrenals stress out easily as cortisol along with SAMe is required in the conversion from nor-epinepherine to epinepherine. However, large doses of SAMe or other direct methyl donors (e.g., methyl-B12) are not recommended, as they can indirectly provide the substrates needed for increased production of epinephrine; in other words, they push the excitatory neurotransmitter pathways when a slow COMT enzyme can't break them down in a timely manner. **(See FIG. 10)** Over time, as the sympathetic nervous system is chronically "on", the adrenal glands are chronically in overdrive until they become sluggish and burned-out (aka, adrenal fatigue), and circadian rhythm and sleep is adversely impacted. It is an intersection of cortisol and norepinephrine and SAMe that creates epinephrine (adrenaline=stress hormone) and it is COMT's job to break it down. In addition, thyroid function is often affected as as it is "downstream" from the adrenals (HPATG axis), and almost every cell in our body has a thyroid hormone receptor. Lack of ability to break down stress hormones takes its toll in the form of higher cancer, autoimmune issues, and heart disease rates. In women, some of the same COMT SNPs may affect their liver's ability to process estrogens, so they may have more extreme PMS symptoms, not do well on BCPs, and tend to feel increased anxiety when estrogen and fight/flight hormones (epinephrine) compete for the same down-regulated enzyme (COMT) to break them down in phase II liver detoxification. In men, these down-regulated enzymes may translate into early prostate issues. There is more specific info in subsequent chapters.

The bottom line is; first support pathways downstream from the folate pathway via a full spectrum of minerals, Krebs cycle support and all B vitamins, except for methylfolate and B-12, initially. Clean up and support the gut as those three to five pounds of gut bacteria and their byproducts do much to signal immune system and modulate neurotransmitter status (e.g., IDO). Address the HPATG axis, including insulin regulation. In some cases, supplementation with lithium orotate may be beneficial in assisting delivery of vitamn B-12 to cells via TCN1 and TCN2. When the foundational minerasl, B vitamins, and Krebs cycle support is in place, then potentially layer in appropriate B12 and methylfolate for methylation support. This is the tricky part and requires support from a practitioner to navigate, especially if one has a homozygous CBS C699T SNP, homoxygous COMT SNPs and/or chronic low vitamin B-6 levels.

Section 1.2 - The Epigenome

Let's shift gears and discuss what is going on with our children and grandchildren with respect to methylation and resulting metabolic issues that were once limited to older folks, but are now expressing in our children.

For those of us over 50 years of age, we would be hard-pressed to identify a childhood friend who was on the spectrum or who had an eating disorder. Now, we have children and grandchildren who have been diagnosed with some sort of neuro issue (e.g., autism spectrum, Aspergers, PANDAS, anorexia/bulimia, and more). Why is this happening when our genetics haven't changed?

The short answer is that our environment and exposures have changed; our epigenome interaction is affecting our gene expression, or phenotype. There is a layer between the outside world and our fixed nuclear DNA called the epigenome. The epigenome interface is capable of toggling segments of our fixed DNA on and off. The toggling is the result of outside influences. Glyphosates we ingest, discussed below, are one BIG example.

How? By way of the epigenome interface, our body's DNA express and subsequent enzyme activity is impacted by the outside world; our food choices where new proteins are introduced through the genetical modification of grains, high frequency electromagnetic waves (think WiFi), plastic byproducts (BPA), viruses, grains and livestock feed that has been saturated by herbicides, pesticides, and more.

It is worth mentioning that our protein biomass from eating cows, chickens, and farm-raised fish can be traced back to genetically modified corn and alfalfa. The corn and soy are genetically modified so that they are able to withstand being doused with organophosphates. Organophosphates are the basis of many insecticides, herbicides, and nerve agents. This includes glyphosates such as Roundup®.
http://www.naturescountrystore.com/roundup/page7.html.

Agent Orange, another herbicide used during the Vietnam War, has been directly linked to a higher incidence of type II diabetes in exposed veterans, birth defects in children born in those sprayed areas, and more.

We eat meat that comes from cows, which eat the genetically modified corn and alfalfa. We eat chicken, which eat the genetically modified corn. We eat fish from a fish farm, which has been fed protein pellets made from chicken parts where the chicken was fed genetically modified corn (See TED talk, How I Fell In Love with a Fish). How much of OUR biomass can be traced back to the same corn and soy and alfalfa, liberally sprayed by organophosphates? How much of these organophosphates are we ingesting through grains in general? What are the cumulative effects on us, via our epigenome, especially if we have a PON1 SNP (serum paraoxonase/arylesterase 1 enzyme responsible for hydrolysing/breaking-down insecticides)? Time is telling us.

In addition, recent research by Alessio Fasano, MD, suggests that besides influencing many systems of the body (e.g., immune system, neurotransmitters, etc.), our gut microbiome may exert influence on our genome, via epigenetics. Again, this is connected to our dietary choices as they dynamically influence our gut microbiome composition. Glyphosates negatively impact our gut microbiome just as they negatively impact the weeds for which they are intended to kill. The United States Patent and Trademark Office (USPTO) website discloses more than six thousand issued patents and published patent applications when you enter "glyphosates AND antimicrobial" in their search engine.

So the question is, by what mechanisms are our DNA segments being toggled on and off? Our DNA expression is toggled on/off by one of two mechanisms. The first method involves attaching a methyl group at a particular location on our DNA in response to outside influences via the epigenome interface. Subsequent copying of a particular segment of DNA that includes an attached methyl group (or a removed methyl group), will affect the resulting enzyme, receptor, or transport protein. The second method involves histone winding or unwinding (think garden hose wrapped tightly around a histone base) so that the wound segment can't be copied and therefore does not express. Alternatively, a segment of the DNA can be unwound and copied via the epigenetic interface. **(See FIG. 1)**

These epigenetic changes can travel with our DNA as we pass them along, generation after generation, by way of sperm and egg, to our offspring. We may now be seeing a cumulative effect, expressing in our children and grandchildren in the form of neuro-issues via GI issues. Similarly, we are seeing a cumulative effect in the form of metabolic disturbances in younger folks (e.g., type II diabetes) that heretofore were typically associated with aging. It is therefore imperative to eat clean, do our best to limit exposures to chemicals, and high frequency RF signals, lower stress, and address methylation enzymatic pathway deficits.

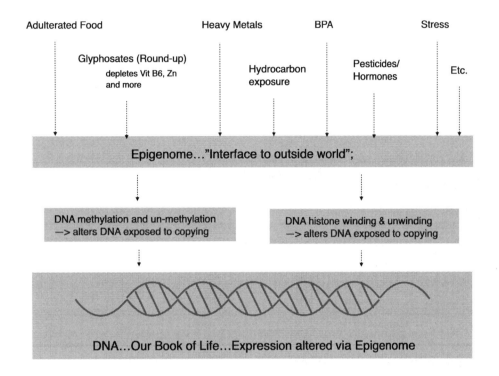

FIGURE 1 - Epigenome

Chapter 2

Liver Detoxification

Section 2.1 - Review of liver detoxification basics

Liver detoxification ("detox") enzymes can be segregated into two primary categories or phases; phase I detox enzymes and phase II detox enzymes.

Phase I detox enzymes include a class of enzymes referred to as, cytochrome P450 enzymes. Although there are dozens of cytochrome P450 enzymes, each cytochrome P450 enzyme performs one of (1) an oxidation reaction, (2) a reduction reaction, (3) a hydrolysis reaction, (4) a hydration reaction, or (5) a de-halogenation reaction. The phase I detox reactions convert a lipid-soluble (nonpolar) molecule, entering the liver, into a more water-soluble intermediary metabolite. The intermediary metabolite is then processed via phase II detox. **(See FIG. 2)** In some cases phase I alone, has the ability to clear the molecule (e.g., caffeine).

The lipid-soluble molecules, entering the liver for phase I detox include steroid hormones, fatty acids, and xenobiotics. Nutrient co-factors for phase II detox enzymes include one or more of B vitamins, glutathione, branch-chain amino acids (e.g., leucine, isoleucine, and valine), flavonoids, and phospholipids.

Phase II detox enzymes include many and carry out one of (1) a sulfation reaction, (2) a glucuronidation reaction, (3) a glutathione conjugation reaction, (4) an acetylation reaction, (5) an amino acid conjugation reaction, or (6) a methylation reaction, in order to convert an intermediary metabolite into an excretory derivative, which is a water-soluble (polar) molecule. The excretory derivative is either (a) passed via bile then feces, or (b) passed via serum to kidneys and urine, and excreted out of the body.

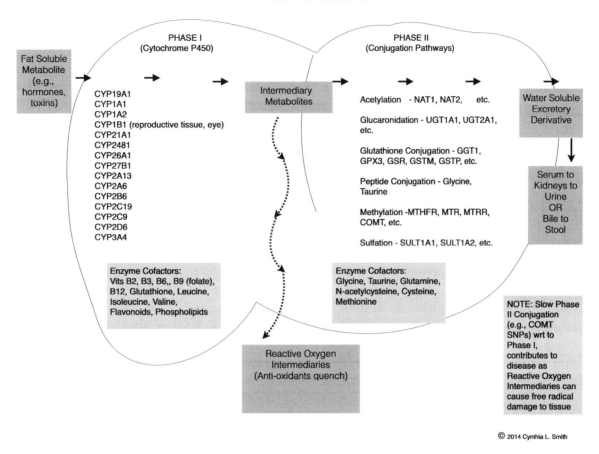

FIGURE 2 – Liver Detox

It should be noted that some intermediary metabolites leaving phase I detox have proven to be toxic over the long term; for example, 4 hydroxy estrones (e.g., 4 OH estrones) generated by CYP1B1. In that case, we want to encourage, through targeted nutritional intervention, quick processing of that intermediate metabolite, via phase II detox, into its non-toxic, water-soluble excretory derivative. For example, magnesium supports COMT function and is needed to convert the toxic 4 OH estrones into safe 4 methoxy-estrones on phase II liver detoxification.

During this process free radicals are produced which, if excessive, can damage the liver cells. Antioxidants reduce the damage caused by these free radicals. If antioxidants are lacking and toxin exposure is high, toxic chemicals become far more dangerous. Some may be converted from relatively harmless substances into potentially carcinogenic substances. Estrone to the intermediary metabolite, 4 OH estrone, is just one example.

Recall from Chapter 1, that the blueprint for making all of our phase I and II detox enzymes, are coded by our own DNA, protected inside of the nucleus of each cell.

As described in Chapter 1, if we analogize the DNA double helix to a ladder, then the nucleotide pairs are the rungs of the ladder. Discrete lengths of DNA, often thousands of nucleotide pairs (i.e., two nucleotides per ladder rung) long, correspond to a blueprint for subsequent manufacturing of a particular enzyme. This is because the sequence of consecutive nucleotides determines which amino acid is selected when building the particular enzyme at a ribosome (assembly plant) outside of the nucleus, but within the cell. Hence we look at potential nucleotide swaps on the DNA ladder rungs, otherwise know as SNPs.

So, for example, when you generate your variant report of SNPs, such as that generated by "Sterling's App", you are looking at a PDF of nucleotide status at particular rungs of the DNA ladder, subsequently associated with assembly of a particular enzyme, receptor, or carrier protein. The particular rungs (identified by "rs numbers") are selected based on extensive research. Some SNPs -> translated to amino acid choices, do not impact the resulting enzyme, receptor, or carrier protein shape/function in a meaningful way. Others do, and they are included in the variant report.

Some SNPs were passed to subsequent generations as a "benefit" to confer a protection based on the current environmental influences at the time the SNPs occurred. For example, sickle cell anemia is thought to confer "protection" from malaria, due to an SNP that induces an alteration in the gene encoding the beta chain of hemoglobin. Swaths of populations, including those whose ancestors were exposed to malaria, have sickle cell anemia in disproportionate percentages.

Section 2.2 - Phase 1 detoxification (cytochrome P450 family)

Susceptibility to toxicants is determined largely by a person's unique ability to biotransform, detoxify, and eliminate endogenous and exogenous toxins. This ability is primarily based on a person's genetic variations and gut microbiome and its DNA, interacting with lifestyle and diet.

A little background...hydrophilic (water soluble) toxins and compounds are excreted through urine and bile, while lipophilic (fat soluble) toxins and compounds are chemically altered into hydrophilic compounds before they can be excreted. Many of the toxic chemicals that enter the body are lipophilic, which means they dissolve only in fatty or oily solutions and not in water. So, for cellular biotransformation of lipophilic compounds, they are first bio-activated (functionalization...phase I detox) and then conjugated to become hydrophilic compounds (phase II detox). In between phase I and phase II detox, active intermediary compounds are generated. Some of the intermediary compounds are highly toxic themselves, so an up-regulation of enzymatic activity in phase I and/or a down-regulation of enzymatic activity in phase II detox, can result in increased build-up of highly toxic compounds. For optimal detoxification, the enzymatic "speed" of phase I and phase II detox should be relatively matched. By understanding whether an SNP is an up-regulation or down-regulation, and how nutrients, drugs, and other chemicals affect the speed of a particular enzyme, it is possible to encourage healthy detoxification, using nutrients such a sulforaphane, milk thistle, and other nutraceuticals.

Also, as most pharmaceuticals influence speed of CYPs in phase I detox, it is best to have an understanding of their affect and interactions with your SNPs. Pharmecogenomics (the interaction of your particular genes with a particular drug) will someday be as easy as a blood spot test prior to surgery or dispensing the drug. In the meantime, it is up to you to understand your personal phase I and II liver detoxification enzyme capabilities and how those capabilities may be affected by pharmaceuticals and other toxins, and vice versa. This will be discussed below.

Drug interactions and their affects on phase I and II clearing/neutralizing speeds, impact many folks, whether subtle or not. There are many Internet sources available for research to determine the impacts of this. I highly recommend doing the research to compare your SNPs and how they may impact clearing of pharmaceuticals to which yourself, your loved ones, or your clients may be exposed. PubMed is a good resource. Also, Wikipedia has some good charts for CYPs. Unitprot is another. Culled research and citations are included with each SNP discussion below. As an aside, many of the anesthesia drugs impact MTR and MTRR (slow them down), so a bit of vitamin B-12 before/after surgery may be warranted in some cases.

It should be noted that many tissues have some ability to detoxify, but phase I and II detoxification enzymes in the liver perform the majority of detoxification reactions. The GI tract, kidney, lungs, skin, and blood-brain barrier also have relatively high activity.

One or both detoxification phases can be inefficient or overloaded. A particularly damaging combination in an ill person is an excessive overload of toxins coming into phase I detox, with an inefficient phase II detox. In some cases this combination is believed to be one of the contributors of marked environmental sensitivities, drug intolerances and interactions that characterize many chronic fatigue and fibromyalgia patients.

Patients with underactive phase I detox may experience an intolerance to caffeine, perfumes, and other environmental chemicals, and an increased risk for liver disease, while those with an overactive system will be relatively unaffected by caffeine drinks. Additionally, inhibition of a CYP450 enzyme, referred to herein as a down-regulation, can increase blood levels of a drug or hormone. Caffeine is an example of a chemical directly neutralized by phase I detox. One way of objectively determining the activity of phase I detox of CYP1A2 is to measure how efficiently a person detoxifies caffeine. Using this test, a surprising fivefold difference in the detoxification rates of apparently healthy adult has been noted.

Substances that activate phase I detoxification:

- Drugs: alcohol; nicotine in cigarette smoke; phenobarbital; sulfonamides; steroids
- Foods: cabbage, broccoli, and brussel-sprouts; charcoal-broiled meats; high-protein diet; oranges and tangerines (but not grapefruits)
- Nutrients: niacin; vitamin B-1; vitamin C
- Herbs: caraway and dill seeds
- Environmental toxins: carbon tetrachloride; exhaust fumes; paint fumes; dioxin; pesticides

Grapefruit juice, which contains naringenin, slows down phase I enzyme activity (CYP3A4 in GI). It decreases the rate of elimination of some drugs (aka, clearing) from the blood and has been found to substantially alter their clinical activity and toxicity. Organic compounds that are furanocoumarin derivatives interfere with the hepatic and intestinal enzyme cytochrome P450 isoform CYP3A4, and are believed to be primarily responsible for the effects of grapefruit on the enzyme. Eight ounces of grapefruit juice contains enough of the furanocoumarin derivatives to decrease cytochrome P450 activity by a remarkable thirty percent. You will see recommendations to abstain from grapefruit juice in many of the package inserts for pharmaceuticals that utilize the CYP3A4 enzyme for their clearing.

After phase I detox, intermediary metabolites produced by phase I CYP450s, enter phase II detox where they are further acted upon by a process referred to as conjugation. In the conjugation pathway, the liver cells add/conjugate another substance (eg. cysteine, glycine, glutathione, taurine, a sulphur molecule, etc.) to a toxic chemical or drug intermediary metabolite, to render it less harmful. This makes the toxin or drug water-soluble, so it can then be excreted from the body via watery fluids such as bile or urine. There are essentially six phase II detox pathways. **(See Section 1.2 for more details on phase II detoxification)**

Switching gears back to glyphosate ready crops – glyphosates have been found to **suppress cytochrome P450 enzyme activity**. This herbicide is used to spray genetically modified and some conventional grain crops. Its commercial name is "Roundup®".

- Corn, soy, wheat, alfalfa, animal feed
    - beef, chicken, farm-raised fish
- All soft drinks and candies sweetened with corn syrup, all chips, cereals, and "power bars" that contain soy fillers.
- Breast milk of American mothers, at anywhere from 760 to 1,600 times the allowable limits in European drinking water.
- The manufacturers of glyphosates claim that it is harmless to humans. However, bacteria, fungi, algae, parasites, and plants use a seven-step metabolic route known as

the "shikimate pathway", for the biosynthesis of aromatic amino acids, and glyphosates inhibit this pathway. This causes the non-resistant weeds to die, which is why it is so effective as an herbicide. The manufacturer argues that since humans do not have this shikimate pathway, glyphosates are safe for humans.

- Dr. Seneff however, points out, "**... our gut bacteria *do* have this pathway, and that's crucial because these bacteria supply our body with important metabolism of amino acids and some B vitamins**". The glyphosates thus (a) kill beneficial gut bacteria, allowing pathogens to grow, (b) interfere with the synthesis of amino acids including methionine, which leads to shortages in critical neurotransmitters and folate, and (c) chelates (removes) important minerals like iron, cobalt and manganese, and much more.
- Children with autism have biomarkers indicative of excessive glyphosate, including zinc and iron deficiency, low serum sulfate, seizures, and mitochondrial disorder.
  - Two key problems in autism that are unrelated to the brain, yet clearly associated with the condition– both of which are linked with glyphosate exposure– are:
    - ✓ <u>Gut dysbiosis</u> (imbalances in gut bacteria, inflammation, leaky gut, food allergies such as gluten intolerance)
    - ✓ <u>Disrupted sulfur metabolism</u> / sulfur and sulfate deficiency
    - – CBS SNPs – vitamin B-6 dependent

http://articles.mercola.com/sites/articles/archive/2013/06/09/monsanto-roundup-herbicide.aspx

  - – Certain microbes in GI break down glyphosate. However, a byproduct of this action is ammonia.
  - – Children with autism tend to have significantly higher levels of ammonia in their blood than the general population. Ditto for those with Alzheimer's disease.
  - – The heaviest use of Roundup® weed-killer began in 1990 and has continued to rise since.
  - – The number of children with autism has gone from 1 in 5,000 in 1975 to 1 in 68 today (based on twelve year olds).

http://themindunleashed.org/2014/10/mit-researchers-new-warning-todays-rate-half-u-s-children-will-autistic-2025.html

  - – Glyphosates affect PON1, CBS, NOS 3, GST, and SOD enzymes

Section 2.2.1 - The CYP1** family

The cytochrome P450 proteins are monooxygenases, which catalyze many reactions involved in drug metabolism and synthesis of cholesterol, steroids, and other lipids.
http://www.ncbi.nlm.nih.gov/pmc/articles/PMC2797837/

http://www.genome.jp/kegg-bin/show_pathway?hsa00980

CYP1 family includes three subfamilies and operates primarily on drug and steroid (especially estrogen) metabolism, benzo(a)pyrene toxification. It includes CYP1A1, CYP1A2, and CYP1B1.

The cofactor of CYPs is heme. Heme is a component of the hemoglobin protein and iron. Thus, anemia affects CYP function.

The human cytochrome P450 (CYP) gene superfamily comprises fifty-seven protein-coding genes in our genomes. One of the eighteen mammalian CYP families is CYP1, which includes three members —CYP1A1, CYP1A2, and CYP1B1.

Both CYP1A1 and CYP1A2 are up-regulated by aryl hydrocarbon receptor (AHR) when activated by ligands, such as polycyclic aromatic hydrocarbons (PAHs), dioxin and β-naphthoflavone, and several dozen possible endogenous ligands.
CYP1A1 is expressed very early during embryogenesis, while CYP1A2 activity does not appear until the neonatal period.
http://www.ncbi.nlm.nih.gov/pmc/articles/PMC3011047/

CYP1A1 is the older gene and few, if any, drugs are metabolized by CYP1A1. Except for eicosanoid metabolism, CYP1A1 substrates most often studied include various halogenated and non-halogenated PAH procarcinogens.

CYP1A2 is the younger gene. It is constitutively highly expressed in the liver; it is inducible (mostly in liver, lung, pancreas, GI tract, and brain), and about two-dozen drugs are metabolized by CYP1A2 (http://medicine.iupui.edu/clinpharm/ddis/table.asp). Endogenous substrates include estradiol-17β, melatonin, uroporphyrinogen III http://www.ncbi.nlm.nih.gov/pmc/articles/PMC2912055/; and eicosanoids; CYP1A2 foreign substrates most often studied include various arylamine and N-heterocyclic procarcinogens.
http://molpharm.aspetjournals.org/content/78/1/46.full.pdf

CYP1A1

+ **<u>Overview for CYP1A1</u>** *Cytochrome P450, Family 1, Subfamily A, Polypeptide 1*
    - CYP1A1 A4889G, rs1048943 (aka, CYP1A1*2C)
    - CYP1A1 C2453A, rs1799814 (aka, CYP1A1*4)
    - CYP1A1 rs4646903 (aka, CYP1A1*2A)

http://meetinglibrary.asco.org/content/114620-132

- Metabolizes xenobiotics – polycyclic aromatic hydrocarbon (PAH), aflatoxins, and food mutagens. PAH emissions are generated by, among other things, charcoal grilling meats.

http://www.gastrojournal.org/article/S0016-5085(99)70554-8/fulltext

- See http://medicine.iupui.edu/clinpharm/ddis/clinical-table for an excellent summary chart of CYP drug interactions.

+ Catalytic activity:
  - RH + reduced flavoprotein + O2 = ROH + oxidized flavoprotein + H2O

+ Cofactor:
  - Heme

http://www.uniprot.org/uniprot/P04798

+ CYP 1A1 enzymes are coupled to glutathione to catalyze bioactivation and detoxification of mutagenic or carcinogenic compounds.

http://labmed.ascpjournals.org/content/42/4/220.full.html

+ CYP1A1*2C polymorphism increase risks of cancer:
  - Leukemia
  - Lung cancer
  - Endometrial cancer
  - Prostate cancer
  - Colorectal cancer
  - Esophageal cancer
  - Oral cancer

+ rs2606345 –
  - Women with CC genotype have tenfold greater odds of depression in Africa compared to AA in Japan.
  - Women with CC and AC genotypes have twofold greater odds of depression in Caucasian
  - Influence breast cancer risk by altering mammographic density.

http://www.ncbi.nlm.nih.gov/pubmed/?term=16949388,
http://www.ncbi.nlm.nih.gov/pubmed/?term=16949393
http://www.ncbi.nlm.nih.gov/pubmed/19630952

+ Whether a CYP1A1 SNP produces a deleterious effect will depend on the habits of the individual. In general, an SNP of CYP1A1 enzymatic activity is an up-regulation. A smoker or someone who consumes charred meat regularly (BBQ or flame-heated meat) or those exposed to xenobiotics from the environment (pesticides, industrial chemicals) have the potential to bio-convert these hazardous compounds to even more carcinogenic substances.

However, this up-regulation can be favorable if the individual can avoid smoking and xenobiotics as much as possible and consumes a diet high in glucosinolate compounds that can further enhance the effect of CYP1A1 SNPs. In that case, an up-regulation of CYP1A1 will increase the "safer" 2 hydroxy-estrone intermediary metabolite. Increasing 2 hydroxy estrogens will be of benefit to both the breast and prostate.

+ CYP1A1 is involved in an NADPH dependent electron transport pathway. It oxidizes compounds including steroids, fatty acids, and xenobiotics.

+ Because the CYP1A1 gene is one of the key enzymes that metabolize estrogen, some polymorphisms have been linked to hormone-related cancers.

+ CYP1A1 C4887A gene may represent a possible genetic risk factor for osteoporosis.

+ CYP1A1 has the potential to convert aromatic hydrocarbons and heterocyclic amines (HCA) to carcinogens. These include substances in tobacco smoke and high temperature cooking of meats.

+ CYP1A1 functions in xenobiotic metabolism including the in-activation of therapeutic agents such as, caffeine, theophylline (COPD drug), phenacetin (pain reliever), and warfarin (blood thinner).

http://informahealthcare.com/doi/abs/10.1080/03602530903112284?journalCode=dmr

+ As a result, if CYP1A1 is compromised (SNPs or not), due to, for example, high caffeine consumption, then an individual may potentially elevate estrogen levels. An increase of estrogen, and its intermediary metabolites have been linked to hormone related cancers such as breast, ovarian, uterine, prostate, and testicular.

+ When should I be concerned about CYP1A1?

- If you have evidence from hormone testing that your estrogen or estrogen intermediate metabolites are elevated, you may want to consider avoiding estrogen mimicking foods and chemicals, genetically modified foods, and conventional foods sprayed with glyphosate.
- Foods/chemicals that may elevate and/or mimic estrogen and/or bind to estrogen receptors (aka, xeno-estrogens) and/or endocrine disruptors:
    ✓ Coffee, black tea, chocolate, soy, dairy, or meat from animals injected with growth hormone, non-organic chicken eggs containing growth hormone, bisphenol A (BPA), flax seed, yucca root, carbonated beverages containing caffeine, dried apricots, dried prunes, dried dates, sesame seeds, chickpeas, beans, peas, tempeh, alfalfa sprouts, bran cereal, tofu, propyl gallate (a preservative used to prevent fats and oils from spoiling), additive, 4-hexyl resorcinol (used to prevent shrimp, lobsters, and other shellfish from discoloring), and phthalates, to name a few.
        - Organic meat from grass-fed animals, bovine growth hormone and antibiotic-free are better choices for an individual with CYP1A1 and elevated estrogen levels.

SNP ID	SNP Name	Risk Allele	Allele Effect
rs1048943	CYP1A1*2C A4889G (aka, Val allele)	C	-Oxidizes steroids, fatty acids, xenobiotics. -Carcinogenic intermediates are not broken down. Increased risk of lung and breast cancer. -Increased activity in CC alleles.
rs1799814	CYP1A1*4	T	-Increase in PAHs. -Slowed by resveratrol. -Slowed by glucosinolates. -Greatest enzymatic activity of all CYP1A1.

http://www.ncbi.nlm.nih.gov/pubmed/18813311?dopt=Abstract

CYP1A2

+ **Overview for CYP1A2** *Cytochrome P450, Family 1, Subfamily A, Polypeptide 2*
- CYP1A2 C164A, rs762551 (aka, CYP1A2*1F or *-163C>A*) - SNP represents increased activity or an up-regulation.
- Metabolizes caffeine.
- Metabolizes xenobiotics – polycyclic aromatic hydrocarbon (PAH), aflatoxins, and food mutagens. PAH emissions are generated by, among other things, charcoal grilling meats.

http://www.gastrojournal.org/article/S0016-5085(99)70554-8/fulltext

- Converts estradiol to 2-OH-estradiol (the "good" form).

+ Catalytic activity:
- RH + reduced flavoprotein + O2 = ROH + oxidized flavoprotein + H2O

+ Cofactor:
- Heme

http://www.uniprot.org/uniprot/P05177

+ CYP1A2 is involved in an NADPH dependent electron transport pathway. It oxidizes compounds including steroids, fatty acids, and xenobiotics.

+ Because the CYP1A2 gene is one of the key enzymes that metabolize estrogen, some polymorphisms have been linked to hormone-related cancers.

+ CYP1A2 C4887A gene may represent a possible genetic risk factor for osteoporosis.

+ CYP1A2 can convert aromatic hydrocarbons and heterocyclic amines to carcinogens. Toxic substances in tobacco smoke and high-temperature cooking of meats containing the HCAs which turn into carcinogens.

+ CYP1A2 functions in xenobiotic metabolism, including the in-activation of therapeutic agents such as, caffeine, theophylline (COPD drug), phenacetin (pain reliever), and warfarin (blood thinner).

http://informahealthcare.com/doi/abs/10.1080/03602530903112284?journalCode=dmr

+ If CYP1A2 is compromised (SNPs or not), due to, for example, high caffeine consumption, then an individual may potentially elevate estrogen levels. An increase of estrogen, and its intermediary metabolites have been linked to hormone related cancers such as breast, ovarian, uterine, prostate, and testicular.

+ When should I be concerned about CYP1A2?

- If you have evidence from hormone testing that your estrogen or estrogen intermediate metabolites are elevated, you may want to consider avoiding estrogen mimicking foods and chemicals, genetically modified foods, and conventional foods sprayed with glyphosate.
- Foods/chemicals that may elevate and/or mimic estrogen and/or bind to estrogen receptors (aka, xeno-estrogens) and/or endocrine disruptors:
    ✓ Coffee, black tea, chocolate, soy, dairy or meat from animals injected with growth hormone, non-organic chicken eggs containing growth hormone, bisphenol A (BPA), flax seed, yucca root, carbonated beverages containing caffeine, dried apricots, dried prunes, dried dates, sesame seeds, chickpeas, beans, peas, tempeh, alfalfa sprouts, bran cereal, tofu, propyl gallate (a preservative used to prevent fats and oils from spoiling), additive, 4-hexyl resorcinol (used to prevent shrimp, lobsters, and other shellfish from discoloring), and phthalates, to name a few.
        § Things that may include BPA:
            ▪ Cash register receipts, BPA is used to line canned goods, canned sodas including "healthy" bubble water, plastics such as storage containers, milk jugs, and water bottles. Also plastic lids used for to-go coffee cups. Do not drink coffee through the plastic lid. There is typically a small triangle at the bottom of plastic bottles that include a number. The numbers one, two, and five at the bottom of plastic bottles are BPA free.

- Organic meat from grass-fed animals, bovine growth hormone and antibiotic-free are better choices for an individual with CYP1A2 and elevated estrogen levels.

SNP ID	SNP Name	Risk Allele	Allele Effect
rs762551	CYP1A2 C164A (aka, CYP1A2*1F)	A C	A=Increased activity- Fast metabolizer -> caffeine. C=Decreased activity- Slow metabolizer with more stimulating effect. AC=Decreased activity- Slow metabolizer.

http://www.ncbi.nlm.nih.gov/pubmed/18813311?dopt=Abstract

CYP1B1

+ **Overview for CYP1B1** *Cytochrome P450, Family 1, Subfamily B, Polypeptide 1*
    - CYP1B1 L432V, rs1056836 (aka, 4326C/G, Val432Leu) is one of the major enzymes involved in the hydroxylation of estrogens, a reaction likely to be relevant in hormonal carcinogenesis.
    - Preferentially oxidizes 17 beta-estradiol to the carcinogenic 4-hydroxy derivative and a variety of procarcinogenic compounds to their activated forms, including polycyclic aromatic hydrocarbons.

http://www.uniprot.org/uniprot/Q16678

    - CYP1B1 N453S, rs1800440 is associated with endometrial cancer and other estrogen fueled cancers. It is susceptible to up-regulation via poor lifestyle. Converts estradiol to 4-OH-estradiol (the "toxic" form). Check COMT SNPs for down-regulation.
    - Metabolizes tamoxifen.
    - Metabolizes xenobiotics – polycyclic aromatic hydrocarbon (PAH), aflatoxins, and food mutagens. PAH emissions are generated by, among other things, charcoal grilling meats.

http://www.gastrojournal.org/article/S0016-5085(99)70554-8/fulltext

    - CYP1B1 R48G, rs10012 is associated with colorectal cancers and prostate cancers. It is susceptible to up-regulation via poor lifestyle. Check COMT SNPs for down-regulation.

http://www.ncbi.nlm.nih.gov/pubmed/21191305

http://www.snpedia.com/index.php/Rs10012

+ Catalytic activity:
- RH + reduced flavoprotein + O2 = ROH + oxidized flavoprotein + H2O
+ Cofactor:
- Heme

http://www.uniprot.org/uniprot/Q16678

+ CYP1B1 is involved in an NADPH dependent electron transport pathway. It oxidizes a variety of structurally unrelated compounds, including steroids, fatty acids, retinoid, and xenobiotics.

+ CYP1B1 oxidizes 17 beta-estradiol to the carcinogenic 4-hydroxy derivative, and a variety of procarcinogenic compounds to their activated forms, including polycyclic aromatic hydrocarbons.

+ In the case of CYP1B1 SNP, an up-regulation of CYP1B1 may increase the toxic 4 hydroxy-estrone intermediary metabolite. Increasing the 4-hydroxy-estrone, especially in combination with a COMT down-regulation (e.g., H62H and V158M), could increase risk of estrogen related cancers, PMS, gallbladder issues, and more. Please see details regarding COMT in Section 2.3.7 for further information.

+ AS noted above, the catalytic activity for CYP1B1 is RH, a protein on red blood cells + reduced flavoprotein + oxygen gas.

+The enzyme activity is increased by liposomes containing anionic phospholipids, phosphatidic acid, and cardiolipin.

+ The CYP1B1 enzyme is active in many tissues, including structures of the eye. More than 140 CYP1B1 gene mutations have been identified to cause early-onset glaucoma. A lack of the CYP1B1 enzyme likely disrupts normal development of the eye.

+ CYP1B1 is an extrahepatic P450 that is overexpressed in many tumours and has been strongly implicated in the activation of carcinogens. 4-hydroxyestrone and 4-hydroxyestradiol have been implicated in hormonal carcinogenesis and CYP1B1 is expressed in target tissues.

+ CYP1B1 is regulated by estradiol via estrogen receptor. This cytochrome P450 gene has been implicated in hormone related cancers, which include ovarian, breast, uterine, testicular, and prostate.

http://joe.endocrinology-journals.org/content/167/2/281.full.pdf

http://www.researchgate.net/publication/8579860_Human_CYP1B1_is_regulated_by_estradiol_via_estrogen_receptor

+ CYP1B1 functions in xenobiotic metabolism, including the in-activation of therapeutic agents, such as caffeine, theophylline (COPD drug), phenacetin (pain reliever), and warfarin (blood thinner).

http://www.nature.com/bjc/journal/v98/n3/full/6604195a.html

+ CYP1B1 is consistently overexpressed in tumor cells as compared to their normal counterparts, but its precise role in drug resistance is yet to be. CYP1B1 overexpression can inactivate flutamide, an antiandrogen used in the treatment of prostate cancer, with high efficiency suggests that this enzyme might play role in chemotherapy resistance.
http://www.nature.com/bjc/journal/v98/n3/full/6604195a.html

+ When should I be concerned about CYP1B1?
- If you have evidence from hormone testing that your estrogen or estrogen intermediate metabolites are elevated, you may want to consider avoiding estrogen mimicking foods and chemicals, genetically modified foods, and conventional foods sprayed with glyphosate.
- Foods/chemicals that may elevate and/or mimic estrogen and/or bind to estrogen receptors (aka, xeno-estrogens) and/or endocrine disruptors.
    - ✓ Coffee, black tea, chocolate, soy, dairy, or meat from animals injected with growth hormone, non-organic chicken eggs containing growth hormone, bisphenol A (BPA), flax seed, yucca root, carbonated beverages containing caffeine, dried apricots, dried prunes, dried dates, sesame seeds, chickpeas, beans, peas, tempeh, alfalfa sprouts, bran cereal, tofu, propyl gallate additive (a preservative used to prevent fats and oils from spoiling), 4-hexyl resorcinol, (used to prevent shrimp, lobsters, and other shellfish from discoloring), and phthalates, to name a few.
    - Organic meat from grass-fed animals, bovine growth hormone and antibiotic-free are better choices for an individual with CYP1B1 and elevated estrogen levels.

SNP ID	SNP Name	Risk Allele	Allele Effect
rs1056836	CYP1B1 L432V (aka, CYP1B1*3)	C G	-C=Increased activity = Lue/Leu -CC=Increase risk of breast, prostat cancer due to increased activty -GG=Val/Val; lung cancer, prostate, endometrial cancer risk. -CG=Higher 2OHe1/16 alpha than wildtype
rs1800440	CYP1B1 N453S (aka, CYP1B1*4)	C	-GG=Associated with decreased levels of urinary 2OHE and 16alpha in premenopausal woman and increased 4OHE in women with breast cancer. -COMT in combo with 2 SNPs above=37% higher 2OHE levels and 26% higher 2OHE/16alpha-OHE1 ratio. -Associated with glycemia and optic disc issues. -GG=Associated with endometrial cancer.
rs10012	CYP1B1 R48G (aka, CYP1B1*2)	C G	-CC=Significant association with endometrial cancer. -GG=Protective for endometrial cancer

http://www.ncbi.nlm.nih.gov/pubmed/?term=16547151

http://www.ncbi.nlm.nih.gov/pubmed/21191305

http://www.ncbi.nlm.nih.gov/pubmed/10426814

Clinical observations associated with CYP1B1 SNPs and estrogen dominance – Cycle issues, fibrocystic breast/ovaries, fluid retention, sleep disturbances, mood disturbances, constipation, heavy periods, PMS.

http://www.ncbi.nlm.nih.gov/pubmed/21191305

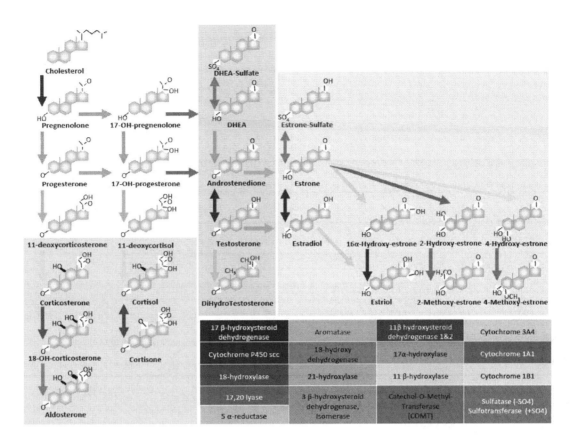

FIGURE 3 - Hormone Schematic

> **Our Two Cents**: On the right side, note the long diagonal (CYP1B1 phase I detox) and bottom right vertical (COMT phase II detox) arrows, and 4-OH estrone therebetween. Also note that cholesterol is a hormone building block, so GI assimilation of fatty acids and good bile production/modulation (liquid and not sludgy) is required. Eighty percent, or so, of cholesterol production is performed by the liver. As you read on, you will see that there are SNPs in key methylation enzymes that contribute to sludgy bile and potential gallbladder "stones" (e.g., BHMT, PEMT, MAT1, SULT2A1 SNPs). I have GI slides on my website that explain the link between SNPs and poor bile production. It is too much to include in this Compendium, but will be included in Compendium II.
> I use Figure 3 extensively with my clients to explain SNPs with respect to estrogen breakdown in the liver, especially in those with the combination of CYP1B1 and COMT V158M and H62H SNPs. That particular combo confers a higher risk for estrogen receptive cancers and estrogen dominance due to the potential build-up of nasty 4-OH estrones as phase I detox (CYP1B1) and phase II detox (COMT; "methylation") speeds are not matched. These pathways however, can be optimized with targeted nutrients.

When I address this combination, I typically replete magnesium, use DIM (or sulforaphane) and calcium-D-glucarate to addess all pathways that support estrogen clearing. Methylation support comes in as a last step in the form of 5MTHF, if needed. Less is more in those with COMT V158M and H62H SNPs. I also use a bit of pulsed (a couple of times per week) lithium orotate if support is needed for TCN1 and TCN2 to move B-12 into cells. A high normal MCV (on standard bloodwork like a CBC with Diff) and/or a high MMA (urine test on Genova Diagnostics NutrEval, and others) is an indication that B-12 may not be making its way into the cells to do its methyl swap with folate. MTHFR and MTR and MTRR work together in this swap.

I also encourage thermography breast scans in those with the CYP1B1/COMT SNP combo, as inflammatory breast cancer is not detected well via mammography or in those with dense breast tissue. I watched my mom suffer and subsequently die at age sixty, after five long years of dealing with the results of inflammatory breast cancer, surgery, chemo, and radiation despite "preventative care" doing yearly mammograms and cyst aspirations. That is the primary reason I left my IP attorney practice and went back to school, completed the IFM series, and continue to study. Figure 9 slowing the link between poor estrogen breakdown and neurotransmitters was prepared with my Mom in mind.

I have had the above drawing for a long time and unfortunately, do not have a citation, as I believe that it is from a slide in the IFM Hormone Module that I took years ago, where my favorite, Bethany Hays, was a speaker.

Section 2.2.2 - The CYP2** Family

The CYP2A family includes 13 subfamilies, and operates primarily on drug and steroid metabolism. Among others, it includes CYP2A6, CYP2C9, CYP2C19, CYP2D6 and CYP2E1.

CYP2A6

+ <u>**Overview for CYP2A6**</u> *Cytochrome P450, family 2, subfamily A, polypeptide 6*
    - CYP2A6, rs1057910 (aka, CYP2C9*3) is a down-regulation or slow metabolizer of substrates via CYP2C9*3.
    - CYP2A6, rs1801272 (aka, CYP2A6*2) is a down-regulation or slow metabolizer of substrates processed via CYP2A6*2.
    - Works in conjuction with the CYP2B6 SNPs in metabolizing nicotine and some xenobiotics.

+ Catalytic activity:

    - 1,4-cineole + NADPH + O_2 = 2-exo-hydroxy-1, 4-cineole + $NADP^+$ + H_2O

+ Cofactor:
- Heme

http://www.uniprot.org/uniprot/P11509

+ CYP2A6 is involved in the metabolism of xenobiotics in the body.

+ CYP2A6 is competent in the metabolic activation of aflatoxin B1. Aflatoxin B1 is derived from both a dedicated fatty acid synthesis and a polyketide synthase, together known as, norsolorinic acid synthase. Aflatoxin B1 can permeate through the skin. Dermal exposure to this aflatoxin in particular environmental conditions can lead to serious health risks.

+ CYP2A6 is the primary enzyme responsible for the oxidation of nicotine and cotinine.

+ CYP2A6 is also involved in the metabolism of several pharmaceuticals, carcinogens, and a number of coumarin-type alkaloids.

+ The following drugs are metabolized by CYP2A6:

Cotinine, coumarin, dexmedetomidine, docetaxal, efavirenz, irinotecan, letrozole, methoxsalen, nicotine, oxaliplatin, pilocarpine, tegafur, valproic acid, and warfarin.

+ CYP2A6 substrates (bind to CYP2D6 active sites; acted upon by CYP2A6 enzyme) include:
- Methyl *tert*-butyl ether which is a gasoline additive
- Methyl-*n*-amylnitrosamine which is known to induce esophageal and nasal tumors in rats
- Nicotine-derived nitrosamine ketone
- Nitrosamines which are used in the manufacture of some cosmetics, pesticides, and in most rubber products
- Aflatoxin which is a mycotoxin
- Coumarin found in cinnamon
- Quinoline extracted from coal tar and used in the manufacture of dyes, the preparation of hydroxyquinoline sulfate, and niacin. It may also be used as a solvent for resins and terpenes
- 1,3 -butadiene, an industrial chemical used in the production of synthetic rubber
- Skatole that is used in fragrance and in many perfumes
- 4,4'-Methylenebis 2-chloroaniline which is a curing agent in polyurethane production
- 2,6-Dichlorobenzonitrile used in herbicides to kill weeds
- Halothane and methoxyflurane which are anaesthetics
- Losigamone which is an anticonvulsant
- Valproic acid which is a mood stabilizer and anticonvulsant
- SM-1252 that is a PAF antagonist. PAF is a platelet-activating factor and a potent phospholipid activator and mediator of many leukocyte functions,

including platelet aggregation and degranulation, inflammation, and anaphylaxis. It is also involved in changes to vascular permeability, the oxidative burst, chemotaxis of leukocytes, as well as augmentation of arachidonic acid metabolism in phagocytes. High PAF levels are associated with allergic reaction, stroke, sepsis, and more.

+ A CYP2A6 inhibitor will cause decreased clearance of a substrate and an associated higher increase in plasma area under the curve (AUC).

+ CYP2A6 inhibitors (reduces activity of CYP2A6) include:
- Isoniazid the first-line medication in prevention and treatment of tuberculosis
- Grapefruit juice
- Methoxsalen (also called xanthotoxin, marketed under the trade names Oxsoralen, Deltasoralen, Meladinine) is a drug used to treat psoriasis, eczema, vitiligo, and some cutaneous lymphomas
- Ketoconazole, an antifungal
- Pilocarpine, which is a muscarinic receptor agonist (activates activity of muscarinic acetylcholine receptor)
- Tranylcypromine, an antidepressant

+ CYP2A6 inducers: (increases metabolic activity of CYP2A6 by binding to and/or activating, or by increasing the expression of the CYP2A6 coding).
- Phenobarbitol (anticonvulsant) and the bactericidal rifampicin

SNP ID	SNP Name	Risk Allele	Allele Effect
rs1801272	CYP2A6*2 A1799T	T	-T=Down regulation/slow metabolizer; Affects nicotine catabolism and coumarins
rs1057910	CYP2A6*3	C	-Down-regulation/slow metabolizer

http://www.ncbi.nlm.nih.gov/pubmed/21191305
https://www.pharmgkb.org/rsid/rs1801272#tabview=tab3&subtab=21

CYP2B6

+ <u>**Overview for CYP2B6**</u> *Cytochrome P450, family 2, subfamily B, polypeptide 6 (aka, CPB6; EFVM; IIB1; P450; CYP2B; CYP2B7; CYP2B7P; CYPIIB6)*
- CYP2B6, rs35303484 (aka, A136G), rs34097093 (aka, C1132T), rs8192719 (aka, C26570T), rs2279344 (G23280A), rs7260329 (aka, G29435A), rs28399499 (aka, I328T), rs2279343 (aka, L262A, rs3745274 (aka, Q172H) rs8192709 (aka, R22C), rs1042389 (aka, T1421C), rs36079186 (aka,

T20715C), rs2279345 (aka, T23499C) is a down-regulation or slow metabolizers of substrates via CYP2C9*3.
- Along with CYP2A6, this enzyme is involved in metabolizing nicotine, along with many other substances.
- This protein localizes to the endoplasmic reticulum and its expression is induced by phenobarbital. The enzyme is known to metabolize some xenobiotics, such as the anti-cancer drugs, cyclophosphamide and ifosfamide.

http://www.ncbi.nlm.nih.gov/pubmed/18781911

+ Catalytic activity:
- 1,4-cineole + NADPH + O2 = 2-exo-hydroxy-1,4-cineole + NADP+ + H2O

+ Cofactor:
- Heme

http://www.uniprot.org/uniprot/P20813

+ This enzyme is involved in an NADPH-dependent electron transport pathway. It oxidizes a variety of structurally unrelated compounds, including steroids, fatty acids, and xenobiotics. Acts as a 1,4-cineole 2-exo-monooxygenase.

http://www.genecards.org/cgi-bin/carddisp.pl?gene=CYP2B6

+ Transcript variants for this gene have been described; however, it has not been resolved whether these transcripts are in fact produced by this gene or by a closely related pseudogene, CYP2B7. Both the gene and the pseudogene are located in the middle of a CYP2A pseudogene found in a large cluster of cytochrome P450 genes from the CYP2A, CYP2B and CYP2F subfamilies on chromosome 19q.

http://www.ncbi.nlm.nih.gov/gene/1555

+ Substrates:
- Alfentanil (opioid)
- Bupropion (antidepressant)
- Cyclophosphamide (NNRTI)
- Ifosfamide (alkylating anti-neoplastic agent)
- Methadone (opiate replacement)
- Nevirapine (NNRTI)
- Propofol (anesthetic)
- Sertraline
- Sorafenib (protein kinase inhibitor)
- Tamoxifen (SERM)
- Valprioc acid (anticonvulsant)

- Methoxetamine

+ Strong inhibitor:
- Orphenadrine (antihistamine)

+ Unspecified potency inhibitor:
- Ticlopidine (antiplatelet)
- ThioTEPA (anticancer)
- Curcumin

+ Inducer:
- Rifampicin (bacterialcidal)
- Carbamazepine (anticonvulsant)
- Phenobarbital (anticonvulsant)
- Phenytoin (antiepileptic)

http://www.uniprot.org/uniprot/P20813

+ Medications/other that can affect CYP2B6 enzymatic function:

- Mephobarbital	- Cyclophosphamide	- Ifosfamide
- Amitriptyline	- Amlodipine	- Amprenavir
- Antipyrine	- Artemether	- Atorvastatin
- Azelastine	- Benzphetamine	- Benzyl alcohol
- Bifonazole	- Brompheniramine	- Bupropion
- Carbamazepine	- Carbinoxamine	- Cholecalciferol
- Cinnarizine	- Cisapride	- Cisplatin
- Citalopram	- Clobazam	- Clofibrate
- Clopidogrel	- Clotiazepam	- Clotrimazole
- Colchicine	- Cyclophosphamide	- Desipramine
- Dexamethasone	- Dextromethorphan	- Diazepam
- Diclofenac	- Diphenhydramine	- Domperidone
- Doxorubicin	- Enzalutamide	- Efavirenz
- Epinastine	- Erythromycin	- Estrone
- Ethanol	- Ethylmorphine	- Flunarizine
- Flunitrazepam	- Fluoxetine	- Fluvastatin
- Fluvoxamine	- Fosphenytoin	- Halothane
- Ifosfamide	- Imipramine	- Irinotecan
- Isoflurane	- Itraconazole	- Ketamine
- Ketobemidone	- Ketoconazole	- Lidocaine
- Loperamide	- Lopinavir	- Lorcaserin
- Malathion	- Memantine	- Methadone

- Methimazole
- Methoxyflurane
- Methylphenobarbital
- Methyltestosterone
- Mexiletine
- Mianserin
- Miconazole
- Midazolam
- Modafinil
- Nelfinavir
- Nevirapine
- Nicardipine
- Nicotine
- Nifedipine
- Nilotinib
- Nitric Oxide
- Orphenadrine
- Ospemifene
- Paroxetine
- Perhexiline
- Permethrin
- Perphenazine
- Pethidine
- Phenobarbital
- Phenytoin
- Prasugrel
- Primidone
- Promethazine
- Propofol
- Quinidine
- Raloxifene
- Regorafenib
- Rifampicin
- Rilpivirine
- Ritonavir
- Ropivacaine
- Roxithromycin
- Selegiline
- Sertraline
- Sevoflurane
- Simvastatin
- Sorafenib
- Sulfaphenazole
- Sulfinpyrazone
- Tamoxifen
- Temazepam
- Testosterone
- Thiotepa
- Ticlopidine
- Tramadol
- Tretinoin
- Valproic Acid
- Venlafaxine
- Verapamil

http://www.ncbi.nlm.nih.gov/pubmed/21301907
http://www.ncbi.nlm.nih.gov/pubmed/17073575

+ Diseases associated with CYP2B6:
- Efavirenz (efavirenz central nervous system toxicity). This is a non-nucleoside reverse transcriptase inhibitor (NNRTI).

http://www.malacards.org/card/efavirenz_poor_metabolism_of

CYP2C9

+ **Overview for CYP2C9** Cytochrome P450, Family 2, Subfamily C, polypeptide 9
- CYP2C9 C430T, rs1799853 (aka, CYP2C9*2) is a down-regulation or slow metabolizer of substrates.
- CYP2C9 A1075C, rs1057910 (aka, CYP2C9*3) is a down-regulation or slow metabolizer of substrates.
- Metabolizes warfarin, ARBs, and many NSAIDs.

+ Catalytic activity:
- (R)-limonene + NADPH + O2 = (+)-trans-carveol + NADP+ + H2O
- (S)-limonene + NADPH + O2 = (-)-trans-carveol + NADP+ + H2O
- (S)-limonene + NADPH + O2 = (-)-perillyl alcohol + NADP+ + H2O

+ Cofactor:
   - Heme

http://www.uniprot.org/uniprot/P11712

+ Individuals with the CYP2C9*2 and/or CYP2C9*3 variant may have increased risk of GI bleeding with use of specific NSAIDs. In addition, those individuals with CYP2C9*2 may have a higher sensitivity to the antiepileptic drug phenytoin and/or warfarin.

+ CYP2C9*1 produces normal enzymatic activity.

+ CYP2C9*2 produces reduced enzymatic activity.

+ CYP2C9 plays a role in the oxidation of xenobiotic and endogenous compounds.

+ CYP2C9 substrates (bind to CYP2C9 active sites; acted upon by CYP2C9 enzyme) include:
   - AM-2201 (a synthetic cannabinoid) Amitriptyline (Elavil®)
   - Apixaban (Eliquis®)
   - Azilsartan (Edarbi®) Bosentan (Tracleer®) Candesartan (Atacand®) Carvedilol (Coreg®)
   - Celecoxib NSAID (nonsteroidal anti-inflammatory) Chlorpropamide [8]
   - Clopidogrel (Plavix®) Cyclophosphamide alkylating agent
   - Dapsone Diclofenac (Voltaren®) NSAID Diphenhydramine (Benadryl®) antihistamine Etodolac
   - Fluoxetine (Prozac®) Flurbiprofen (Ansaid®) Fluvastatin (Lescol®) Statin Formoterol (Foradil®)
   - Glibenclamide Sulfonylurea Glimepiride (Amaryl®) Sulfonylurea Glipizide (Glucotrol®) Sulfonylurea Glyburide (Diabeta®, Glynase®)
   - Ibuprofen (Motrin®, Advil®) Indomethacin (Indocin®) Irbesartan (Avapro®) Angiotensin II blocker
   - JWH-018 (an analgesic used in synthetic cannabis) ketamine (used in anesthetics and pain killers)
   - Lornoxicam NSAID Losartan (Cozaar®) Angiotensin II blocker
   - Meloxicam (Mobic®) NSAID Mestranol (Norinyl®)
   - Naproxen (Naprosyn®, Aleve®) NSAID Nateglinide (Starlix®)
   - Olodaterol (Striverdi Respimat®) Ospemifene (Osphena®) Phenobarbital
   - Piroxicam (Feldene®) Prasugrel (Effient®) Rosiglitazone (Avandia®)
   - Sildenafil (ED drug)
   - Tamoxifen (anti-estrogen) Terbinafine (Lamisil®) Tetrahydrocannabinol (THC found in the cannabis plant) Tolbutamide Sulfonylurea Torsemide (Demadex®)

Valproic acid (Depakote®) Voriconazole (Vfend®) Zafirlukast (Accolate®) Zileuton (Zyflo®)
- Minor/sensitive substrates:
    - Ramelteon (Rozerem®)
    - Rosuvastatin (Crestor®)
    - Celecoxib known as Celebrex
    - Phenytoin known as Dilantin
    - Warfarin known as Coumadin

+ CYP2C9 inducers (increases metabolic activity of CYP2C9 by binding to and/or activating, or by increasing the expression of the CYP2C9 coding).

Strong Inducers:
- Rifampicin
- Secobarbital

Weak Inducers:
- Aprepitant
- Phenobarbital

- Bosentan
- St John's Wort

Moderate inducer:
- Carbamaze

Additional inducers (class uncertain):
- Peginterferon alfa-2b (PegIntron®)
- Rifapentine (Priftin®)
- Tocilizumab (Actemra®)
- Tumor Necrosis Factor inhibitors - (adalimumab, Humira®, certolizumab, Cimzia®, etanercept, Enbrel®, golimumab, Simponi®, infliximab, Remicade®)

+ A CYP2C9 inhibitor will cause decreased clearance of a substrate and an associated higher increase in plasma area under the curve (AUC).

+ CYP2C9 inhibitors (reduces activity of CYP2C9) include:
- Fluconazole (Diflucan®)
- Miconazole (antifungal)
- Amentoflavone (constituent of ginkgo biloba and St. John's Wort)
- Sulfaphenazole (antibacterial)
- Valproic acid (anticonvulsant, mood-stabilizing)
- Apigenin
- Fluvoxamine (Luvox®)
- Miconazole
- Metronidazole (Flagyl®)
- Many more

+ CYP2C9 inhibitors (class uncertain)
- Antihistamines (H1-receptor antagonist)

- Cyclizine
- Promethazine
- Chloramphenicol
- Fenofibrate
- Flavones
- Flavonols
- Fluvastatin (statin)
- Fluvoxamine (SSRI)
- Isoniazid
- Lovastatin (statin)
- Phenylbutazone (NSAID)
- Probenecid
- Sertraline (SSRI)
- Sulfamethoxazole (antibiotic)
- Teniposide (chemo)
- Voriconazole (antifungal)
- Zafirlukast (leukotriene)
- Quercetin (anti-inflammatory)
- Metronidazole (Flagyl®)

SNP ID	SNP Name	Risk Allele	Allele Effect
rs1799853	CYP2C9*2 C430T	T	-TT=Down-regulation/slow metabolizer. Adverse drug reactions e.g., Increased GI bleeding with NSAIDs.
rs1057910	CYP2C9*3 A1075C	C	-CC= Down-regulation/slow metabolizer. Adverse drug reactions.

http://www.ncbi.nlm.nih.gov/pubmed/21191305

https://www.pharmgkb.org/rsid/rs1801272#tabview=tab3&subtab=21

CYP2C19

+ **Overview for CYP2C19** *Cytochrome P450, Family 2, Subfamily C, polypeptide 19*
  - CYP2C19, rs3814637 (aka, C1418T), rs12767583 (aka, C5709T), rs4986894 (aka, T98C), rs17878459 (aka, G276A), rs4986893 (aka, G636A), rs28399504 (aka, A5001G), rs72552267 (aka, G395A), rs72558186 (aka, T24294A),

rs41291556 (aka, T358C), rs17884712 (aka, G17784A), rs3758581 (aka, V331I), encodes the enzyme cytochrome P450, family 2, subfamily C, and polypeptide 19.
- CYP2C19*17, rs12248560 encodes an ultra-rapid up-regulation of the enzyme resulting in extensive metabolization of CYP2C19 substrates. For example, a person taking an antiplatelet medication may be at increased risk of bleeding.
- CYPC19*17 metabolizes xenobiotics (i.e., chemical substances in the body, not made by the body, such as a pharmaceutical drug), including proton pump inhibitors and some antiepileptic. Approximately five to ten percent are metabolized by CYP2C19, including Plavix (antiplatelet), Omeprazole (anti-ulcer), Mephenytoin (antiseizure), Proguanil (antimalarial), and Diazepam (anti-anxiety), as well as some steroid hormones such as progesterone.

http://circ.ahajournals.org/content/121/4/512.full

+ Catalytic activity:
- $^+$-(R)-limonene + NADPH + O2 = (+)-trans-carveol + NADP+ + H2O
- $^-$-(S)-limonene + NADPH + O2 = (-)-trans-carveol + NADP+ + H2O
- $^-$-(S)-limonene + NADPH + O2 = (-)-perillyl alcohol + NADP+ + H2O

+ Cofactor:
- Heme

http://www.uniprot.org/uniprot/P33261#ptm_processing

+ CYP2C19*1 produces normal enzymatic activity.

+ CYP2C19*2 (rs4244285) produces reduced enzymatic activity.

+ CYP2C19 substrates (bind to CYP2C19 active sites; acted upon by CYP2C19 enzyme) include:
- Antidepressants
  - TCAs
  - SSRIs
  - Moclobemide
  - Bupropion
- Antiepileptics
- Proton pump inhibitors
- Clopidogrel (antiplatelet)
- Proguanil (antimalarial)
- Propranolol (beta-blocker)
- Gliclazide (sulfonylurea)
- Carisoprodol (muscle relaxant)

- Chloramphenicol (bacterial antimicrobial)
- Cyclophosphamide
- Indomethacin (NSAID)
- Nelfinavir (anti-retroviral)
- Nilutamide (anti-androgen)
- Progesterone
- Teniposide (chemo)
- Warfarin (anticoagulant)

+ A CYP2C19 inhibitor will cause decreased clearance of a substrate and an associated higher increase in plasma area under the curve (AUC).

+ CYP2C19 inhibitors (reduces activity of CYP2C19) include:
- Strong
    - Moclobemide (antidepressant)
    - Fluvoxamine (SSRI)
    - Chloramphenicol (bacteriostatic antimicrobial)
- Weak
    - Anticonvulsants
- Unspecified
    - Proton pump inhibitors
    - Cimetidine (H2-receptor antagonist)
    - Fluoxetine (SSRI)
    - Indomethacin (NSAID)
    - Ketoconazole (antifungal)
    - Modafinil (eurgeroic)
    - Probenecid (uricosuric)
    - Ticlopidine (anti-platelet)
    - Isoniazid

+ CYP2C19 inducers: (increases metabolic activity of CYP2C19 by binding to and/or activating or by increasing the expression of the CYP2C19 coding).
- Rifampicin (bactericidal)
- Artemisinin
- Carbazepine (anticonvulsant, mood stabilizing)
- Norethisterone (contraceptive)
- Prednisone (corticosteroid)
- Aspirin

SNP ID	SNP Name	Risk Allele	Allele Effect
rs12248560	CYP2C19*17 806C>T	T	-T=Ultra rapid metabolizer – breaks down associated drugs too quickly, especially PPIs.
rs4244285	CYP2C19*2	A	-Down-regulation; reduced enzymatic activity.

http://www.ncbi.nlm.nih.gov/pubmed/21191305

https://www.pharmgkb.org/rsid/rs1801272#tabview=tab3&subtab=21

http://www.medscape.com/viewarticle/745300_4

CYP2D6

+ **Overview for CYP2D6** *Cytochrome P450, Family 2, Subfamily D, polypeptide 6*
    - CYP2D6 S486T, rs1135840 (aka, CYP2D6*2xN) represents an up-regulation; aka, increased enzymatic activity.
  ❖ **NOTE**: the C allele is actually an up-regulation.
      - Avoid codeine. Consider an alternative analgesic, e.g., morphine or a non-opioid. Consider avoiding tramadol.

http://www.ncbi.nlm.nih.gov/books/NBK100662/

    - CYP2D6 T100C, rs1065852 (aka, CYP2D6*10) is considered a non-functioning or partially functioning variant, so it confers reduced activity and clearing of substrates.
    - CYP2D6 C2850T, rs16947 (aka, CYP2D6*2); GG normal, AG common variant with normal activity, AA: increased risk for up-regulation.
      - Coexists with other polymorphisms.

http://www.ncbi.nlm.nih.gov/pubmed/16835697

    - CYP2D6*4 produces no enzyme activity; poor metabolizer
    - CYP2D6 S486T, rs1135840 (aka, 4180G>C or S486T); G risk allele confers an up-regulation or increased activity.
    - Responsible for the metabolism of many drugs and environmental chemicals that it oxidizes. It is involved in the metabolism of drugs such as anti-arrhythmics, adrenoceptor antagonists, and tricyclic antidepressants.
    - Metabolizes xenobiotics - herbicides and insecticides.

http://hmg.oxfordjournals.org/content/early/2013/09/04/hmg.ddt417.full.pdf

https://www.pharmgkb.org/rsid/rs16947#tabview=tab3&subtab=21

http://www.pharmacytimes.com/publications/issue/2008/2008-07/2008-07-8624

http://www.ncbi.nlm.nih.gov/pubmed/16007002

https://www.pharmgkb.org/gene/PA128

http://www.consumer-health.com/services/NewGeneticTestsHelpDoctorsPrescribetheRightMedicineforYou.php

http://en.wikipedia.org/wiki/CYP2D6

+ Catalytic activity:
  - RH + reduced flavoprotein + O2 = ROH + oxidized flavoprotein + H2O

+ Cofactor:
  - Heme

http://www.uniprot.org/uniprot/P10635

+ CYP2D6 is primarily expressed in the liver. It is also highly expressed in areas of the CNS, including the substantia nigra.

+ CYP2D6 is one pathway for phase I detoxification of insecticides and herbicides.

+ CYP2D6 is responsible for the metabolism and elimination of approximately twenty-five percent of clinically used drugs in a process referred to as, O-demethylation.

+ Another study found that twenty to thirty percent of all drugs are metabolized by CYP2D6, including dextromethorphan (a key ingredient in products such as Nyquil), beta-blockers, antiarrhythmics, and antidepressants.

+ Individuals with the CYP2C9*2 and/or CYP2C9*3 variant may have increased risk of GI bleeding with use of specific NSAIDs. In addition, those individuals with CYP2C9*2 may have a higher sensitivity to the antiepileptic drug phenytoin and/or warfarin.

+ Over 100 CYP2D6 allelic variants have been identified (http://www.imm.ki.se/CYPalleles), with CYP2D6 enzyme activity ranging from no activity to ultra-rapid activity. Four CYP2D6 metabolizer phenotypes have been defined among European populations, with poor metabolizers representing five to ten percent of the population, intermediate metabolizer ten to fifteen percent, extensive metabolizer seventy-five to eighty-five percent, and ultra-rapid metabolizer one to ten percent.

http://link.springer.com/article/10.1007/s00228-003-0657-4?no-access=true

+ CYP2D6 substrates (bind to CYP2D6 active sites; acted upon by CYP2D6 enzyme) include:
  - Sensitive:
    - Aripiprazole (Abilify)
    - Atomoxetine (Strattera®)
    - Desipramine (Norpramin®)
    - Dextromethorphan (Robitussin DM®)
    - Iloperidone (Fanapt®)
    - Metoprolol (Toprol®)

- Nebivolol (Bystolic®)
- Perphenazine
- Propafenone (Rythmol®)
- Risperdal
- Risperidon
- Venlafaxine (Effexor®)
- Vortioxetine (Brintellix®)
- Thioridazine (Mellaril®, Sonapax)

+ Additional CYP2D6 substrates:
- Alprenolol, alfeprol, alpheprol, and alprenololum (Gubernal, Regletin, Yobir, Apllobal, Aptine, Aptol Duriles)
- Amitriptyline (Elavil®)
- Amphetamine
- Arformoterol (Brovana®)
- Bufuralol
- Carvedilol (Coreg®)
- Chlorpheniramine (Chlor-Trimeton®)
- Chlorpromazine (Thorazine®)
- Ciclesonide (Alvesco®, Omnaris®)
- Clomipramine (Anafranil®)
- Clonidine (Catapres®)
- Clozapine (Clozaril®)
- Codeine or 3-methylmorphine
- Debrisoquine
- Dextromethorphan found in over-the-counter cold medications
- Donepezil (Aricept®)
- Doxazosin (Cardura®, Cardura XL®)
- Doxepin
- Duloxetine (Cymbalta®)
- Encainide (Enkaid)
- Flecainide (Tambocor®)
- Fluoxetine (Prozac®)
- Fluphenazine
- Fluvoxamine (Luvox®)
- Formoterol (Foradil®)
- Haloperidol (Haldol®)

- Hydrocodone
- Imipramine (Tofranil®)
- Ivermectin (Stromectol®)
- Levomepromazine also known as methotrimeprazine, Lidocaine xylocaine, or lignocaine
- Mianserin (Depnon, Lantanon, Lerivon, Lumin, Norval, Tolvon, Tolmin)
- Metoclopramide (Reglan®)
- Mexiletine
- Mirtazapine (Remeron®)
- Minaprine (Brantur, Cantor)
- Nortriptyline (Pamelor®)
- Olanzapine (Zyprexa®) (minor substrate)
- Ondansetron (Zofran®)
- Oxycodone (Oxycontin®)
- Paliperidone (Invega®) (minor substrate)
- Paroxetine (Paxil®)
- Perhexiline
- Phenacetin
- Phenformin
- Promethazine (Phenergan®)
- Propranolol (Inderal®)
- Remoxipride (Roxiam)
- Sparteine
- Tamoxifen
- Tamsulosin (Flomax®)
- Timolol maleate
- Tiotropium (Spiriva®) (minor substrate)
- Tramadol (Ultram®)
- Trimipramine (Surmontil®)
- Tropisetron
- Umeclidinium (Anoro Ellipta®)
- Zuclopenthixol (Cisordinol, Clopixol, Acuphase) also known as zuclopentixol

+ A CYP2D6 inhibitor will cause decreased clearance of a substrate, and an associated higher increase in plasma area under the curve (AUC).

- Strong inhibitors
    - Bupropion (Wellbutrin®)

- Fluoxetine (Prozac®)
- Metoclopramide (Reglan®)
- Paroxetine (Paxil®)
- Quinidine
- Moderate inhibitors
    - Cinacalcet (Sensipar®)
    - Dronedarone (Multaq®)
    - Duloxetine (Cymbalta®)
    - Mirabegron
    - (Myrbetriq®)
    - Terbinafine (Lamisil®)
- Weak inhibitors
    - Amiodarone (Cordarone®)
    - Asenapine (Saphris®)
    - Buprenorphine
    - Celecoxib (Celebrex®)
    - Cimetidine (Tagamet®)
    - Clemastine, also known as meclastin
    - Desipramine (Norpramin®)
    - Desvenlafaxine (Pristiq®)
    - Diltiazem (Cardizem®)
    - Diphenhydramine (Benadryl®)
    - Echinacea
    - Escitalopram (Lexapro®)
    - Febuxostat (Uloric®)
    - Gefitinib (Iressa®)
    - Hydralazine (Apresoline®)
    - Hydroxychloroquine (Plaquenil®)
    - Imatinib (Gleevec®)
    - Imipramine (Tofranil®)
    - Methadone
    - Nortriptyline (Pamelor®)
    - Oral contraceptive pills
    - Propafenone (Rythmol®)
    - Ranitidine (Zantac®)
    - Ritonavir (Norvir®)

- Sertraline (Zoloft®)
- Telithromycin (Ketek®)
- Venlafaxine (Effexor®)
- Verapamil (Calan®, Isoptin®, etc.)
- Unspecified inhibitors:
    - Bicalutamide (Casodex, Cosudex, Calutide, Kalumid)
    - Chlorpheniramine (Chlor-Trimeton®)
    - Chlorpromazine (Thorazine®)
    - Citalopram (Celexa®)
    - Clomipramine (Anafranil®
    - Cobicistat (part of Stribild®)
    - Cocaine
    - Diphenhydramine
    - Doxepin
    - Doxorubicin (Adriamycin Doxil Myocet)
    - Fluphenazine
    - Fluvoxamine (Luvox®)
    - Halofantrine (Halfan)
    - Haloperidol (Haldol®)
    - Hydroxychloroquine (Plaquenil®)
    - Hydroxyzine (Vistaril® Atarax)
    - Hyperforin (St. John's Wort)
    - Levomepromazine also known as methotrimeprazine
    - Lorcaserin (Belviq®)
    - Methadone
    - Mibefradil (Posicor)
    - Midodrine (Amatine, ProAmatine, Gutron)
    - Moclobemide (Amira, Aurorix, Clobemix, Depnil, and Manerix)
    - Niacin (Niaspan®, Slo-Niacin®)
    - Perphenazine
    - Promethazine
    - Risperidone (Risperdal)
    - Sertraline (Zoloft®)
    - Thioridazine (Mellaril®)
    - Tripelennamine (Pyribenzamine)
    - Vilazodone (Viibryd®)

- Zuclopenthixol (Cisordinol, Clopixol, Acuphase)

+ CYP2D6 inducers (increases metabolic activity of CYP2D6 by binding to and/or activating, or by increasing the expression of the CYP2D6 coding) include:
- Dexamethasone
- Rifampicin
- Glutethimide (strong inducer)

CYP2D6 allele and enzyme activity[9]

Allele	CYP2D6 activity
*CYP2D6*1*	normal
*CYP2D6*2*	increased
*CYP2D6*3*	none
*CYP2D6*4*	none
*CYP2D6*5*	none
*CYP2D6*9*	decreased
*CYP2D6*10*	decreased
*CYP2D6*17*	decreased

https://en.wikipedia.org/wiki/CYP2D6

SNP ID	SNP Name	Risk Allele	Allele Effect
rs1135840	CYP2D6 S486T CYP2D6*2xN	G C	-GG=Normal activity -CC=Increase activty
rs1065852	CYP2D6 T100C CYP2D6*10	T	-TT=Associated with non-functioning or partially functioning – reduced activity and clearing of substrates. -T allele higher in Asian populations.
rs16947	CYP2D6 C2850T	A	-AA=Significant upregulation – fast activity

http://www.ncbi.nlm.nih.gov/pubmed/21191305

https://www.pharmgkb.org/rsid/rs1801272#tabview=tab3&subtab=21

http://www.medscape.com/viewarticle/745300_4

CYP2E1

+ **Overview for CYP2E1** *Cytochrome P450, Family 2, Subfamily E, Polypeptide 1*
    - CYP2E1 G9896C, rs2070676 (aka, CYP2E1*1B) is, inter alia located in dopamine containing neurons in the substantia nigra, has been hypothesized to be of importance for the pathophysiology of Parkinson's disease via its capability to detoxify putative neurotoxins. Can increase production of ROS in the presence of chemicals that further down-regulate. Coffee and smoking exacerbate. Research seems to indicate that this is a down-regulation, thus increased ROS.
    - CYP2E1 A4768G, rs6413419 (aka, CYP2E1*4 or 4768G>A or V179I). Acrylamide is formed in heat-treated carbohydrate rich foods in the so-called, Maillard reaction, and is readily absorbed in the body and converted to glycidamide by epoxidation by the CYP2E1 (cytochrome P450 2E) enzyme. Look at GSTM1, GSTT1, and GSTP1 SNPs, as well.
    - Metabolizes drugs - acetaminophen, halothane, and chlorzoxazone.
    - Metabolizes xenobiotics - alcohol, ketones, nitrosamines, and food mutagens.

http://www.ncbi.nlm.nih.gov/pubmed/19381774?dopt=Abstract
http://www.ncbi.nlm.nih.gov/pubmed/18798002?dopt=Abstract
http://www.researchgate.net/publication/242017880_Acetaldehyde_and_parkinsonism_role_of_CYP450_2E1
http://www.ncbi.nlm.nih.gov/pubmed/19131562?dopt=Abstract

+ Catalytic activity:
    - 4-nitrophenol + NADPH + O2 = 4-nitrocatechol + NADP+ + H2O
+ Cofactor:
    - Heme

http://www.uniprot.org/uniprot/P05181

+ CYP2E1 is involved in the metabolism of xenobiotics.
+ CYP2E1 substrates (bind to CYP2E1 active sites; acted upon by CYP2E1 enzyme) include:
    - Acetaminophen
    - Aniline
    - Benzine
    - Chlorzoxazon
    - Dacarbazine
    - Enflurane

- Ethanol
- Eszopiclonne
- Halothane
- Isoflurane
- Isoniazid
- Methoxyflurane
- Paracetamol
- Sevoflurane
- Theophylline
- Trimethadione
- Zopiclone

+ A CYP2E1 inhibitor will cause decreased clearance of a substrate and an associated higher increase in plasma area under the curve (AUC).

- Alosetron
- Amitriptyline
- Bromazepam
- Chlorpromazine
- Chlorzoxazone
- Cimetidine
- Clotrimazole
- Clozapine
- Desipramine
- Diclofenac
- Diethyldithiocarbamate
- Disulfiram
- Econazole
- Entacapone
- Fluphenazine
- Flurazepam
- Imipramine
- Interferon-g1b
- Isoniazid
- Methimazole
- Methoxsalen
- Miconazole
- Modafinil

- Nicotine
- Nortriptyline
- Orphenadrine
- Pilocarpine
- Pimozide
- Propofol
- Ritonavir
- Selegiline
- Sildenafil
- Sulconazole
- Thioridazine
- Ticlopidine
- Tioconazole
- Tranylcypromine

+CYP2E1 inducers: (increases metabolic activity of CYP2E1 by binding to and/or activating, or by increasing the expression of the CYP2E1 coding).

- Ethanol
- Isoniazid
- Tobacco

SNP ID	SNP Name	Risk Allele	Allele Effect
rs2070676	CYP2E1*1B C9896G	G C	-GG=Induced by alcohol, coffee, smoking. -CC=Wild type, no definitive up or down-regulation but works with other CYP genes in regulating detox pathways.
rs6413419	CYP2E1*4 A4768G	A	-AA=AS above. Works with other CYP genes to detoxify carcinogens.

http://www.ncbi.nlm.nih.gov/pubmed/19381774

Section 2.2.3 - The CYP3** Family

CYP3A4

+ **Overview for CYP3A4** *Cytochrome P450, Family 3, Subfamily A, Polypeptide 4*

- CYP3A4 392G>A, rs2740574 (aka, CYP3A4*1B) is involved in androgen metabolism and confers a ~ tenfold higher risk of aggressive prostate cancer in African American males, as it facilitates the oxidative deactivation of testosterone. Along with CYP3A5*3; SNP rs776746 may increase risk for hypertension in pregnancy. It appears to be a down-regulation based on research.
- Forty to forty-five percent of pharmaceutical drugs are metabolized in phase 1 via this enzyme.
- Metabolizes xenobiotics - aflatoxin, food mutagens
- CYP3A4 M445T, rs4986910 (aka, CYP3A4*3 and 1334T>C, 23171T>C) affects colorectal cancer risk by determining the genotoxic impact of exogenous carcinogens and levels of sex hormones.

http://www.ncbi.nlm.nih.gov/pubmed/16414488?dopt=Abstract
http://www.ncbi.nlm.nih.gov/pubmed/20617557?dopt=Abstract
http://www.ncbi.nlm.nih.gov/pubmed/19214745?dopt=Abstract
http://www.ncbi.nlm.nih.gov/pubmed/17615053?dopt=Abstract

+ CYP3A4 oxidizes xenobiotics such as, toxins and drugs.

http://www.uniprot.org/uniprot/Q6GRK0

+ The expression of CYP3A4 has been linked to estrogen related cancers.

+ Caffeine can elevate estrogen levels up to seventy percent, if CYP3A4 SNPs are present.

+ CYP3A4 substrates (bind to CYP3A4 active sites; acted upon by CYP3A4 enzyme) include:
- Alfentanil (Alfenta)
- Alfuzosin (Uroxatral)
- Almotriptan (Axert)
- Alprazolam (Xanax)
- Amiodarone (Cordarone)
- Amitriptyline
- Amlodipine (Norvasc)
- Anastrozole
- Aprepitant (Emend)
- Aripiprazole
- Astemizole
- Atazanavir (Reyataz)
- Atorvastatin (Lipitor)
- Bepridil (Vascor)
- Bexarotene (Targretin)

- Bicalutamide
- Bosentan (Tracleer)
- Bromocriptine (Parlodel)
- Budesonide (Entocort)
- Buprenorphine (Subutex)
- Bupropion (Buspar)
- Buspirone
- Caffeine
- Carbamazepine (eg, Tegretol)
- Cerivastatin
- Cevimeline (Evoxac)
- Chlorphenamine
- Cilostazol (Pletal)
- Cisapride (Propulsid)
- Citalopram
- Clarithromycin (Biaxin)
- Clomipramine
- Clonazepam (Klonopin)
- Clopidogrel (Plavix) Cocaine
- Codeine
- Colchicine
- Cyclobenzaprine
- Cyclophosphamide (Cytoxan)
- Cyclosporine (Neoral)
- Dapsone (Avlosulfon)
- Darunavir (Prezista)
- Dasatinib (Sprycel)
- Delavirdine (Rescriptor)
- Dexamethasone (Decadron)
- Dextromethorphan
- Diazepam
- Dihydroergotamine
- Diltiazem (Cardizem)
- Disopyramide (Norpace)
- Docetaxel (Taxotere)
- Domperidone

- Donepezil (Aricept)
- Doxorubicin (Adriamycin)
- Droperidol
- Dutasteride (Avodart)
- Ebastine (Kestine)
- Efavirenz (Sustiva)
- Eletriptan (Relpax)
- Eplerenone (Inspra)
- Ergotamine (Ergomar)
- Erlotinib (Tarceva)
- Erythromycin
- Estazolam (ProSom)
- Eszopiclone (Lunesta)
- Ethinyl
- Ethinylestradiol
- Estradiol
- Ethosuximide (Zarontin)
- Etoposide (Vepesid)
- Exemestane (Aromasin)
- Felodipine (Plendil)
- Fentanyl (Sublimaze)
- Finasteride (Proscar)
- Flurazepam (Dalmane)
- Fosamprenavir (Lexiva)
- Galantamine (Reminyl)
- Gefitinib (Iressa)
- Granisetron (Kytril)
- Halofantrine (Halfan)
- Haloperidol
- Hydrocortisone
- Ifosfamide (Ifex)
- Imatinib (Gleevec)
- Imipramine
- Indinavir (Crixivan)
- Irinotecan (Camptosar)
- Isradipine (DynaCirc)

- Itraconazole (Sporanox)
- Ixabepilone (Ixempra)
- Ketoconazole (Nizoral)
- Lapatinib (Tykerb)
- Lercanidipine
- Levacetylmethadol
- Levomethadyl (Orlaam)
- Lidocaine
- Loperamide (Imodium)
- Lopinavir (Kaletra)
- Loratadine (Claritin)
- Lovastatin (Mevacor)
- Maraviroc (Selzentry)
- Mefloquine (Lariam)
- Methadone
- Methoxetamine
- Methylprednisolone
- Midazolam (Versed)
- Mifepristone (Mifeprex)
- Mirtazapine (NaSSA)
- Modafinil (Provigil)
- Nateglinide
- Nefazodone
- Nelfinavir
- Nevirapine (Viramune)
- Nicardipine (Cardene)
- Nifedipine (Adalat)
- Nimodipine (Nimotop)
- Nisoldipine (Sular)
- Nitrendipine (Baypress)
- Norfluoxetine
- Omeprazole
- Ondansetron
- Oxybutynin (Ditropan)
- Oxycodone (Percodan)
- Paclitaxel (Taxol)

- Paricalcitol (Zemplar)
- Pimozide (Orap)
- Pioglitazone
- Praziquantel (Biltricide)
- Prednisolone Prednisone
- Progesterone
- Propranolol Propoxyphene (Darvon)
- Quazepam (Doral)
- Quetiapine (Seroquel)
- Quinacrine
- Quinidine
- Quinine
- Ranolazine (Ranexa)
- Reboxetine
- Repaglinide (Prandin)
- Rifabutin (Rimactane)
- Risperidone
- Ritonavir (Norvir)
- Salmeterol
- Saquinavir (Invirase)
- Sertraline
- Sibutramine (Meridia)
- Sildenafil (Viagra)
- Simvastatin (Zocor)
- Sirolimus (Rapamune)
- Solifenacin (Vesicare)
- Sorafenib
- Sufentanil (Sufenta)
- Sunitinib (Sutent)
- Tacrolimus (Prograf)
- Tadalafil (Cialis)
- Tamoxifen (Nolvadex)
- Tamsulosin (Flomax)
- Telithromycin
- Temsirolimus
- Teniposide (Vumon)

- Terfenadine
- Testosterone
- Tiagabine (Gabitril)
- Tinidazole (Tindamax)
- Tipranavir (Aptivus)
- Topiramate (Topamax)
- Toremifene
- Tramadol
- Trazodone
- Triazolam (Halcion)
- Vardenafil (Levitra)
- Vemurafenib
- Venlafaxine
- Verapamil (Calan)
- Vinblastine (Velbane)
- Vincristine (Oncovin)
- Vindesine
- Warfarin (Coumadin)
- Zaleplon
- Ziprasidone (Geodon)
- Zolpidem (Ambien)
- Zonisamide (Zonegran)
- Zopiclone (Imovane)

+ A CYP3A4 inhibitor will cause decreased clearance of a substrate and an associated higher increase in plasma area under the curve (AUC).

- Amiodarone
- Amprenavir
- Aprepitant
- Atazanavir
- Avalox
- Bergamottin (Grapefruit)
- Bicalutamide
- Buprenorphine
- Cafestol (in unfiltered coffee)
- Chloramphenicol
- Cimetidine

- Cipro
- Ciprofloxacin
- Clarithromycin
- Conivaptan
- Cyclosporine
- Darunavir
- Dasatinib
- Delavirdine
- Diltiazem
- Dithiocarbamate
- Erythromycin
- Fluconazole
- Fluoroquinolone (cipro, ciprofloxacin, levequin, avalox, floxacin)
- Fluoxetine
- Fluvoxamine
- Fosamprenavir
- Gestodene
- Ginkgo biloba
- Grapefruit juice
- Imatinib
- Indinavir
- Isoniazid
- Itraconazole
- Ketoconazole
- Lapatinib
- Mibefradil
- Miconazole
- Mifepristone
- Milk thistle
- Nefazodone
- Nelfinavir
- Norfloxacin
- Norfluoxetine
- Orphenadrine
- Piperine
- Posaconazole

- Ritonavir
- Quinupristin
- Saquinavir
- Star fruit
- Tamoxifen
- Telithromycin
- Troleandomycin
- Valerian
- Verapamil
- Voriconazole

+ CYP3A4 inducers: (increases metabolic activity of CYP3A4 by binding to and/or activating, or by increasing the expression of the CYP3A4 coding)

- Aminoglutethimide
- Bexarotene
- Bosentan
- Butalbital
- Carbamazepine
- Dexamethasone
- Efavirenz
- Fosphenytoin
- Griseofulvin
- Modafinil
- Nafcillin
- Nevirapine
- Oxcarbazepine
- Phenobarbital
- Phenytoin
- Pioglitazone
- Primidone
- Rifabutin
- Rifampin
- Rifapentine
- St. John's wort
- Troglitazone

SNP ID	SNP Name	Risk Allele	Allele Effect
rs2740574	CYP3A4*1B 392G>A	G	-GG=Involved in androgen metabolism (oxidative deactivation of testosterone) -GG/AG alleles 10x higher risk of aggressive prostate cancer in African American men (>54%)
rs4986910	CYP3A4*3 M445T	C	-Estrogen metabolism. -Significantly decreased risk of breast cancer with the minor allele T.

http://www.ncbi.nlm.nih.gov/pubmed/19127255?dopt=Abstract

http://www.ncbi.nlm.nih.gov/pubmed/16414488?dopt=Abstract

CYP3A5

+ Overview for CYP3A5 *Cytochrome P450, Family 3, Subfamily A, Polypeptide 5*

- CYP3A5, CYP3A5*2 rs28365083 (aka, C2899A), CYP3A5*3 rs776746 (aka, G237A), CYP3A5*6 rs10264272 (aka, G624A,) CYP3A5*9 rs28383479 (aka, G1009A) is expressed in the prostate and the liver. It is also expressed in epithelium of the small intestine and large intestine for uptake and in small amounts in the bile duct, nasal mucosa, kidney, adrenal cortex, epithelium of the gastric mucosa with intestinal metaplasia, gallbladder, intercalated ducts of the pancreas, chief cells of the parathyroid, and the corpus luteum of the ovary (at protein level).

http://www.uniprot.org/uniprot/P08684

- CYP3A5*2 rs28365083 – nonfunctional allele
- CYP3A5*3 rs776746 - most common nonfunctional allele
- CYP3A5*9 rs28383479 – nonfunctional allele

❖ **NOTE:** CYP3A5*1 - in terms of phenotypes, individuals are 'expressors' of CYP3A5 if they carry at least one CYP3A5*1 allele, and 'nonexpressors' if they don't.

http://www.snpedia.com/index.php/CYP3A5

❖ **NOTE:** Metabolizer variations in CYP3A5, depending on alleles:
- Extensive metabolizers have diplotype *1/*1
- Intermediate metabolizers have diplotypes *1/*3, *1/*6, or *1/*7
- Poor metabolizers have diplotypes *3/*3, *6/*6, *7/*7, *3/*6, *3/*7, *6/*7

https://www.pharmgkb.org/guideline/PA166124619

+ Catalytic activity:
- RH + reduced flavoprotein + O2 = ROH + oxidized flavoprotein + H2O

+ Cofactor:
- Heme

http://www.uniprot.org/uniprot/P20815

+ In liver microsomes, CYP3A5 is involved in an NADPH-dependent electron transport pathway. It oxidizes a variety of structurally unrelated compounds, including steroid hormones, fatty acids, and xenobiotics.

http://ghr.nlm.nih.gov/gene/CYP3A5

+ CYP3A5 metabolizes drugs such as olanzapine, tacrolimus, nifedipine, and cyclosporine, as well as the steroid hormones testosterone, progesterone, and androstenedione.

+ Catalytic activity:
- RH + reduced flavoprotein + O2 = ROH + oxidized flavoprotein + H2O.

+ CYP3A5 is responsible for the metabolism of tacrolimus, which is an inhibitor of calcineurin that has been used widely to prevent organ rejection since its approval in the United States in 1994. Despite this effort to individualize tacrolimus therapy, a large percentage of patients suffer from adverse effects, especially nephrotoxicity. "In vitro to in vivo scaling using both liver microsomes and recombinant enzymes yielded higher predicted in vivo tacrolimus clearances for patients with a CYP3A5*1/*3 genotype compared with those with a CYP3A5*3/*3 genotype. In addition, formation of 13-DMT was 13.5-fold higher in human kidney microsomes with a CYP3A5*1/*3 genotype compared with those with a CYP3A5*3/*3 genotype. These data suggest that CYP3A5 contributes significantly to the metabolic clearance of tacrolimus in the liver and kidney."
http://dmd.aspetjournals.org/content/34/5/836.full

"The CPIC dosing guideline for tacrolimus recommends increasing the starting dose by 1.5 to 2 times the recommended starting dose in patients who are CYP3A5 intermediate or extensive metabolizers, though total starting dose should not exceed 0.3 mg/kg/day. Therapeutic drug monitoring should also be used to guide dose adjustments."
https://www.pharmgkb.org/gene/PA131

+ This gene may be an important contributor to individual and inter-racial variation in CYP3A mediated metabolism of drugs including antipsychotics (olanzapine), antiestrogen (tamoxifen), anticancer (irinotecan, docetaxel, vincristine), antimalarial (mefloquine, artemether, lumefantrine), immunomodulators (tacrolimus, cyclosporine), antihistamines (chlorpheniramine, terfenadine, astemizole), antiplatelets (clopidogrel), antihypertensives (nifedipine, amlodipine, felodipine, verapamil), antivirals (indinavir, nelfinavir, ritonavir, saquinavir), HMG-CoA reductase inhibitors (atorvastatin, cerivastatin, lovastatin) antibiotics (clarithromycin), and steroids (testosterone, estradiol, progesterone and androstenedione).
http://www.ncbi.nlm.nih.gov/pubmed/24604039?dopt=Abstract

+ Medications/other that may affect CYP3A5 enzymatic function:

- Alfentanil
- Alprazolam
- Alprazolam
- Amiodarone
- Amitriptyline
- Amlodipine
- Amprenavir
- Aripiprazole
- Aprepitant
- Argatroban
- Atorvastatin
- Artemether
- Astemizole
- Axitinib
- Azelastine
- Beclomethasone
- Boceprevir
- Brentuximab vedotin
- Buprenorphine
- Buspirone
- Cabazitaxel
- Caffeine
- Carbamazepine
- Chloramphenicol
- Chloroquine
- Chlorphenamine
- Cilostazol
- Cimetidine
- Ciprofloxacin
- Cisapride

- Clarithromycin
- Clonidine
- Clopidogrel
- Cocaine
- Codeine
- Crizotinib
- Cyclophosphamide
- Cyclosporine
- Dapsone
- Dasatinib
- Daunorubicin
- Delavirdine
- Dexamethasone
- Diazepam
- Diltiazem
- Disulfiram
- Docetaxel
- Dolutegravir
- Domperidone
- Dutasteride
- Enzalutamide
- Eplerenone
- Erlotinib
- Estradiol
- Estrone
- Ethosuximide
- Etoposide
- Felodipine
- Fentanyl
- Finasteride
- Fluconazole
- Fluoxetine
- Flutamide
- Fluticasone
- Fluvoxamine
- Gestodene
- Gefitinib
- Fluvastatin
- Granisetron
- Halofantrine
- Haloperidol
- Hydrocortisone
- Ifosfamide
- Iloperidone
- Imatinib
- Indinavir
- Irinotecan
- Itraconazole
- Ketoconazole
- Lapatinib
- Lercanidipine
- Levomethadyl
- Lidocaine
- Losartan
- Lovastatin
- Methadone
- Midazolam
- Modafinil
- Mycophenolate
- Nateglinide
- Nefazodone
- Nelfinavir
- Flutamide
- Nicardipine
- Nifedipine
- Nevirapine
- Nimodipine
- Nisoldipine
- Nitrendipine
- Norethindrone
- Norfloxacin
- Nortriptyline
- Ondansetron
- Oxazepam
- Oxcarbazepine
- Oxybutynin
- Oxycodone
- Paclitaxel
- Paliperidone
- Pentamidine
- Perampanel
- Phenelzine
- Phenobarbital
- Phenytoin
- Pimozide
- Ponatinib
- Pravastatin
- Praziquantel
- Progesterone
- Propranolol
- Quetiapine
- Quinacrine
- Quinine
- Ranitidine
- Reserpine
- Rifampicin
- Nimodipine
- Nisoldipine
- Nitrendipine
- Rifapentine
- Risperidone
- Ritonavir
- Rivaroxaban
- Rosuvastatin
- Salmeterol
- Saquinavir
- Saxagliptin
- Sildenafil

- Simvastatin
- Sirolimus
- Sorafenib
- Sulfasalazine
- Sunitinib
- Tamoxifen
- Telithromycin
- Temsirolimus
- Teniposide
- Testosterone
- Thalidomide
- Trazodone
- Tretinoin
- Triazolam
- Troleandomycin
- Udenafil
- Valproic Acid
- Vardenafil
- Verapamil
- Vincristine
- Voriconazole
- Zalcitabine
- Zaleplon
- Ziprasidone
- Zolpidem

SNP ID	SNP Name	Risk Allele	Allele Effect
rs28365083	CYP3A5*2	T	-Non-functioning allele
rs776746	CYP3A5*3	A G	-Most common non-functioning allele -Low activity

http://www.ncbi.nlm.nih.gov/pubmed/17521857

Section 2.2.4 - The CYP4** Family

CYP4A11

+ **Overview for CYP4A11** *Cytochrome P450, Family 4, Subfamily A, Polypeptide 11*
    - CYP4A11, rs9333025 (aka, G921A)
    - CYP4A11 localizes to the endoplasmic reticulum and hydroxylates medium-chain fatty acids such as laurate and myristate, and is involved in drug metabolism and synthesis of cholesterol, steroids, and other lipids.

+ Catalyzes the omega- and (omega-1)-hydroxylation of various fatty acids such as laurate, myristate, and palmitate. Has little activity toward prostaglandins A1 and E1. Oxidizes arachidonic acid to 20-hydroxyeicosatetraenoic acid (20-HETE).

http://www.genecards.org/cgi-bin/carddisp.pl?gene=CYP4A11

+ Catalytic activity:
    - Octane + 2 reduced rubredoxin + O2 + 2 H+ = 1-octanol + 2 oxidized rubredoxin + H2O

+ Cofactor:
    - Heme

http://www.uniprot.org/uniprot/Q02928

+ Medications/other that may affect CYP4A11 enzymatic function:
    - Cisplatin
    - Clofibrate
    - Dexamethasone

- Estrone
- Pegvisomant
- Rifampicin
- Ethanol
- Pentamidine
- Tretinoin
- Lansoprazole
- Phenobarbital

Section 2.2.5 – SNPs Related to Phase I Detoxification

HFE

+ **Overview for HFE** *Human Hemochromatosis protein*
  - HFR, rs1800562 (aka, C282Y), rs1800708 (aka, 110795T>C), rs2071302 (aka, 11622T>C); rs2794719 (aka, 6382T>G); rs9366637 (aka, 6590C>T); rs2071303 (aka, 8828T>C); rs1799945 (aka, H63D).
  - HFE C282Y: This gene encodes human hemochromatosis protein, which is thought to regulate iron absorption by regulating the interaction of the transferrin receptor with transferrin.

+ The protein encoded by this gene is a membrane protein that is similar to MHC class I-type proteins and associates with beta-2 microglobulin (beta2M).

+ HFE is responsible for regulating the absorption of iron

+ The iron storage disorder hereditary hemochromatosis (HHC) is an autosomal recessive genetic disorder that usually results from defects in this gene.

+ HFE is related to positive regulation of T-cell mediated cytotoxicity.

http://www.uniprot.org/uniprot/Q6B0J5

+ Hereditary hemochromatosis, also called HH, is an iron storage disorder where excess iron is not effectively removed from the blood. In serious cases, this excess iron will cause iron overload and if untreated can lead to cirrhosis of the liver, diabetes, hypermelanotic pigmentation of the skin, heart disease, liver cancer, depression, fatigue, and other problems.

+ Those with two copies of hereditary hemochromatosis alleles will very likely have some trouble processing iron, but won't necessarily have hemochromatosis. Hemochromatosis is only diagnosed when blood iron levels exceed certain thresholds. Depending on which alleles and other factors, iron processing deficiency may not reach the level of formally being diagnosed as hemochromatosis. Women are less likely to have hemochromatosis because menstruation will regularly eliminate excess iron, but may become affected after menopause. Similarly, regular blood donors are unlikely to be affected. Diet, alcohol consumption, and supplement use all can affect blood iron levels.

http://www.snpedia.com/index.php/Hemochromatosis

+ The mutation or polymorphism most commonly associated with hemochromatosis is p. C282Y. About one in two hundred people of Northern European origin have two copies of this variant, particularly males. They are at high risk of developing hemochromatosis.

http://www.niddk.nih.gov/health-information/health-topics/liver-disease/hemochromatosis/Pages/facts.aspx

+ The HFE protein has been shown to interact with transferrin receptor protein 1 (TFRC).

http://www.ncbi.nlm.nih.gov/pubmed/6270680

+ Its primary mode of action is then through regulation of the iron storage hormone hepcidin.

http://www.ncbi.nlm.nih.gov/pubmed/16848710

❖ **NOTE**: If low ferritin, then could have oxalate issues (which inhibits iron absorption) BMP2.

http://www.ncbi.nlm.nih.gov/pubmed/17847004

+ The following tests can be used to detect an overload of iron in the body:

| Serum ferritin | Total iron binding capacity |
| Serum iron | Serum transferrin saturation |

+ If any of these are out of range, your practitioner may suggest additional testing, such as:

Liver function tests	Blood sugar levels
Lyme	SIBO (small bacterial overgrowth)
Alpha-fetoprotein levels	Electrocardiogram
CT Scan	Ultrasound
MRI	

+ Possible treatments include:
- Phlebotomy (drawing blood will remove excess iron)
- Calcium supplementation (Calcium binds with iron)
- Higher oxalate diet (Oxalates bind with iron. When treating someone with a vitamin B-6 deficiency, low lysine, pyroluria, calcium oxalate stones, elevated oxalates, and the patient has a hereditary hemochromatosis SNP compromised, you may then start seeing an elevation in ferritin.)

http://www.irondisorders.org/Websites/idi/files/Content/854256/DietRecommendations.pdf

- Consuming tea or coffee with the chemical tannin (tannin binds with iron). Unlike other alcohol, red wine contains tannins. Tannins are not recommended if there is liver damage.

http://www.irondisorders.org/Websites/idi/files/Content/854256/DietRecommendations.pdf

❖ **NOTE**: Some of these treatments can be dangerous and cause other health issues. This should only be done under the supervision of a qualified practitioner.

+ Many practitioners suggest avoiding the following:

- Supplements that include iron
- Alcohol
- Sugar
- Artificial ascorbic acid (vitamin C-rich foods instead)
- Foods enriched with iron, like cereals and flours, that are fortified
- Avoid shellfish because people with hereditary hemochromatosis are more prone to infection. Shellfish contain vibrio vulnificus, which can be fatal to people with high levels of iron

http://www.irondisorders.org/Websites/idi/files/Content/854256/DietRecommendations.pdf
http://www.hemochromatosisdna.com/about-the-disease/treatment#.VT7NELmUCUk

+ Symptoms of iron overload:
- hearing loss
- osteoporosis
- liver disease
- metabolic syndrome
- enlarged liver or spleen
- hairloss
- cirrhosis
- hypothyroidism
- liver cancer
- hypogonadism
- elevated liver enzymes
- premature death
- heart attack
- testicular failure
- cardiomyopathy
- impotence
- heart failure
- infertility
- diabetes mellitus
- depression
- elevated blood sugar
- hypopituitarism
- elevated iron (serum iron, serum ferritin)
- osteoarthritis
- adrenal function problems
- joint pain
- grayish colored skin
- bone pain
- jaundice
- loss of period
- yellowing of the eyes
- loss of interest in sex

+ Iron mismanagement resulting in overload can accelerate neurodegenerative diseases such as, Alzheimer's, early-onset Parkinson's, Huntington's, epilepsy, and multiple sclerosis.

http://www.irondisorders.org/iron-overload

+ Some genetic mutations to look at in association with HFE SNPs:
- SOD2 A16V (SOD 2 is iron binding) and HFE together can cause a tenfold increase for heart disease.

http://www.ncbi.nlm.nih.gov/pubmed/15591282?dopt=Abstract

- G6PD Folks with G6PD deficiency typically have too much iron in their blood.

http://g6pddeficiency.org/wp/faq/good-bad-iron/

- <u>RAB6B</u> Some HFE SNPs in combination with RAB6B SNPs have been associated with elevated serum transferrin saturation.

http://www.ncbi.nlm.nih.gov/pubmed/19084217?dopt=Abstract

+ Molecular function:
- Antigen binding

+ Biological process:
- Antigen processing and presentation
- Antigen processing and presentation of peptide antigen via MHC class I

http://www.uniprot.org/uniprot/Q6B0J5

SNP ID	SNP Name	Risk Allele	Allele Effect
rs1800562	HFE C282Y	A	-Key gene. Prevents the altered HFE protein from reaching the cell surface, so it cannot interact with Hepcidin and transferrin receptors. -Increased risk of Porphyria cutanea tarda. -Increased risk of Sideroblastic anemia when SNPs in ALAS2.
rs1799945	HFE H63D	G	-Works with HFE C282Y to increase risk.

http://ghr.nlm.nih.gov/gene/HFE
http://www.ncbi.nlm.nih.gov/pubmed/17521857

PON1

+ **<u>Overview for PON1</u>** *Paraoxonase 1 protein* (aka, arylamine N-acetyltransferase)
- PON1, rs662 (aka, Q192R) is an arylesterase that mainly hydrolyzes paroxon to produce p-nitrophenol. Paroxon is an organophosphorus anticholinesterase compound that is produced in vivo by oxidation of the insecticide, parathion. Polymorphisms in this gene are a risk factor in coronary artery disease.

+ The majority of organophosphate pesticides (OP) in current use are phosphorothioates (P = S), which are activated by the cytochromes P450 to the oxon (P = O), that inhibit acetylcholinesterase in the nervous system and neuromuscular junctions to cause acute toxicity. http://dmd.aspetjournals.org/content/35/2/315.full

+ PON1 hydrolyzes the toxic metabolites of a variety of organophosphorus insecticides and nerve gasses.

http://www.uniprot.org/uniprot/P27169

+ Insecticides:
- parathion
- diazinon
- chlorpyrifos

+ A number of organophosphorothioate insecticides are detoxified in part via a two-step pathway involving bioactivation of the parent compound by the cytochrome P450 systems, then hydrolysis of the resulting oxygenated metabolite (oxon) by serum and liver paraoxonases (PON1).

+ The expression of PON1 is developmentally regulated. Newborns have very low levels of PON1.

http://www.ncbi.nlm.nih.gov/pubmed/10794389

+ PON1 is important in the prevention of vascular disease. The wide acceptance of the oxidation theory of atherogenesis has prompted attention to antioxidant mechanisms, particularly the prevention of lipid oxidation by high-density lipoprotein-associated proteins like paraoxonase 1 (PON1) enzyme. There is a growing interest in the enzyme's importance in cardiovascular health prompted by evidence that it may have a role in lipid metabolism and the development of atherosclerosis via its antioxidant effects. PON1 is capable of hydrolyzing homocysteine thiolactone, a metabolite of homocysteine, which can impair protein function leading to endothelial dysfunction and vascular damage.

http://www.ncbi.nlm.nih.gov/pubmed/22673025

+ Sporadic amyotrophic lateral sclerosis (SALS) causes progressive muscle weakness because of the loss of motor neurons. SALS has been associated with exposure to environmental toxins, including pesticides and chemical warfare agents, many of which are organophosphates. http://www.sciencedirect.com/science/article/pii/S0161813X06003007

+ Catalytic activity:
- A phenyl acetate + H2O = a phenol + acetate
- An aryl dialkyl phosphate + H2O = dialkyl phosphate + an aryl alcohol
- An N-acyl-L-homoserine lactone + H2O = an N-acyl-L-homoserine

+ Cofactor:
- Calcium. It binds two calcium ions per subunit.

+ Molecular function:
- Aromatic compound catabolic process
- Carboxylic acid catabolic process
- Dephosphorylation
- Organophosphate catabolic process
- Positive of binding

- Positive regulation of cholesterol efflux
- Positive regulation of cholesterol activity
- Response to external stimulau
- Response to fatty acids
- Response to fluoride
- Response to nutrient level
- Response to toxic substance

+ Subcellular location:
- Secreted > extracellular space

+ Cellular component:
- Blood microparticle
- Extracellular exosome
- Extracellular region
- High-density lipoprotein particle
- Intracellular membrane-bounded organelle
- Sperical high-density lipoprotein particle

http://www.uniprot.org/uniprot/P27169

+ Associated disease:
- Microvascular complications of diabetes - pathological conditions that develop in numerous tissues and organs as a consequence of diabetes mellitus. They include diabetic retinopathy, diabetic nephropathy leading to end-stage renal disease, and diabetic neuropathy. Diabetic retinopathy remains the major cause of new-onset blindness among diabetic adults. It is characterized by vascular permeability and increased tissue ischemia and angiogenesis. Disease susceptibility is associated with variations affecting the gene represented in this entry. Homozygosity for the Leu-55 allele is strongly associated with the development of retinal disease in diabetic patients.

http://www.omim.org/entry/612633

RAB6B

+ **Overview for RAB6B** *Ras-related protein Rab-6B*
- rs2280673 (aka, C282Y)
- rs2280673 is relevant to hemochromatosis as it is associated with serum transferrin levels. The risk allele appears to be C. **(See HFE write-up above)**

http://www.snpedia.com/index.php/Hemochromatosis
http://www.ncbi.nlm.nih.gov/pubmed/19084217?dopt=Abstract

+ Ras-related protein has a role in retrograde membrane traffic at the level of the Golgi complex and may function in retrograde transport in neuronal cells.

http://www.sciencedirect.com/science/article/pii/S0014482707002923

+ The molecular functions for RAB6B are:
- GTPase activity
- GTPase binding
- Myosin V binding

+ Biological processes:
- Intracellular protein transport
- Intra-Golgi vesicle-mediated transport
- Rab protein signal transduction
- Retrograde transport, endosome to Golgi
- Retrograde vesicle-mediated transport, Golgi to ER

http://hmg.oxfordjournals.org/content/early/2011/06/22/hmg.ddr272.full.pdf

+ Subcellular location:
- Golgi apparatus membrane; lipid anchor
- Cytoplasmic vesicle

+ Cellular component:
- Cytoplasmic membrane-bounded vesicle
- Golgi apparatus
- Golgi membrane

http://www.uniprot.org/uniprot/Q9NRW1

SOD3

+ **Overview for SOD3** *Superoxide Dismutase 3*, Extracellular
- SOD3, rs2855262 (aka, 489 C>T) is a member of the superoxide dismutase (SOD) protein family. SODs are antioxidant enzymes that catalyze the dismutation of two superoxide radicals into hydrogen peroxide and oxygen. The product of this gene is thought to protect the brain, lungs, and other tissues from oxidative stress. The protein is secreted into the extracellular space and forms a glycosylated homotetramer that is anchored to the extracellular matrix (ECM) and cell surfaces through an interaction with heparan sulfate proteoglycan and collagen.

http://www.ncbi.nlm.nih.gov/gene/6649

+ SOD3 protects the extracellular space from toxic effect of reactive oxygen intermediates by converting superoxide radicals into hydrogen peroxide and oxygen.

+ The product of this SOD3 is thought to protect the brain, lungs, and other tissues from oxidative stress.

http://www.ncbi.nlm.nih.gov/gene/6649

+ Diseases related to SOD3 are coronary artery disease, pulmonary emphysema, prostate cancer, keratopathy and usual interstitial pneumonia.
  - Keratopathy is related to cataract and bullous keratopathy. The compounds *uric acid* and *manganese superoxide* have been mentioned in the context of this disorder. Affiliated tissues include endothelial, eye, and brain.

+ SOD3 plays a role in therapeutic effects in tissue damage recovery.

+ Foods rich in superoxide dismutase are sprouts and algae.

+ Catalytic activity:
  - 2 superoxide + 2 H+ = O_2 + H_2O_2

+ Cofactor:
  - Copper (Cu cation)   Binds one copper ion per subunit.
  - Zinc (Zn^{2+})   Binds one zinc ion per subunit

+ Molecular function:
  - Copper ion binding
  - Heparin binding
  - Superoxide dismutast activity
  - Zinc ion binding

+ Biological process:
  - Removal of superoxide radicals
  - Response to copper ions
  - Response to hypoxia
  - Response to reactive oxygen species
  - Retrograde vesicle-mediated transport, Golgi to ER

+ Subcellular location:
  - Secreted > extracellular space
  ❖ **NOTE**: ninety-nine percent of EC-SOD is anchored to heparan sulfate proteoglycans in the tissue interstitium, and one percent is located in the vasculature in equilibrium between the plasma and the endothelium.

+ Cellular component
  - Cytoplasm
  - Extracellular exosome
  - Extracellular matrix
  - Extracellular region

- Extracellular space
- Golgi lumen
- Nucelus
- Trans-Golgi network

http://www.uniprot.org/uniprot/P08294

SNP ID	SNP Name	Risk Allele	Allele Effect
rs2855262	SOD3 489>T	T	-Copper and zinc in it catalytic center. -No research in this particular variant. Other research suggests and -15 fold increase in SOD3 in plasma

http://www.ncbi.nlm.nih.gov/pubmed/12126755

Section 2.3 - Phase II detoxification

- ❖ **NOTE**: Recall from Section 2.1 that the toxic chemicals that enter the body generally are fat-soluble, which means they dissolve only in fatty or oily solutions and not in water. This makes them difficult for the body to excrete. Phase I detox either directly neutralizes a toxin (e.g., caffeine) or modifies the toxic chemical to form activated intermediates (e.g., estrone) that are then neutralized by one or more of the several phase II detox enzyme systems. In phase I detox, a toxic chemical is converted into a less harmful chemical. Some may be converted from relatively harmless substances into potentially carcinogenic substances. Phase II detox is called the conjugation pathway, whereby the liver cells add another substance (e.g., cysteine, taurine, glutathione, glycine, or a sulphur molecule) to a toxic chemical or drug, to render it less harmful. This makes the toxin or drug water-soluble, so it can then be excreted from the body via watery fluids such as bile or urine. Individual xenobiotics and metabolites usually follow one or two distinct pathways.

  There are essentially six phase II detox pathways:
  - Glutathione conjugation
  - Acetylation
  - Glucuronidation
  - Amino acid conjugation (glycine, taurine)
  - Sulfation
  - Methylation

I have grouped SNPs in their phase II categories, in alphabetical order. I have also included SNPs "related" to that category. For example, under the "glutathione" category, you will find the SNPs that encode for glutathione (e.g., GSTM1), as well as, SNPs that are related to glutathione (e.g., GGT1, which catalyzes the transfer of the glutamyl moiety of glutathione to a variety of amino acids and dipeptide acceptors). Through conjugation, the liver is able to turn drugs, intermediary metabolites of hormones, and various toxins into excretable substances. For efficient phase II detox, the liver cells require sulphur-containing amino acids such as, taurine and cysteine. Nutrient cofactors such as, glycine, glutamine, choline, and inositol are also required for efficient phase II detox. The rate at which phase I detox produces activated intermediary metabolites must be balanced by the rate at which phase II detox finishes its processing. People with a very active phase I detox (e.g., up-regulated CYP1B1), coupled with slow or inactive phase II detox enzymes (e.g., down-regulated COMT enzyme), may find themselves with ongoing health issues such as premenstrual syndrome. In that case, removing substances that up-regulate phase I detox and support, via nutrient cofactors, the down-regulated phase II detox enzymes, may result in improvement in liver detoxification. An imbalance between phase I and phase II can also occur when a person is exposed to large amounts of toxins or exposed to toxins for a long period of time. In these situations, the critical nutrients needed for phase II detox become depleted, which allows the highly toxic activated intermediates to build up. Proper functioning of the liver's detoxification systems is especially important for the prevention of cancer. Up to ninety percent of all cancers are thought to be due to the effects of environmental carcinogens, such as those in cigarette smoke, food, water, and air, combined with deficiencies of the nutrients the body needs for proper functioning of the detoxification and immune systems. When working properly, the liver clears ninety-nine percent of the bacteria and other toxins during the first pass. However, when the liver is damaged, such as in alcoholics, the passage of toxins increases by over a factor of ten.

Section 2.3.1 – Glutathione conjugation – our body's master anti-oxidant

Glutathione:

Cytosolic and membrane-bound forms of glutathione S-transferase are encoded by two distinct supergene families. Currently, eight distinct classes of the soluble cytoplasmic mammalian glutathione S-transferases have been identified: alpha, kappa, mu, omega, pi, sigma, theta, and zeta.

Glutathione recycling - Reduced glutathione is converted to its oxidized form, GSSG via GSH peroxidase, using H2O2 (from SOD enzyme). GSSG is converted back to reduced GSH via GSH reductase using NADPH (from pentose phosphate pathway).

Nutrients needed - Glutathione precursors (cysteine, glycine, glutamic acid, and co-factors), essential fatty acids (black currant seed oil, flax seed oil, EPA), parathyroid tissue, and vitamin B-6.

- ❖ **NOTE**: Although ethyl alcohol is cleared via glutathion conjugation and sulfation, ethyl alcohol associated SNPs are listed in the Section 2.3.7.2.

+Some drugs cleared/conjugated by glutathione:
- Acetaminophen
- Penicillin
- Ethacrynic acid
- Tetracycline

+Some Xenobiotics cleared/conjugated by Glutathione:
- Styrene
- Acroiein
- Ethylene oxide
- Benzo pyrenes
- Methylparathion
- Chlorobenzene
- Anthracene
- Toxic metals
- Petrolem distillates
- Napthalene

+Some substances of dietary and endogenous origin cleared/conjugated by glutathione:
- Bacterial toxins
- Aflotoxin
- Lipid peroxides
- Ethyl alcohol
- Quercitin
- N-acetylcysteine
- Prostaglandins
- Billirubin

GGT1

+ <u>**Overview for GGT1**</u> *Gamma-glutamyltransferase 1*

- GGT1, rs6519519 (aka, C17146T), rs5760485 (aka, T11756C), rs5751901 (aka, T17549C)
- GGT/FAM211B rs4820599
- Aka, CD224 (Cluster of Differentiation 224)

http://en.wikipedia.org/wiki/GGT1

- Human gamma-glutamyltransferase catalyzes the transfer of the glutamyl moiety of glutathione to a variety of amino acids and dipeptide acceptors and is present in tissues involved in absorption and secretion.
- Its main physiological function is to make cysteine available for regeneration of intracellular glutathione and hence, to protect against oxidative stress.

http://www.ncbi.nlm.nih.gov/pmc/articles/PMC3276286/

+ This enzyme is a member of the gamma-glutamyltransferase protein family, of which many members have not yet been fully characterized. This gene encodes several transcript variants; studies suggest that many transcripts of this gene family may be non-functional or represent pseudogenes. The functional transcripts that have been fully characterized have been grouped and classified as type I gamma-glutamyltransferase. Complex splicing events may take place in a tissue-specific manner, resulting in marked dissimilarity in the 5' UTRs. Several 5' UTR transcript variants of the type I gene have been identified in different tissues and cancer cells.

http://www.ncbi.nlm.nih.gov/pubmed/10392451

+ GGT1 SNPs may contribute to diabetes and other metabolic disorders.

http://www.ncbi.nlm.nih.gov/gene/2678

+ Exposure to tetrachloroethylene resulted in a significant increase in total GGT serum levels.

https://www.wikigenes.org/e/ref/e/1351699.html

+ Gamma-glutamyltransferase 1 cleaves the gamma-glutamyl bond of extracellular glutathione (gamma-Glu-Cys-Gly), glutathione conjugates, and other gamma-glutamyl compounds. The metabolism of glutathione releases free glutamate and the dipeptide, cysteinyl-glycine, which is hydrolyzed to cysteine and glycine by dipeptidases. In the presence of high concentrations of dipeptides and some amino acids, can also catalyze a transpeptidation reaction, transferring the gamma-glutamyl moiety to an acceptor amino acid to form a new gamma-glutamyl compound. Initiates extracellular glutathione (GSH) breakdown, provides cells with a local cysteine supply and contributes to maintain intracellular GSH level. It is part of the cell antioxidant defense mechanism. Isoform 3 seems to be inactive.

+ Serum GGT activity is an independent predictor of morbidity and mortality, and increases in obesity and metabolic syndrome. These associations are strengthened by our discovery that SNPs affecting GGT, even at suggestive, rather than genome-wide-significant levels, include a highly significant excess of those affecting cardiovascular disease and diabetes. The direction of association between SNPs at the *GGT1* locus (and potentially elsewhere) and serum GGT activity changes with age and differences in allelic effects on GGT between health and disease deserves further study.

http://www.ncbi.nlm.nih.gov/pmc/articles/PMC3276286/

+ Hepatic GGT activity is elevated in some liver diseases. GGT is released into the bloodstream after liver damage, and an elevated level of the enzyme may be a useful early sign of hepatocellular carcinoma.

http://www.omim.org/entry/231950

+ GGT1 catalyzes the transfer of the glutamyl moiety of glutathione to a variety of amino acids and dipeptide acceptors. GGT1 also initiates extracellular glutathione (GSH) breakdown, provides cells with a local cysteine supply and contributes to maintain intracellular GSH level. As part of the cell antioxidant defense mechanism, GGT1 can be detected in fetal and adult kidney and liver, adult pancreas, stomach, intestine, placenta, and lung.

http://www.sinobiological.com/GGT1-Protein-Antibody-a-5487.html?gclid=CjwKEAjw7YWrBRCThIyogcGymQsSJAAmz_ndDAyaqdjoJsJoXRcWj_G9Is1vXmM7mntrDvclkiG1ZRoCgO_w_wcB

+ Catalytic activity:
- A (5-L-glutamyl)-peptide + an amino acid = a peptide + a 5-L-glutamyl amino acid
- Glutathione + H_2O = L-cysteinylglycine + L-glutamate.
- Leukotriene C_4 + H_2O = leukotriene D_4 + L-glutamate

+ Enzyme regulation:
- Activated by autocatalytic cleavage

+ Pathway:
- Sulfur metabolism
- Glutathione metabolism

+ Molecular function:
- Gamma-glutamyltransferase activity
- Glutathione hydrolase activity

+ Biological process:
- Arachidonic acid metabolic process
- Cysteine biosynthetic process
- Glutathione biosynthetic process
- Glutathione derivative biosynthesis process
- Leukotriene biosynthetic process
- **Regulation of Immune system process**
- **Regulation of inflammatory response**

- Small molecule metabolic process
- Xenobiotic metabolic process
- Cellular amino acid metabolic process
- Glutamate metabolic process
- Glutathione catabolic process
- Glutathione metabolic process
- Leukotriene metabolic process
- Spermatogenesis
- Zymogen activation

http://www.uniprot.org/uniprot/P19440

+ Associated disease:
- Glutathionuria
- Glutathioninuria

http://www.genecards.org/cgi-bin/carddisp.pl?gene=GGT1

+ GGT1 may contribute to diabetes and other metabolic disorders.

http://www.ncbi.nlm.nih.gov/gene/2678

+ People exposed to tetrachloroethylene showed a significant increase in total GGT serum levels.

https://www.wikigenes.org/e/ref/e/1351699.html

GPX3

+ **Overview for GPX3** *Glutathione peroxidase 3* (aka, Extracellular Glutathione Peroxidase, Plasma Glutathione Peroxidase)
- GPX3, rs8177412 (aka, 129T>C). This gene encodes plasma glutathione peroxidase (GPx-P) or extracellular glutathione peroxidase, which functions in the detoxification of hydrogen peroxide. It contains a selenocysteine (Sec) residue at its active site. The selenocysteine is encoded by the UGA codon, which normally signals translation termination. The 3' UTR of Sec-containing genes have a common stem-loop structure, the Sec insertion sequence (SECIS), which is necessary for the recognition of UGA as a Sec codon rather than as a stop signal.
- This gene product belongs to the glutathione peroxidase family and protects cells and enzymes from oxidative damage by catalyzing the reduction of hydrogen peroxide, lipid peroxides, and organic hydroperoxide, by glutathione.
- Simply put, GPX3 scavenge peroxides.

http://www.ncbi.nlm.nih.gov/gene?Db=gene&Cmd=ShowDetailView&TermToSearch=2878

- GPX3 is a selenocysteine-containing antioxidant enzyme that reacts with hydrogen peroxide and soluble fatty acid hydroperoxides, thereby helping to maintain redox balance within cells.

http://www.ovarianresearch.com/content/4/1/18
http://www.ncbi.nlm.nih.gov/pmc/articles/PMC2693281/

- Expressed in kidney, lung, breast, placenta, catabolic pathway of activated oxygen species, and free radical detoxification.
- Function: Protects cells and enzymes from oxidative damage by catalyzing the reduction of hydrogen peroxide, lipid peroxides, and organic hydroperoxide by glutathione.

http://www.genecards.org/cgi-bin/carddisp.pl?gene=GPX3
http://www.mybiosource.com/prods/Protein/GLUTATHIONE-PEROXIDASE-GPX-Human/datasheet.php?products_id=173097

+ This gene is often down-regulated in cancer.

+ There were some relationships between rs8177412 of promoter polymorphisms in the plasma glutathione peroxidase (GPX-3) gene and arterial ischemic stroke and they may be an important risk factor for stroke.

http://en.cnki.com.cn/Article_en/CJFDTOTAL-NJYK200902012.htm

+ GPX3 has been found to be positively regulated by 17β-estradiol in skeletal muscle.

http://www.ncbi.nlm.nih.gov/pmc/articles/PMC2854140/
http://journals.plos.org/plosone/article?id=10.1371/journal.pone.0010164

+ Selenium-methylselenocysteine has been shown to increase GPX3 expression.

+ GPX3 was found to be down-regulated by high-fat diet and appears to be decreased in human prostate cancers, suggesting that GPX3 may have a possible role in modulating carcinogenesis.

http://www.ncbi.nlm.nih.gov/pmc/articles/PMC3132426/

+ GPX3 dysfunction occurs commonly in thyroid, prostate, cervical, gastric, and colon cancers.

+ Catalytic activity:
  - 2 glutathione + H_2O_2 = glutathione disulfide + 2 H_2O

+ Molecular function:
  - Glutathione peroxidase activity
  - Selenium binding
  - Transcription factor binding

+ Biological process:
  - Hydrogen peroxide catabolic process
  - Protein homotetramerization

- Response to lipid hydroperoxide
- Response to reactive oxygen species

+ Subcellular location:
- Secreted

+ Cellular component:
- Extracellular exosome
- Extracellular region
- Extracellular space

http://www.uniprot.org/uniprot/P22352

GSR

+ **Overview for GSR** *Glutathione Reductase, Mitochondrial*
- GSR, rs2551715 (aka, A43851G), rs3594 (aka, G*1377T)
- This gene encodes a member of the class-I pyridine nucleotide-disulfide oxidoreductase family. This enzyme is a homodimeric flavoprotein. It is a central enzyme of cellular antioxidant defense and reduces oxidized glutathione disulfide (GSSG) to the sulfhydryl form GSH, which is an important cellular antioxidant. Rare mutations in this gene result in hereditary glutathione reductase deficiency. Multiple alternatively spliced transcript variants encoding different isoforms have been found.
- GSR (glutathione reductase) is a protein-coding gene. Diseases associated with GSR include pyridoxine deficiency and hemolytic anemia due to glutathione reductase deficiency.

http://www.genecards.org/cgi-bin/carddisp.pl?gene=GSR

+ Function: Maintains high levels of reduced glutathione in the cytosol.

+ Glutathione plays a key role in maintaining proper function and preventing oxidative stress in human cells. It can act as a scavenger for hydroxyl radicals, singlet oxygen and various electrophiles. Reduced glutathione reduces the oxidized form of the enzyme glutathione peroxidase, which in turn reduces hydrogen peroxide (H_2O_2), a dangerously reactive species within the cell. In addition, it plays a key role in the metabolism and clearance of xenobiotics, acts as a cofactor in certain detoxifying enzymes, participates in transport, and regenerates antioxidants such and vitamins E and C to their reactive forms. The ratio of GSSH/GSH present in the cell is a key factor in properly maintaining the oxidative balance of the cell, that is, it is critical that the cell maintains high levels of the reduced glutathione and a low level of the oxidized glutathione disulfide. This narrow balance is maintained by glutathione reductase, which catalyzes the reduction of GSSG to GSH.

http://www.sciencedirect.com/science/article/pii/S0304416512002735

+ GSH is a key cellular antioxidant and plays a major role in the phase 2 metabolic clearance of electrophilic xenobiotics.

+ **Link to G6PD** - In Favism, patients lack (or have a much lower) glucose-6-phosphate dehydrogenase, an enzyme in their pentose phosphate pathway that reduces $NADP^+$ to NADPH while catalyzing the conversion of glucose-6-phosphate to 6-Phosphogluconolactone. Glucose-6-phosphate dehydrogenase deficient individuals have less NADPH available for the reduction of oxidized glutathione via glutathione reductase. Thus, their basal ratio of oxidized to reduced glutathione, is significantly higher than that of patients who express glucose-6-phosphate dehydrogenase, normally, making them unable to effectively respond to high levels of reactive oxygen species, which cause cell lysis.

http://www.ncbi.nlm.nih.gov/pubmed/18177777

+ In a recent study, an SNP in the glutathione reductase gene was found to be highly associated with lupus in African Americans in the study.

http://www.ncbi.nlm.nih.gov/pubmed/23637325

+ Mutations in this GSR may result in hereditary glutathione reductase deficiency, pyridoxine deficiency, and hemolytic anemia due to glutathione reductase deficiency.

http://www.genecards.org/cgi-bin/carddisp.pl?gene=GSR

+ Catalytic activity:

    2 glutathione + NADP (+) = glutathione disulfide + NADPH

+ Cofactor:

    Binds one FAD per subunit

+ Molecular function:
- Electron carrier activity
- Flavin adenine dinucleotide binding
- Glutathione-disulfide reductase activity
- NADP binding

+ Biological process:
- Cell redox homeostasis
- Gene expression
- Glutathione metabolic process
- Nucleobase-containing small molecule interconversion
- Nucleobase-containing small molecule metabolic process
- Response to reactive oxygen speciaes (ROS)
- Small molecule metabolic process
- Transcription initiation from RNA polymerase II promoter

+ Cellular component:
- Cytosol
- External side pf plasma membrane
- Extracellular exosome
- Mitochondria matrix

http://www.uniprot.org/uniprot/P00390

+ Associated disease:
- Kwashiokor
- Glioma
- African sleeping sickness
- Heart disease
- Oriental sore
- Oral cancer
- Sarcoidosis

https://www.wikigenes.org/e/gene/e/2936.html

GSS

+ **Overview for GSS** *Glutathione synthetase*
- GSS, rs22273684 (aka, A18836C), rs6088659 (aka, A5997G), rs2236270 (aka, C25447A, rs28936396 (aka, C373T), rs6060124 (aka, G11705T)
- The GSS gene provides instructions for making an enzyme called glutathione synthetase. Glutathione synthetase participates in a process called the gamma-glutamyl cycle. The gamma-glutamyl cycle is a sequence of chemical reactions that takes place in most of the body's cells. These reactions are necessary for the production of glutathione, a small molecule made of three protein building blocks (amino acids). Glutathione protects cells from damage caused by unstable oxygen-containing molecules, which are byproducts of energy production. Glutathione is called an antioxidant because of its role in protecting cells from the damaging effects of these unstable molecules. Glutathione also helps process medications and cancer causing compounds (carcinogens), and helps build DNA, proteins, and other important cellular components.

http://ghr.nlm.nih.gov/gene/GSS.

+ More than thirty mutations in the GSS gene have been identified in people with glutathione synthetase deficiency. Characteristic features of this condition include, the abnormal destruction of red blood cells (hemolytic anemia), the release of large amounts of a compound called 5-oxoproline in the urine (5-oxoprolinuria), and elevated acidity in the blood and tissues (metabolic acidosis). Severely affected individuals may also have neurological problems.

+ Most of the GSS mutations involved in glutathione synthetase deficiency change single amino acids in glutathione synthetase. Other mutations disrupt how genetic information from the GSS gene is pieced together to make a blueprint for producing the enzyme. The altered glutathione synthetase enzyme may be unstable, shorter than usual, or the wrong shape. All of these changes reduce the activity of the enzyme and disrupt the gamma-glutamyl cycle, preventing adequate production of glutathione.

+ Low levels of glutathione affect other chemical reactions in the body, leading to the overproduction of 5-oxoproline. Accumulation of this compound in red blood cells and other tissues causes hemolytic anemia and metabolic acidosis, and its release leads to 5-oxoprolinuria.

+ Glutathione synthetase deficiency is related to an increased rate of hemolysis and defective function of the central nervous system.

http://www.uniprot.org/uniprot/P48637

+ Characteristic features of this condition include, the abnormal destruction of red blood cells (hemolytic anemia), the release of large amounts of a compound called 5-oxoproline in the urine (5-oxoprolinuria), and elevated acidity in the blood and tissues (metabolic acidosis). Severely affected individuals may also have neurological problems.

http://ghr.nlm.nih.gov/gene/GSS

+ Neutropenia has been observed in children with GSS deficiency.

https://www.wikigenes.org/e/gene/e/2937.html

+ Catalytic activity:
- ATP + gamma-L-glutamyl-L-cysteine + glycine = ADP + phosphate + glutathione.

+ Cofactor:
- Magnesium   Binds one Mg^{2+} ion per subunit

+ Pathway:
- Sulfur metabolism
- Glutathione biosynthesis
- Glutathione from L-cystein and -glutamate

+ Molecular function:
- ATP binding
- Glutathiones synthase activity
- Magnesium ion binding
- Glutathione binding
- Glycine binding

- Protein homodimerization activity

+ Biological process:
- Aging
- Cellular amino acid metabolic process
- Glutathion biosynthetic process
- Nervous system development
- Response to amino acids
- Response to nutrient levels
- Response to tumor necrosis factor
- Response to cadmium ion
- Response to oxidative stress
- Small molecule metabolic process
- Glutathione derivative biosynthetic process
- Xenobiotic metabolic process

http://www.uniprot.org/uniprot/P48637

GSTM1

+ **Overview for GSTM1** *Glutathione S-transferase Mu 1*
- GSTM1, rs2740574 (aka, 5419C>T) this gene encodes a cytoplasmic glutathione S-transferase that belongs to the mu class. The mu class of enzymes functions in the detoxification of electrophilic compounds, including carcinogens, therapeutic drugs, environmental toxins, and products of oxidative stress, by conjugation with glutathione.
- Additional rs numbers in "Sterling's App" include, rs4147565 (aka, 6360G>A); rs4147567 (aka, 7107A>G); rs4147568 (aka, 7175T>A); rs1056806 (aka, 7730C>T); rs12562055 (aka, 8048T>A; rs2239892 (aka, 8869A>G).

http://www.ncbi.nlm.nih.gov/gene?Db=gene&Cmd=ShowDetailView&TermToSearch=2944

+ The GSTM1 enzyme is biosynthesized in the body from amino acids L-cysteine, L-glutamic acid, and glycine, so all must be available. The limiting amino acid is typically cysteine; so many folks will take N-Acetyl cysteine as a supplement to build their glutathione pool.

+ Glutathione exists in both reduced (GSH) and oxidized (GSSG) states. In the reduced state, the thiol group of cysteine is able to donate a reducing equivalent ($H^+ + e^-$) to other unstable molecules, such as reactive oxygen species. In donating an electron, glutathione itself becomes reactive, but readily reacts with another reactive glutathione to form glutathione disulfide (GSSG). GSH can then be regenerated from GSSG by the enzyme glutathione reductase (GSR) using NADPH as an electron donor. The ratio of reduced glutathione to oxidized glutathione within cells is often used as a measure of cellular toxicity.

+ Glutathione levels may be reduced due to SNPs, lack of one or more of the three required amino acids (from poor diet or malabsorption), stress, aging, and toxicity. Some health conditions commonly associated with low glutathione levels include, autoimmune disease where, when toxins enter the body and glutathione is low, Th-17 may become upregulated. The upregulated Th-17 produces interleukin 17 (IL-17) and determines the *severity* of the autoimmune flare-up. Thus down-regulating Th-17 via increasing glutathione levels is something to be considered.

http://www.ncbi.nlm.nih.gov/pmc/articles/PMC3254057/

http://www.ncbi.nlm.nih.gov/pmc/articles/PMC3555796

+ Proper glutathione levels are also required so that the other antioxidants such as vitamin C, vitamin E, selenium, and carotenoids, can be properly utilized within the body.

http://blog.radiantlifecatalog.com/bid/62226/7-Ways-to-Boost-Your-Glutathione-raw-foods-vital-whey-and-more

+ Glutathione is important for ATP to function properly.

+ Supplements that may be utilized to support glutathione production:
- Curcumin
- Selenium
- Silymarin (milk thistle)
- Vitamin C
- Vitamin E
- MSM
- NAC
- B vitamins
- Glutathione cream
- Oral glutathione
- IV glutathione, but care must be taken.

+ Foods and herbs that are known to boost glutathione:

(For optimal glutathione boosting, fruits and vegetables are best consumed fresh, not cooked or processed; however, be mindful of goitrogens if thyroid disease.)

- broccoli
- cauliflower
- milk thistle
- curcumin
- kale
- watermelon
- parsley
- whey protein
- raw milk
- raw eggs

- cabbage
- avocado
- spinach
- onion
- turmeric
- red meat
- organ meats
- garlic

+ Catalytic activity:
    - RX + glutathione = HX + R-S-glutathione
+ Molecular function:
    - Enzyme binding
    - Glutathione binding
    - Glutathione transferase activity
    - Protein homodimerization activity
+ Biological process:
    - Cellular detoxification of nitrogen compound
    - Glutathione derivative biosynthetic process
    - Glutathione metabolic process
    - Nitrobenzene metabolic process
    - Small molecule metabolic process
    - Xenobiotic catabolic process
    - Xenobiotic metabolic process
+ Cellular component:
    - Cytoplasm
    - Cytosol

http://www.uniprot.org/uniprot/P09488

GSTM3

+ **Overview for GSTM3** *Glutathione S-transferase Mu 3* (brain)
    - *GSTM3*, rs7483 (aka, V2241) this gene encodes a cytoplasmic glutathione S-transferase that belongs to the mu class. The mu class of enzymes functions in the detoxification of electrophilic compounds, including some carcinogens, therapeutic drugs, environmental toxins, and products of oxidative stress, by conjugation with glutathione.
    - Conjugation of reduced glutathione to a wide number of exogenous and endogenous hydrophobic electrophiles. May govern uptake and detoxification of both endogenous compounds and xenobiotics at the testis and blood-brain barriers.

http://www.genecards.org/cgi-bin/carddisp.pl?gene=GSTM3

+ Catalytic activity:
- RX + glutathione = HX + R-S-glutathione

+ Kinetics:
- KM=1.1 mM for 1-chloro-2, 4-dinitrobenzene
- KM=0.084 mM for glutathione

+ Molecular function:
- Enzyme binding
- Glutathione binding
- Glutathione transferase activity
- Identical protein binding
- Protein homodimerization activity

+ Biological process:
- Cellular detoxification of nitrogen compound
- Establishment of blood-nerve barrier
- Glutathione derivative biosynthetic process
- Glutathione metabolic process
- Nitrobenzene metabolic process
- Response to estrogen
- Small molecule metabolic process
- Xenobiotic catabolic process
- Xenobiotic metabolic proces

+ Cellular component:
- Cytoplasm
- Cytosol
- Extracellular exosome
- Nucleus
- Sperm fibrous sheath

http://www.uniprot.org/uniprot/P21266

GSTP1

+ **Overview for GSTP1** *Glutathione S-transferase Pi 1*
- *GSTP1*, rs1138272 (aka, A114V) this gene is expressed in many human tissues, particularly in the biliary tree and renal distal convoluted tubules.

http://www.ncbi.nlm.nih.gov/pubmed/1977319

- Additional rs numbers in Sterling's App include, rs1695 (aka, I105V).

- GSTP1 known for its ability to catalyze the conjugation of the reduced form of glutathione (GSH) to exogenous and endogenous hydrophobic electrophiles for the purpose of detoxification. It regulates negatively CDK5 activity via p25/p35 translocation to prevent neurodegeneration.

http://www.uniprot.org/uniprot/P09211.

- The GST family consists of three superfamilies: the cytosolic, mitochondrial, and microsomal.

http://www.ncbi.nlm.nih.gov/pubmed/15717864

- This GST family member is a polymorphic gene encoding active, functionally different GSTP1 variant proteins that are thought to function in xenobiotic metabolism and play a role in susceptibility to cancer and other diseases.

http://www.genecards.org/cgi-bin/carddisp.pl?gene=GSTP1

- One study suggested that GSTP1 methylation is a major event in breast carcinogensis and may act as a tumor specific biomarker.

http://www.ncbi.nlm.nih.gov/pmc/articles/PMC3494109/

+ GSTP1 is found in the following tissues and anatomical compartments:

- bone marrow
- whole blood
- white blood cells
- lymph nodes
- thymus brain
- cortex
- cerebellum
- retina
- spinal cord
- heart
- smooth muscle
- skeletal muscle
- small intestine
- colon
- adipocyte
- kidney
- liver
- lung
- pancreas
- thyroid
- salivary gland
- adrenal gland
- breast
- skin
- ovary
- uterus
- placenta
- prostate
- testes
- tonsil
- myeloid
- monocytes
- dentritic cells
- NK (natural killer) cells
- CD4 T-cells
- CD8 T-cells
- B lymphoblasts
- B cells
- endothelial
- fetal brain

- cingulate cortex
- prefrontal cortex
- parietal lobe
- occipital lobe
- temporal lobe
- ciliary ganglion
- cerebellum peduncles
- globus pallidus
- olfactory bulb
- thalamus
- hypothalamus
- subthamalic nucleus
- caudate nucleus
- amygdala
- pons
- medulla oblongata
- sub-cervical ganglion
- dorsal root ganglion
- trigerminal ganglion
- cardiac myocytes
- atrioventricular node
- tongue
- fetal liver
- fetal lung
- trachea
- bronchial epithelium
- appendix
- fetal thyroid
- pancreatic islet
- day pineal
- night pineal
- pituitary
- uterus corpus
- testis seminif tubule
- testis germ
- testis interstitial
- testes leydig

+ Catalytic activity:
- RX + glutathione = HX + R-S-glutathione

+ Molecular function:
- Dinitrosyl-iron complex binding
- Glutathione transferase activity
- JUN kinase binding
- Kinase regulator activity
- Mitric oxide binding
- S-nitrosoglutathione binding

+ Biological process:
- Cellular response to lipopolysaccharid
- Central nervous system development
- Common myeloid progenitor cell proliferation
- Glutathione derivative biosynthetic process
- Glutathione metabolic process
- Negative regulation of acute inflammatory response
- Negative regulation of apoptotic process

- Negative regulation of biosynthetic process
- Negative regulation of ERK1 and ERK2 cascade
- Negative regulation of fibroblast proliferation
- Negative regulation of 1-kappaB kinase/NF-kappaB signaling
- Negative regulation of interleukin-1beta production
- Negative regulation of JUN kinase activity
- Negative regulation of monocyte chemotactic protein-1 production
- Negative regulation of nitri-oxide synthase biosynthetic process
- Negative regulation of protein kinase activity
- Negative regulation of stress-activated MAPK cascade
- Negative regulation of tumor necrosis factor-mediated signaling pathway
- Negative regulation of tumor necrosis factor production
- Nitric oxide storage
- Positive regulation of superoxide anion generation
- Regulation ERK1 and ERK2 cascade
- Regulation of stress-activated MAPK cascade
- Response to reactive oxygen species
- Small molecule metabolic process
- Xenobiotic metabolic process

+ Cellular component:
- Cytoplasm
- Cytosol
- Extracellular exosome
- Extracellular space
- Intracellular
- Mitochondrion
- Nucleus
- Plasma membrane
- TRAF2-GSTP1 complex
- Vesicle

http://www.uniprot.org/uniprot/P09211

Section 2.3.2 – Acetylation – conjugation with acetyl-CoA

+Nutrients needed - Acetyl-CoA, molybdenum, iron, niacinamide (B-3), vitamin B-2

+Some drugs cleared/conjugated by acetylation:
- Clonazepam

- Dapsone
- Mescaline
- Isoniazid
- Hydralazine
- Procainamide
- Benzidine
- Sulfonamides
- Promizole

+Some Xenobiotics cleared/conjugated by acetylation:
- 2 Aminofluorine
- Anilines

+Some substances of dietary and endogenous origin cleared/conjugated by acetylation:
- Serotonin
- PABA
- Histamine
- Tryptamine
- Caffeine
- Choline
- Tyramine
- Coenzyme A

NAT1

+ **Overview for NAT1** *N-acetyltransferase 1 protein* (aka, arylamine N-acetyltransferase)
- *NAT1*, rs4986782 (aka, R187Q) is a phase II xenobiotic metabolizing enzyme involved in the biotransformation of many aromatic amines and heterocyclic amines. It also catalyzes the N- or O- acetylation of various arylamine and heterocyclic amine substrates and is able to bioactivate several known carcinogens. This gene detoxifies hydrazine and arylamine drugs. It is considered the most common "slow acetylator" arylamine NAT1 genetic variant.

+ NAT1 metabolizes drugs and other xenobiotics and functions in folate catabolism.

http://www.cancerindex.org/geneweb//NAT1.htm

http://www.genecards.org/cgi-bin/carddisp.pl?gene=NAT1

+ NAT1, rs4986782 is associated with a higher frequency of smoking-induced lung cancer, head, and neck cancers.

+ NAT1, rs4986782 is associated with a reduced N-acetylation phenotype. For example, in peripheral blood mononuclear cells, NAT1 14B was reported to result in reduced *N*-acetyltransferase activities and protein levels.

http://dmd.aspetjournals.org/content/40/1/198.full.pdf+html

+ Many drugs and chemicals found in the environment, such as those in cigarette smoke, second hand cigarette smoke, carbon fuel emissions, and burnt charcoaled meat, can be either detoxified by NATs and eliminated from the body or bioactivated to metabolites that have the potential to cause toxicity and/or cancer.

+ NAT polymorphisms are a risk factor for several different types of cancers. Hydrazine sulfate is detoxified by NAT. In addition to being used as jet fuel, it is also used in treating colon, rectal, lung, brain, Hodgkin's, and other cancers and requires NAT for its breakdown.

+ NAT1 affects the growth and drug resistance of breast cancer cells. 1 Arylamine N-acetyltransferase is a marker in human estrogen receptor-positive breast cancer.

http://dmd.aspetjournals.org/content/40/1/198.full

+ Catalytic activity:
- Acetyl-CoA + an arylamine = CoA + an N-acetylarylamine

+ Molecular function:
- Arylamine N-acetyltransferase activity

+ Biological process:
- Small molecule metabolic process
- Xenobiotic metabolic process

+ Cellular component:
- Cytoplasm
- Cytosol

http://www.uniprot.org/uniprot/P18440

NAT2

+ **Overview for NAT2** *N-acetyltransferase 2 protein* (aka, arylamine N-acetyltransferase)
- *NAT2*, rs1041983 (aka, C282T), rs1799929 (aka, C481T), rs1801279 (aka, G191A), rs1799931 (aka, G286E), rs1801280 (aka, I114T), rs1208 (aka, K268R), rs1799930 (aka, R197Q), rs1805158 (aka, R64W).
- NAT2 is a phase II xenobiotic metabolizing enzyme involved in the biotransformation of many aromatic amines and heterocyclic amines. It also catalyzes the N- or O- acetylation of various arylamine and heterocyclic amine substrates and is able to bioactivate several known carcinogens. This gene

detoxifies hydrazine and arylamine drugs. NAT2 metabolizes drugs and other xenobiotics, and functions in folate catabolism.

+ N-acetyltransferases are enzymes acting primarily in the liver to detoxify a large number of chemicals, including caffeine and several prescribed drugs. The NAT2 acetylation polymorphism is important because of its primary role in the activation and/or deactivation of many chemicals in the body's environment, including those produced by cigarettes, as well as, aromatic amine and hydrazine drugs used medicinally. In turn, this can affect an individual's cancer risk.

+ Individuals can be classified as either rapid, or slow, metabolizers (i.e., detoxifiers). In general, slow metabolizers have higher rates of certain types of cancer and are more susceptible to side effects from chemicals metabolized by NAT2.

http://www.ncbi.nlm.nih.gov/pubmed/10667461?dopt=Abstract

+ Drugs reported to be metabolized by NAT2 include; isoniazid, sulfadimidine, hydralazine, dapsone, procaine amide, sulfapyridine, nitrazepam, and some sulfa drugs.

http://www.ncbi.nlm.nih.gov/pmc/articles/PMC1049571/

+ It takes two slow metabolizer alleles to give rise to a slow metabolizer phenotype, or to put it another way, the rapid metabolizer allele is dominant to the slow metabolizer, and you therefore only need one to be a rapid metabolizer.

+ The most common alleles are then defined as follows:
- NAT2*4: considered to be the wild-type allele and the exemplar rapid metabolizer; consists of the first nucleotide shown in the "aka" (also known as) names listed above for these seven NAT2 SNPs, i.e., an allele in question is NAT2*4 if it is rs1801279 (G) and rs 1041983 (C) and rs1801280 (T) and ... etc.

+Almost all of the remaining common alleles are slow metabolizers, such as:
- NAT2*5A: 341C + 481T, i.e., rs1801280(C) + rs1799929(T)
- NAT2*5B: 341C + 481T + 803G, i.e., rs1801280(C) + rs1799929(T) + rs1208(G)
- NAT2*5C: 341C + 803G, i.e., rs1801280(C) + rs1208(G)
- NAT2*5D: 341C, i.e., rs1801280(C)
- NAT2*5E: 341C + 590A, i.e., rs1801280(C) + rs1799930(A)
- NAT2*5G: 282T + 341C + 481T + 803G, i.e., rs1041983(T) + rs1801280(C) + rs1799929(T) + rs1208(G)
- NAT2*5J: 282T + 341C + 590A, i.e., rs1041983(T) + rs1801280(C) + rs1799930(A)
- NAT2*6A: 282T + 590A, i.e., rs1041983(T) + rs1799930(A)
- NAT2*6B: 590A (only), i.e., no variation compared to NAT2*4 except rs1799930(A)
- NAT2*6C: 282T + 590A + 803G, i.e., rs1041983(T) + rs1799930(A) + rs1208(G)
- NAT2*6E: 481T + 590A, i.e., rs1799929(T) + rs1799930(A)

- NAT2*7A: 857A (only), i.e., rs1799931(A)
- NAT2*7B: 282T + 857A, i.e. rs1041983(T) + rs1799931(A)
- NAT2*14A: 191A, i.e., rs1801279(A)
- NAT2*14B: 191A + 282T, i.e., rs1801279(A) + rs1041983(T)
- NAT2*14C: 191A + 341C + 481T + 803G, i.e., rs1801279(A) + rs1801280(C) + rs1799929(T) + rs1208(G)
- NAT2*14D: 191A + 282T + 590A, i.e., rs1801279(A) + rs1041983(T) + rs1799930(A)
- NAT2*14E: 191A + 803G, i.e., rs1801279(A) + rs1208(G)
- NAT2*14F: 191A + 341C + 803G, i.e., rs1801279(A) + s1801280(C) + rs1208(G)
- NAT2*14G: 191A + 282T + 803G, i.e., rs1801279(A) + rs1041983(T) + rs1208(G)

+However there are also a few rapid (i.e., normal) metabolizer variants as well:
- NAT2*11A: 481T, i.e., rs1799929(T)
- NAT2*12A: 803G, i.e., rs1208(G)
- NAT2*12B: 282T + 803G, i.e., rs1041983(T) + rs1208(G)
- NAT2*12C: 481T + 803G, i.e., rs1799929(T) + rs1208(G)
- NAT2*13: 282T (only), i.e., rs1041983(T) http://www.snpedia.com/index.php/NAT2

+ The proportion of slow and rapid metabolizers is known to differ between different ethnic populations. In general, the slow metabolizer phenotype is most prevalent (>80%) in Northern Africans and Scandinavians, and lowest (5%) in Canadian Eskimos and Japanese. Intermediate frequencies are seen in Chinese populations (around 20% slow metabolizers), whereas 40 - 60% of African-Americans and most non-Scandinavian Caucasians are slow metabolizers.

+ Many drugs and chemicals found in the environment, such as those in cigarette smoke, second hand cigarette smoke, carbon fuel emissions and burnt charcoaled meat, can be either detoxified by NATs and eliminated from the body or bioactivated to metabolites that have the potential to cause toxicity and/or cancer. NAT 2 has been implicated in some adverse drug reactions and is a risk factor for several different types of cancers. Further, NAT polymorphisms are a risk factor for several different types of cancers. Hydrazine sulfate is detoxified by NAT. In addition to being used as jet fuel, it is also used in treating colon, rectal, lung, brain, Hodgkin's, and other cancers and requires NAT for its breakdown.

+ NAT2 metabolism has been associated with adverse reactions to amine drugs such as sulfonamides, codeine, zoloft, setraline, repaglinide, methadone, flomax, tamsulosin, sibutramine, cinacalcet, rivastigmine, lariam, ethambutol, lopinavir, isoniazid, dapsone, procainamide, and acetaminophen.

+ NAT2 has been shown to play roles in the catabolism of folate, which is required for the synthesis of S-adenosylmethionine, the methyl donor for cellular methylation reactions (methyl transferases).

+ Catalytic activity:
- Acetyl-CoA + an arylamine = CoA + an N-acetylarylamine

+ Molecular function:
- Arylamine N-acetyltransferase activity

+ Biological process:
- Small molecule metabolic process
- Xenobiotic metabolic process

+ Cellular component:
- Cytoplasm
- Cytosol

http://www.uniprot.org/uniprot/P11245

Section 2.3.3 – Glucuronidation – UDP-glucuronic acid covalently linked

+Nutrients needed - glucuronic acid, magnesium, B-vitamins

http://www.balancedconcepts.net/liver_phases_detox_paths.pdf

+Some drugs cleared/conjugated by glucuronidation:
- Salicylates
- Morphine
- Acetaminophen
- Benzodiazepines
- Meprobamate
- Clofibric acid
- Naproxen
- Digoxin
- Phenylbutazone
- Naproxen
- Digoxin
- Phenylbutazon
- Valproic acid
- Steroids
- Lorazepam
- Ciramadol
- Propranoiol

- Oxazepam

+Some xenobiotics cleared/conjugated by glucuronidation:
- Carbamate
- Phenols
- Thiophenol
- Aniline

+Some substances of dietary and endogenous origin cleared/conjugated by glucuronidation:
- Billirubin
- Estrogens
- Melatonin
- Bile acid
- Vitamin E
- Vitamin A
- Vitamin K
- Vitamin D
- Steroid hormone

UGT1A1

+ **Overview for UGT1A1** *UDP-glucuronosyltransferase 1-1* (aka, UDPGT and UDP glucuronosyltransferase 1 family, polypeptide A1)

- *UGT1A1*, rs6717546 (aka, A188730G), rs887829 (aka, C175181T), rs4148325 (aka, C179920T), rs6742078 (aka, G179250T), rs62625011 (aka, G182349A), rs4148323 (aka, G211A), rs72551348 (aka, G328A), rs72551351 (aka, L175G), rs72551341 (aka, L175G), rs34547608 (aka, T175439C) encodes UDP-glucuronosyltransferase, an enzyme of the glucuronidation pathway that that provides instructions for making enzymes called UDP-glucuronosyltransferases. These enzymes perform a chemical reaction called glucuronidation, in which a compound called glucuronic acid is attached (conjugated) to one of a number of different substances

http://www.ncbi.nlm.nih.gov/gene/54658

+ The protein produced from the UGT1A1 gene, called the bilirubin uridine diphosphate glucuronosyl transferase (bilirubin-UGT) enzyme, is the only enzyme that glucuronidates bilirubin, a substance produced when red blood cells are broken down. This enzyme converts the toxic form of bilirubin (unconjugated bilirubin) to its nontoxic form (conjugated bilirubin), making it able to be dissolved and removed from the body.

The bilirubin-UGT enzyme is primarily found in cells of the liver, where bilirubin glucuronidation takes place. Conjugated bilirubin is dissolved in bile, a fluid produced in the liver, and excreted with solid waste.

http://ghr.nlm.nih.gov/gene/UGT1A1

+ UGT1A1 is of major importance in the conjugation and subsequent elimination of potentially toxic xenobiotics and endogenous compounds. It is able to catalyze the glucuronidation of 17beta-estradiol, 17alpha-ethinylestradiol, 1-hydroxypyrene, 4-methylumbelliferone, 1-naphthol, paranitrophenol, scopoletin, and umbelliferone.

http://www.uniprot.org/uniprot/P22309#P22309

+ UGT1A1*80 A188730G is related to beta-Thalassemia, HIV and hyperbilirubinemia.

https://www.pharmgkb.org/rsid/rs887829#tabview=tab3&subtab=22

+ UGT1A1*6 G211A is related to angina pectoris, non-small-cell-lung carcinoma, diarrhea, drug toxicity, Gilbert's syndrome, heart failure, drug toxicity, genital female neoplasms, hepatitis, HIV, hyperbilirubinemia, neonatal jaundice, neoplasms, neutropenia, overall survival, thrombocytopenia, and tuberculosis.

https://www.pharmgkb.org/rsid/rs4148323#tabview=tab4&subtab=22

+ Can induce via sulforaphane, EGCG, flavenoids.

+ The preferred substrate of this enzyme is bilirubin, although it also has moderate activity with simple phenols, flavones, and C18 steroids.

+ Mutations in this gene result in Crigler-Najjar syndromes types I and II, and in Gilbert syndrome.

http://www.ncbi.nlm.nih.gov/gene?Db=gene&Cmd=ShowDetailView&TermToSearch=54658&ordinalpos=2&itool=EntrezSystem2.PEntrez.Gene.Gene_ResultsPanel.Gene_RVDocSum

+ Irinotecan is a camptothecin analog used as an anticancer drug. Severe, potentially life-threatening toxicities can occur from irinotecan treatment. People with certain UGT1A1's may experience toxicity with is drug.

http://www.ncbi.nlm.nih.gov/pubmed/20602618

+ Catalytic activity:

    - UDP-glucuronate + acceptor = UDP + acceptor beta-D-glucuronoside

+ Molecular function:

    - Enzyme binding
    - Enzyme inhibitor activity
    - Glucuronosyltransferase activity
    - Protein heterodimerization activity
    - Protein homodimerization activity
    - Retinoic acid binding

- Steroid binding

+ Biological process:
- Acute-phase response
- Bilirubin conjugation
- Biphenyl catabolic process
- Cellular glucuronidation
- Cellular response to ethanol
- Cellular response to glucocorticoid stimulus
- Cellular response to hormone synthesis
- Digestion
- Drug metabolic process
- Flavone metabolic process
- Flavonoid biosynthetic process
- Flavondoid glucuronidation
- Heme catabolic process
- Heterocycle metabolic process
- Liver development
- Negative regulation of catalytic activity
- Negative regulation of cellular glucuronidation
- Negative regulation of fatty acid mmetabolic process
- Negative regulation of glucuronosyltransferase activity
- Negative regulation of steroid metabolic process
- Organ regeneration
- Porphyrin-containing compound metabolic process
- Response to drug
- Response to lipopolysaccharide
- Response to nutrient
- Response to starvation
- Retinoic acid metabolism
- Small molecule metabolic process
- Xenobiotic glucuronidation
- Xenobiotic metabolic process

+ Subcellular location:
- Microsome
- Endoplasmic reticulum membrane

+ Cellular component:
- Cytochrome complex
- Endoplasmic reticulum
- Endoplasmic reticulum chaperone complex
- Endoplasmic reticulum membrane
- Integral component of plasm membrane

http://www.uniprot.org/uniprot/P22309

+ Associated disease:
- Gilbert syndrome - occurs as a consequence of reduced bilirubin transferase activity and is often detected in young adults with vague non-specific complaints.

http://www.ncbi.nlm.nih.gov/pubmed/11013440

UGT2A1, UGT2A2

+ **Overview for UGT2A1 and UGT2A2** *UDP-glucuronosyltransferase 2A1* and *UDP-glucuronosyltransferase 2A2*

- *UGT2A1*, rs1347046 (aka, R75K), encodes UDP-glucuronosyltransferase, an enzyme of the glucuronidation pathway that provides instructions for making enzymes called UDP-glucuronosyltransferases. These enzymes perform a chemical reaction called glucuronidation, in which a compound called glucuronic acid is attached (conjugated) to one of a number of different substances.. Isoform 2A1 is mainly expressed in the brain, fetal lung, olfactory epithelium. Isoform 2A2 is mainly expressed in colon, intestine, liver and stomach.

http://www.ncbi.nlm.nih.gov/gene/54658

+ Characterizes the expression and glucuronidation activities of the human uridine 5'-diphospho (UDP)-glucuronosyltransferase. UGT2A1/2a2 has glucuronidation activity towards several different endobiotic and xenobiotic substrates.

http://www.uniprot.org/citations/19858781

+ The biological processes for UGT2A1/2A2 are the following:
- Cellular glucuronidation
- Detection of chemical stimulus
- Flavonoid glucuronidation
- Sensory perception of smell
- Cellular response to hormone stimulus
- Flavonoid biosynthetic process
- Metabolic process

http://www.uniprot.org/uniprot/Q9Y4X1

+ UGT2A1/2A2 plays a role in the olfactory perception and in protection of the neural system against airborne hazardous chemicals.

http://www.uniprot.org/citations/10359671

+ It is also mainly expressed in the nasal mucosa and it has glucuronidation activity towards several different endobiotic and xenobiotic substrates.

http://www.uniprot.org/citations/19858781

Section 2.3.4 – Peptide conjugation – glycine/ taurine

+Nutrients needed -arginase enzyme, glycine, gly co-factors (folate, manganese, B-2, B- 6/P-5-P)

Section 2.3.4.1 – Glycine peptide conjugation - most commonly utilized in amino acid detoxification

+Some drugs cleared/conjugated by peptide conjugation; glycine:

- Salicylates
- Nicotinic acid
- Chlorpheniramine
- Brompheniramine

+Some xenobiotics cleared/conjugated by peptide conjugation; glycine:

- Benzoic acid
- Phenylacetic acid
- Naphylacetic acid
- Aliphatic amines
- Organic acids

+Some substances of dietary and endogenous origin cleared/conjugated by peptide conjugation; glycine:

- Bile acid
- PABA
- Plant acids

Section 2.3.4.2 – Taurine peptide conjugation

+Some drugs cleared/conjugated by peptide conjugation; taurine:

- Ibuprofen (minor)
- Levocetirizine Dihydrochloride (minor, mostly renal elimination)

+Some xenobiotics cleared/conjugated by peptide conjugation; taurine:

- Propionic acid
- Caprylic acid

+Some substances of dietary and endogenous origin cleared/conjugated by peptide conjugation; taurine:
- Bile acid
- Stearic acid
- Palmitic acid
- Myristic acid
- Lauric acid
- Butyric acid

Section 2.3.5 – Sulfation- conjugation with sulfur containing compounds

The human cytosolic sulfotransfases (hSULTs) comprise a family of twelve phase II enzymes involved in the metabolism of drugs and hormones, the bioactivation of carcinogens, and the detoxification of xenobiotics. They are grouped into four gene families: SULT1, SULT2, SULT4, and SULT6. The SULT1 family is further divided into four subfamilies: SULT1A, 1B, 1C, and 1E. The SULT1A subfamily consists of "phenol sulfotransferases"; SULT1E1 is a high-affinity estrogen sulfotransferase, but the substrate specificities of the human SULT1B and SUL1C enzymes are less well defined. The SULT1C subfamily includes three human genes, named SULT1C2, SULT1C3, and SULT1C4. SULT1C3 is essentially an orphan enzyme.
http://www.ncbi.nlm.nih.gov/pmc/articles/PMC3935139/

+Nutrients needed - molybdenum, cysteine, and its precursor methionine, co-factors (vitamin B-12, folic acid (B-9), methyl donors, magnesium, B-6/P-5-P), MSM, SAMe, taurine.

+Some drugs cleared/conjugated by sulfation:
- Acetaminophen
- Methyl dopa
- Minoxidil
- Metaraminol

+Some xenobiotics cleared/conjugated by sulfation:
- Aniline
- Pentachlorophelon
- Terpenes
- Hydroylamines
- Phenols

+Some substances of dietary and endogenous origin cleared/conjugated by sulfation:
- DHEA

- Quercitin
- Bile acids
- Safrole
- Tyramine
- Thyroxine
- Estrogens
- Testosterone
- Cortisol
- Catecholamines
- Melatonin
- 3-hydroxy coumarin
- 25 hydroxy Vitamin D
- Ethyl alcohol
- CCK
- Cerebrosides

SULT1C3

+ <u>**Overview for SULT1C3**</u> *Sulfotransferase Family, Cytosolic, 1C, Member 3 (aka, Sulfotransferase 1C3, ST1C3)*

- SULT1C3, rs1470874 (aka, A108878711G), rs10209928 (aka, C13537727T), rs13392744 (aka, C13545841T), rs17035962 (aka, G13554307A), rs2219078 (aka, G535A), rs6722745 (aka, M194T), rs17035911 (aka, T148C), encodes a sulfotransferase 1C3 enzyme of the sulfation pathway that is expressed in the small intestine.
- Sulfotransferase enzymes catalyze the sulfate conjugation of many hormones, neurotransmitters, drugs, and xenobiotic compounds. These cytosolic enzymes are different in their tissue distributions and substrate specificities. The gene structure (number and length of exons) is similar among family members.

http://www.ncbi.nlm.nih.gov/gene/54658

+ Sulfotransferase utilizes 3'-phospho-5'-adenylyl sulfate (PAPS) as a sulfonate donor and has low sulphotransferase activity towards various substrates with alcohol groups (in vitro).

http://www.nextprot.org/db/entry/NX_Q6IMI6

+ Catalytic activity:

- 3'-phosphoadenylyl sulfate + an alcohol = adenosine 3',5'-bisphosphate + an alkyl sulfate

+ Molecular function:

- Alcohol sulfotransferase activity
- Aryl sulfotransferase activity

+ Biological process:
- Sulfur compound metabolic activity

http://www.uniprot.org/uniprot/Q6IMI6

+ Cellular component:
- Cytoplasm

SULT2A1

+ **Overview for SULT2A1** *Sulfotransferase family, cytosolic, 2A, dehydroepiandrosterone (DHEA)-preferring, member 1 (aka, bile salt transferase)*
- SULT2A1, rs2910393 (aka, A13527G), rs2547242 (aka, A15550G), rs296366 (aka, A20117G), rs11083907 (aka, C90C), rs4149452 (aka, G17136A), rs296365 (aka, 20104C), rs11569679 (aka, G781A), rs2547231 (aka, G9598T), rs4149449 (aka, G9696A), rs8113396 (aka, T15557C), rs4149448 (aka, T8298C), encodes a Sulfotransferase 2A1 enzyme of the sulfation pathway.
- Sulfotransferases aid in the metabolism of drugs and endogenous compounds by converting these substances into more hydrophilic water-soluble sulfate conjugates for excretion. This enzyme encoded by SULT2A1 catalyzes the sulfation of steroids and bile acids in the liver and adrenal glands and may have a role in the inherited adrenal androgen excess in women with polycystic ovary syndrome. It is present in the liver, adrenals, and at lower level, also in the kidneys.

http://www.ncbi.nlm.nih.gov/gene/6822

+ Present in liver, adrenal, and at lower level, in the kidney.

+ Sulfotransferase utilizes 3'-phospho-5'-adenylyl sulfate (PAPS) as a sulfonate donor and has low sulphotransferase activity towards various substrates with alcohol groups (in vitro).

http://www.nextprot.org/db/entry/NX_Q6IMI6

+ Catalytic activity:
- 3'-phosphoadenylyl sulfate + glycolithocholate = adenosine 3',5'-bisphosphate + glycolithocholate 3-sulfate.
- 3'-phosphoadenylyl sulfate + taurolithocholate = adenosine 3',5'-bisphosphate + taurolithocholate sulfate.

+ Molecular function:
- Bile salt sulfotransferase activity
- Sulfotransferase activity

+ Biological process:
- Bile acid catabolic process
- Cellular lipid metabolic process
- Cellular lipid metabolism process
- Digestion
- Small molecule metabolic process
- Steroid metabolic process
- Sulfation
- Xenobiotic metabolic process

http://www.uniprot.org/uniprot/Q06520

Section 2.3.6 – Methylation

Nutrients needed - methionine, magnesium, folate, vitamin B-12, methyl donors, choline, betaine

+Some drugs cleared/conjugated by methylation:
- Thiouracil
- Isoetharine
- Rimiterol
- Dobutamine
- Butanephrin
- Eluophed
- Morphine
- Levaphanol
- Nalorphine

+Some xenobiotics cleared/conjugated by methylation:
- Peraquat
- Beta carbolines
- Isoquinolines
- Mercury
- Lead
- Arsenic
- Thallium
- Tin
- Pyridine

+Some substances of dietary and endogenous origin cleared/conjugated by methylation:
- Dopamine (Methylation -> COMT)

- Epinepherine
- Histamine
- Norepinepherine
- L-dopa
- Apomorphine
- Hydroxyestradiols

Section 2.3.6.1 – Methylation Figures

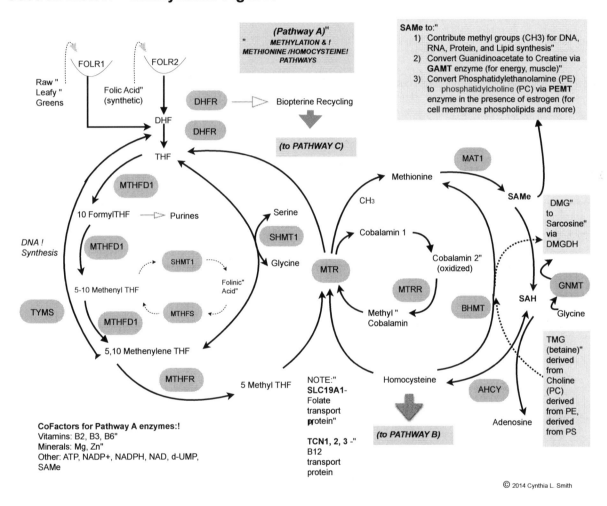

FIGURE 4 – Folate and Methionine/Homocysteine Pathway

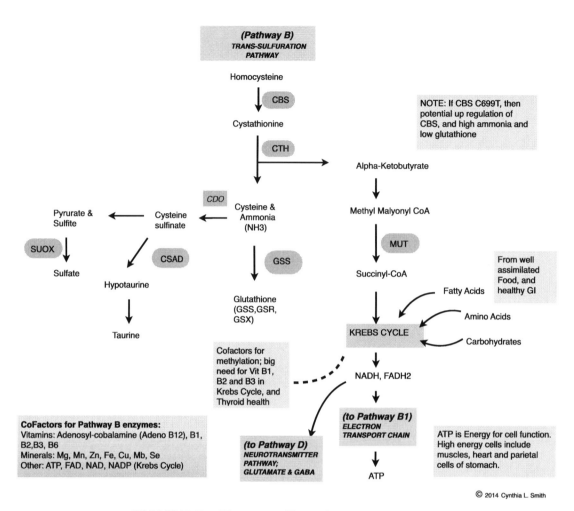

FIGURE 5 – Trans-sulfuration Pathway

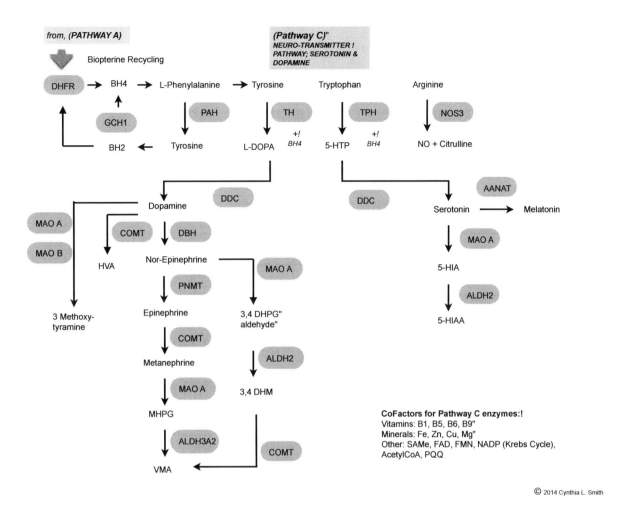

FIGURE 6 – Neurotransmitter Pathway

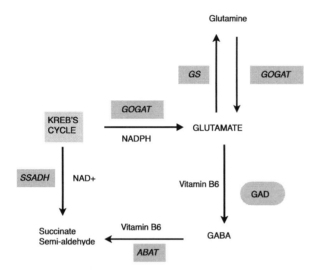

FIGURE 7 – Glutamate/GABA Pathway

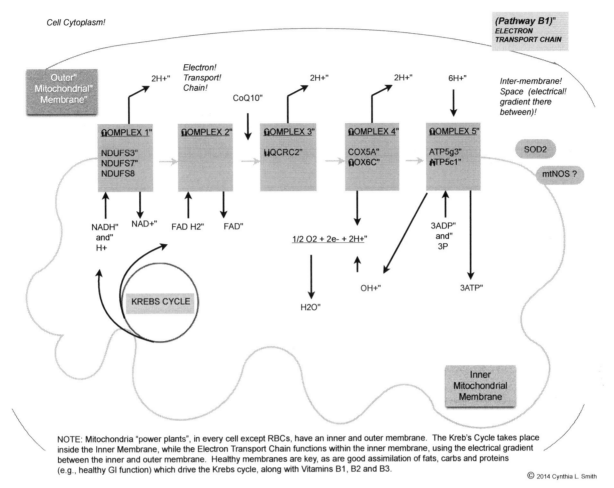

FIGURE 8 – Mitochondria; Electron Transport Chain

Section 2.3.6.2 – Methylation SNPs

ACAT1

+ <u>Overview for ACAT1</u> *Acetyl-Coenzyme A acetyltransferase1* (aka, Sterol O-acyltransferase 1)

- *ACAT1*, rs3741049 (aka, G22670A), encodes Acetyl-CoA acetyltransferase, mitochondrial, also known as, acetoacetyl-CoA thiolase.
- This enzyme plays an essential role in breaking down proteins and fats from the diet. Specifically, it helps process isoleucine, an amino acid that is a building block of many proteins.

http://ghr.nlm.nih.gov/gene/ACAT1

- This gene encodes a mitochondrially-localized enzyme that catalyzes the reversible formation of acetoacetyl-CoA from two molecules of acetyl-CoA. During the breakdown of proteins, the ACAT1 enzyme is responsible for the last step in processing isoleucine. It converts 2-methyl-acetoacetyl-CoA into two smaller molecules, propionyl-CoA and acetyl-CoA, that can be used to produce energy.

https://en.wikipedia.org/wiki/ACAT1#cite_note-entrez-1

- Catalyzes the formation of fatty acid-cholesterol esters, which are less soluble in membranes than cholesterol. Plays a role in lipoprotein assembly and dietary cholesterol absorption. In addition to its acyltransferase activity, it may act as a ligase (an enzyme that brings about ligation of DNA or another substance).

http://www.uniprot.org/uniprot/P35610

- Acetyl-CoA acetyltransferase, mitochondrial is activated by potassium ions binding near the CoA binding site and the catalytic site.
- Acetyl-CoA acetyltransferase expression is promoted transcriptionally (up-regulated) by leptin, angiotensin II, and insulin in human monocytes/macrophages.

https://www.ncbi.nlm.nih.gov/pubmed/19625677
https://www.ncbi.nlm.nih.gov/pubmed/18971559
https://www.ncbi.nlm.nih.gov/pubmed/23564383

- ❖ **NOTE**: Angiotensin II is known to accelerate the progression of macrophage-driven atherosclerotic lesions. Acetyl-CoA acetyltransferase converts intracellular free cholesterol into cholesterol ester for storage in lipid droplets and promotes foam cell formation in atherosclerotic lesions.
- ❖ Insulin resistance characterized by hyperinsulinemia is associated with increased risk of atherosclerosis. Acetyl-CoA acetyltransferase is involved in cellular cholesterol homeostasis and in atherosclerotic foam cell formation.

+ It is thought that ACAT1 (and/or SHMT) SNPs confer a higher tendancy for gut dysbiosis.
+ Defects in this gene are associated with 3-ketothiolase deficiency, an inborn error of isoleucine catabolism characterized by urinary excretion of 2-methyl-3-hydroxybutyric acid, 2-methylacetoacetic acid, tiglylglycine, and butanone.

http://www.genecards.org/cgi-bin/carddisp.pl?gene=ACAT1

+ ACAT1 is present ubiquitously in many cell types; ACAT2 is enriched mainly in intestinal enterocytes.
+ rs1044925 appears to be the primary SNP associated with Acetyl-Coenzyme A acetyltransferase 1 deficiency.
+ ACAT1 plays a major role in ketone body metabolism. Defects may cause a 3-ketothiolase deficiency. Dr Yasko believes it will cause an increase in gut bugs (particularly clostridia), as well as, elevated fatty acid metabolites.

+ If a mutation in the ACAT1 gene reduces the activity of this enzyme, the body is unable to process isoleucine and ketones properly. As a result, harmful compounds can build up and cause the blood to become too acidic, which impairs tissue function, especially in the CNS.

+ "Further assessment of ACAT1 on human castration-resistant metastatic prostate cancer tissues revealed substantially elevated expression of ACAT1 in these specimens. Taken together, our results indicate that enzymes of the ketogenic pathway are up-regulated in high-grade prostate cancer and could serve as potential tissue biomarkers for the diagnosis or prognosis of high-grade disease".

http://www.ncbi.nlm.nih.gov/pubmed/23443136

+ The results show that the enzyme activity of ACAT1 with Gln526 is less active than that of ACAT1 with Arg526 by forty percent.

http://www.ncbi.nlm.nih.gov/pubmed/24517390

> **Our Two Cents**: Acetyl-CoA acetyltransferase contributes to cholesterol synthesis. Cholesterol is a building block for many hormones, and bile, among other things. Bile creation requires taurine and often folks with ACAT1 SNP will spill/waste taurine in their urine due to lack of bile acids for conjugation. In that case, supplementing with bile salts may be helpful when eating higher fat foods. Also, because acetyl CoA enters the Krebs cycle (aka, the citric acid cycle) as one of its first steps, the addition of supplemental support of vitamins B-2 and B-5 will support the reaction between puyruvate and the Kreb's cycle. Other supplements that may be helpful are, benfotiamine (derived from vitamin B-1) and low dose ALA. If there are SNPs in both ACAT1 and SHMT, address SHMT first. (Recall that SHMT catalyzes the reversible reaction of serine and tetrahydrofolate (THF) to glycine and 5,10-methylene THF).

+ Catalytic activity:
- Acyl-CoA + cholesterol = CoA + cholesterol ester

+ Molecular function:
- Cholesterol binding
- Cholesterol O-acyltransferase activity
- Fatty-acyl-CoA binding
- Sterol O-acyltransferase activity

+ Biological process:
- Cholesterol efflux
- Cholesterol esterification
- Cholesterol homeostasis
- Cholesterol metabolic process
- Cholesterol storage

- Macrophage derived foam cell differentiation
- Positive regulation of amyloid precursor protein biosynthetic process
- Very-low-density lipoprotein particle assembly

+ Subcellular location:
- Endoplasmic reticulum membrane

+ Cellular component:
- Endoplasmic reticulum
- Endoplasmic reticulum membrane
- Integral component of membrane

http://www.uniprot.org/uniprot/P35610

ACE

+ **Overview for ACE** *Angiotensin converting enzyme* (aka, ACE Del 16)
- ACE, rs4343 (aka, G2328A)
- The protein encoded by ACE converts angiotensin I to angiotensin II. This results in an increase of the vasoconstrictor activity of angiotensin. The protein is also able to inactivate bradykinin, a potent vasodilator.
- Angiotensin converting enzyme therefore regulates blood pressure and the balance of fluids and salts in the body. ACE also stimulates production of the hormone, aldosterone, which triggers the absorption of salt and water by the kidneys.

http://ghr.nlm.nih.gov/gene/ACE

+ The catalytic activity for ACE is conversion of angiotensin I to angiotensin II, with increase in vasoconstrictor activity, but no action on angiotensin II.

+ The enzyme regulation is strongly activated by chloride, and specifically inhibited by lisinopril, captopril and enalaprilat.

+ The enzyme may promote high levels of angiotensin II and cause an increase in aldosterone. High aldosterone leads to increase potassium loss in the urine and increased sodium retention. Decreased potassium can lead to fatigue and decreased energy production as cellular membrane activation, particularly for the brain and peripheral nervous system, dependent upon sodium/potassium balance. Animal studies show a correlation between high angiotensin II with increased anxiety and decreased learning and memory. Blood pressure regulation, low frustration threshold, and increased anxiety may result. The effects are worsened by stress, and a MAOA mutation may exacerbate.

http://www.snpedia.com/index.php/Yasko_Methylation

+ + The "G" allele at rs4343 translates to a likely deletion at ACE Del16 and therefore increased ACE activity.

+ ACE SNPs are associated with an increased susceptibility to hypertension, cardiovascular disease, and atherosclerosis. These genes will indicate if the individual is sensitive to sodium via the renin-angiotensin-aldosterone system.

+ ACE SNPs, may influence numerous disparate conditions or phenotypes, including:

- Diabetic nephropathy

https://www.ncbi.nlm.nih.gov/pubmed/?term=17376814

- Renal disease

https://www.ncbi.nlm.nih.gov/pubmed/?term=16791616

- Cancer (incl. survival and tumor burden)

https://www.ncbi.nlm.nih.gov/pubmed/?term=17898867

- Athletic performance

https://www.ncbi.nlm.nih.gov/pubmed/?term=17885020

  o (A;A) better endurance vs. strength; (G;G) better strength vs. endurance.

+ Perhaps the best-studied ACE SNP is actually not a single nucleotide polymorphism at all; instead, it is an insertion/deletion of an Alu repetitive element in an intron of the ACE gene. Alleles containing the insertion are called "I" alleles, and "D" alleles lack the repetitive element. Homozygotes are (I;I).

+ Catalytic activity:

- Release of a C-terminal dipeptide, oligopeptide-|-Xaa-Yaa, when Xaa is not Pro, and Yaa is neither Asp nor Glu. Thus, conversion of angiotensin I to angiotensin II, with increase in vasoconstrictor activity, but no action on angiotensin II.

+ Cofactor:

- Zinc (ZN^{2+})   Binds two Zn^{2+} ions per subunit
- Chloride   Binds three chloride ions per subunit

+ Molecular function:

- Actin binding
- Bradykinin receptor binding
- Carboxypeptidase
- Chloride ion binding
- Drug binding
- Endopeptidase activity
- Metallopeptidase activity
- Mitogen-activated protein kinase binding
- Peptidyl-dipeptidase activity

- Tripeptidyl-peptidase activity
- Zinc ion binding

+ Biological process:
- Angiotensin catabolic process in blood
- Angiotensin maturation
- Antigen processing and presentation of peptide
- Arachidonic acid secretion
- Beta-amyloid metabolic process
- Blood vessel remodeling
- Cell proliferation in bone marrow
- Cellular protein metabolic process
- Heart contraction
- Hematopoitic stem cell differentiation
- Hormone catabolic process
- Kidney development
- Mononuclear cell proliferation
- Negative regulation of gap junction assembly
- Neutrophil mediated immunity
- Peptide catabolic process
- Positive regulation of peptidy-cysteine S-nitrosylation
- Positive regulation of peptidyl-tyrosine autophosphorylation
- Positive regulation of protein tyrosine kinase activity
- Regulation of angiotensin metabolic process
- **Regulation of blood pressure**
- Regulation of hematopoitic stem cell proliferation
- Regulation of renal output by angiotensin
- Regulation of smooth muscle cell migration
- Regulation of systemic arterial blood pressure by renin-angiotensin
- Regulation of vasoconstriction
- Regukation of vasodilation
- Spermatogenesis

+ Subcellular location:
- Soluble form, secreted
- Cell membrane
- Cytoplasm

+ Cellular component:

- Endosome
- External side of plasma membrane
- Extracellularexosome
- Extracellular region
- Extracellular space
- Integral component of membrane
- Lysosome

❖ **NOTE**: Detected in both cell membrane and cytoplasm in neurons

http://www.uniprot.org/uniprot/P12821

ADA

+ <u>**Overview for ADA**</u> *Adenosine Deaminase* (aka, Adenosine aminohydrolase)
- *ADA*, rs2299686 (aka, A10376G), rs11555566 (aka, A239G), rs244076 (aka, A534G), rs6031692 (aka, C10783T), rs452159 (aka, C14275A), rs447833 (aka, G22021A), rs73598374 (aka, G22A)
- The ADA enzyme is involved in purine metabolism. It is needed for the breakdown of adenosine from food and for the turnover of nucleic acids in tissues.

http://www.ncbi.nlm.nih.gov/pubmed/1925539

- Present in virtually all mammalian cells, its primary function in humans is the development and maintenance of the immune system. However, the full physiological role of ADA is not yet completely understood.

http://www.ncbi.nlm.nih.gov/pubmed/11223861

+ The high degree of amino acid sequence conservation suggests the crucial nature of ADA in the purine salvage pathway.
- Recall that purines are biologically synthesized as nucelotides and in particular as ribotides, i.e., bases attached to ribose 5-phosphate. Purines from turnover of nucleic acids (or from food) can also be salvaged and reused in new nucleotides.

+ Primarily, ADA in humans is involved in the development and maintenance of the immune system. However, ADA association has also been observed with epithelial cell differentiation, neurotransmission, and gestation maintenance.

http://www.ncbi.nlm.nih.gov/pubmed/10506947

+ The ADA enzyme is produced in all cells, but the highest levels of adenosine deaminase occur in immune system cells called lymphocytes, which develop in lymphoid tissues. This defends the body against potentially harmful invaders, such as viruses or bacteria.

+ The adenosine deaminase enzyme is meant to eliminate a molecule called deoxyadenosine.

+ Mutations result in the absence or deficiency of the adenosine deaminase enzyme in cells, preventing the normal breakdown of deoxyadenosine. This can result in severe combined immunodeficiency.

+ Treatment for ADA deficiency is gene therapy and bone marrow transplant.

http://en.wikipedia.org/wiki/Adenosine_deaminase_deficiency

+ Most ADA deficiency is found in infants. Adenosine deaminase deficiency can be late onset in childhood and a milder form in adulthood.

http://www.ncbi.nlm.nih.gov/pmc/articles/PMC1377486/

+ Catalytic activity:
- Adenosine + H2O = inosine + NH3

+ Cofactor:
- Zinc (ZN^{2+})   Binds one Zn^{2+} ion per subunit

+ Molecular function:
- Adenosine deaminase activity
- Purine nucleoside binding
- Zinc ion binding

+ Biological process:
- Adenosine catabolic process
- Aging
- dATP catabolic process
- Deoxyadenosine catabolic process
- Embryonic digestive tract development
- Germinal center B cell differentiation
- Histamine secretion
- Hyposanthine salvage
- Iosone biosynthetic process
- Liver development
- Lung alveolus development
- Negative regulation of adenosine receptor signaling pathway
- Negative regulation of circadian cycle, non-REM sleep
- Negative regulation of inflammatory response
- Negative regulation of leukocyte migration
- Negative regulation of mature B cell apoptotic process
- Negative regulation of mucus secretion
- Negative regulation of penile erection

- Negative regulation of of thymocyte apoptotic process
- Peyer's patch development
- Positive regulation of alpha-beta T-cell differentiation
- Positive regulation of B cell proliferation
- Positive regulation of calcium-mediated signaling
- Positive regulation of germinal center formation
- Positive regulation of heart rate
- Positive regulation of smooth muscle contraction
- Positive regulation of T-cell receptor signaling pathway
- Purine-containing compound salvage
- Purine nucleobase metabolic process
- Purine ribonucleoside monophosphate biosynthetic process
- Regulation oc cell-adhesion mediated by integrin
- Response to drug
- Response to hydrogen peroxide
- Response to hypoxia
- Response to morphine
- Response to vitamin E
- T-cell activation
- Trophectodermal cell differentiation
- Xanthine biostnthetic process

+ Subcellular location:
- Cell membrane; peripheral membrane protein; extracellular side
- Cell junction
- Cytoplasmic vesicle lumen
- Cytoplasm

+ Cellular component:
- Cell junction
- Cell surface
- Cytoplasm
- Cytoplasmic membrane-bounded vesicle lumen
- Cytosol
- Dendrite cytoplasm
- External side of plasma membrane
- Extracellular space
- Lysosome

- Membrane
- Neuronal cell body
- Plasma membrane

http://www.uniprot.org/uniprot/P00813

ADD1

+ **Overview for ADD1** Adducin 1 (alpha) [Homo sapiens (humans)]
    - *ADD1*, rs4961 (aka, G460W) or (Gly460Trp) encodes a change from a glycine to a tryptophan.
    - Adducins are a family of cytoskeleton proteins encoded by three genes (alpha, beta, gamma).

+ Adducin 1 is related to essential hypertension
    - Essential hypertension is elevated blood pressure of unknown origin.

http://ghr.nlm.nih.gov/gene/ADD1

+ A study of 477 Italian patients indicated that carriers of one or two rs4961(T) alleles were at 1.8 times increased risk for hypertension (CI: 1.32-2.43). This study also indicated that carriers of the risk (T) allele responded better to diuretics and sodium-restricted diets, in that they tended to lower their blood pressure by ~10 mmHg points compared to rs4961(G;G) homozygotes similarly treated.

http://www.ncbi.nlm.nih.gov/pubmed/9149697?dopt=Abstract

+ Beta-adducin is expressed at high levels in brain and hematopoietic tissues. Adducin binds with high affinity to Ca(2+)/calmodulin and is a substrate for protein kinases A and C.

http://www.ncbi.nlm.nih.gov/gene/118

+ Molecular function:
    - Actin binding
    - Actin filament binding
    - Poly(A) RNA binding
    - Protein heterodimerzation activity
    - Protein homodimerazation binding
    - Spectrin binding
    - Structural molecular activity
    - Transcription factor binding

+ Biological process:
    - Actin cytoskeleton organization
    - Actin filament bundle assembly
    - Apoptotic process

- Barbed-end actin filament capping
- Cell morphogenesis
- Cellular component disassembly involved in aptosis
- Cellular protein metabolic process
- Endoplasmic reticulum unfolded protein response
- Ethrocyte differentiation
- Hemoglobin metabolic process
- Homeostasis of number of cells within tissue
- In utero embryonic development
- IRE1-mediated unfolded protein response
- Multicellular organism growth
- Positive regulation of protein binding
- Programmed cell death
- Transmembrane transport

+ Subcellular location:
- Cytoplasm
- Cell membrane

+ Cellular component:
- Cytosol
- F-actin capping protein complex
- Focal adhesion
- Intermediate filament cytoskeleton
- Nucleoplasm
- Nucleus
- Plasma membrane

http://www.uniprot.org/uniprot/P35611

ADK

+ **Overview for ADK** *Adenosine Kinase*
- *ADK*, rs4746181 (aka, A48021G), rs946185 (aka, A517797G), rs1538311, (aka, G509567T).
- This gene encodes an enzyme adenosine kinase that catalyzes the transfer of the gamma-phosphate from ATP to adenosine, thereby serving as a regulator of concentrations of both extracellular adenosine and intracellular adenine nucleotides.

- Adenosine kinase is a phosphotransferase, the enzyme that catalyzes the interconversion of adenine nucleotides, and plays an important role in cellular energy homeostasis.
- ATP dependent phosphorylation of adenosine and other related nucleoside analogs to monophosphate derivatives. http://www.uniprot.org/uniprot/P55263

+ Adenosine has widespread effects on the cardiovascular, nervous, respiratory, and immune systems and inhibitors of the enzyme could play an important pharmacological role in increasing intravascular adenosine concentrations and acting as anti-inflammatory agents. Multiple transcript variants encoding different isoforms have been found for this gene.

http://www.genecards.org/cgi-bin/carddisp.pl?gene=ADK
http://www.ncbi.nlm.nih.gov/gene/132

+ Catalytic activity:
- ATP + adenosine = ADP + AMP

+ Nutrient cofactor:
- Magnesium   Binds three Mg^{2+} ions per subunit

+ Pathway: AMP biosynthesis via salvage pathway
- This protein is involved in step one of the subpathway that synthesis AMP from adenosine.
- This subpathway is part of the AMP biosynthesis salvage pathway, which is part of purine metabolism.

+ Molecular function:
- Adenosine kinase activity
- ATP binding
- Metal ion binding
- Phosphotransferase activity, alcohol group as an acceptor
- Poly(A) NA binding

+ Biological process:
- AMP salvage
- dATP biosynthetic process
- Nucleobase-containing small molecule metabolic process
- Purine-containing compound salvage
- Purine nucleobase metabolic process
- Ribonucleoside monophosphate biosynthetic process
- Small molecule metabolic process

+ Subcellular location:
- Nucleus

- Cytoplasm
+ Cellular component:
    - Cytoplasm
    - Cytosol
    - Nucleoplasm

http://www.uniprot.org/uniprot/P55263

AGT

+ **Overview for AGT** *Angiotensinogen* (serpin peptidase inhibitor)
    - *AGT*, rs699 (aka, M235T/C4072T)
    - The enzyme encoded by AGT, angiotensinogen, is essential component of the renin-angiotensin system (RAS), and a potent regulator of blood pressure, body fluid, and electrolyte homeostasis.
    - Angiotensin-2 acts directly on vascular smooth muscle as a potent vasoconstrictor, affects cardiac contractility and heart rate through its action on the sympathetic nervous system, and alters renal sodium and water absorption through its ability to stimulate the zona glomerulosa cells of the adrenal cortex to synthesize and secrete aldosterone.
    - When looking at AGT SNPs, consider the staus of ACE generated enzyme, which converts angiotensin I to angiotensin II.
    - Angiotensin-3: stimulates aldosterone release.
    - Angiotensin 1-7: is a ligand for the G protein-coupled receptor MAS1. It has vasodilator and antidiuretic effects, and an antithrombotic effect that involves MAS1-mediated release of nitric oxide from platelets.

http://www.uniprot.org/uniprot/P01019

+ This protein is part of the renin-angiotensin system, which regulates <u>blood pressure</u> and the balance of fluids and salts in the body. In the first step of this process, angiotensinogen is converted to angiotensin I. With an additional step, angiotensin I is converted to angiotensin II. Angiotensin II causes blood vessels to narrow (constrict), which results in increased blood pressure. This molecule also stimulates production of the hormone aldosterone, which triggers the absorption of salt and water by the kidneys. The increased amount of fluid in the body also increases blood pressure. Proper blood pressure during fetal growth, which delivers oxygen to the developing tissues, is required for normal development of the kidneys, particularly of structures called the proximal tubules, and other tissues. In addition, angiotensin II may play a more direct role in kidney development, perhaps by affecting growth factors involved in the development of kidney structures.

+ When AGT is not functioning properly it can lead to essential hypertension and renal tubular dysgenisis.

http://ghr.nlm.nih.gov/gene/AGT

+ Angiotensin-1 is a substrate of the ACE gene.

+ AGT M235T/C4072T rs699 is associated with essential hypertension and pre-eclampsia.

+ Molecular functions:
- Growth factor activity
- Hormone activity
- Serine-type endopeptidase inhibitor activity
- Sodium channel regulator activity
- Superoxide-generatine NADPH oxidase activator activity
- Type 1 angiotensin receptor binding
- Type 2 angiotensin receptor binding

+ Biological process:
- Please refer to http://www.uniprot.org/uniprot/P01019 for a complete list of biological processes related to AGT, as the list is extensive.

+ Subcellular location:
- Secreted

+ Cellular component:
- Blood microparticle
- Cytoplasm
- Extracellular exosome
- Extracellular region
- Extracellular space

http://www.uniprot.org/uniprot/P01019

+ Diseases related to AGT are:
- Acute coronary artery syndrome
- Coronary artery disease
- Type II diabetes
- Essential hypertension
- Hypertension
- Left ventricular hypertrophy
- Cirrhosis
- Myocardial infarction
- Peptic ulcer hemorrhage and
- Stroke

AHCY

+ **Overview for AHCY-01** *Adenosylhomocysteinase*
    - *AHCY*, rs819147 (aka, G14905A)
    - The AHCY gene provides instructions for producing the enzyme S-adenosylhomocysteine hydrolase. This enzyme is involved in a multi-step process that breaks down the protein building block (amino acid), methionine.

+ The cofactor for AHCY is NAD+, derived from nitamin B3.

http://www.uniprot.org/uniprot/P23526

+ S-adenosylhomocysteine hydrolase belongs to the adenosylhomocysteinase family. It catalyzes the reversible hydrolysis of S-adenosylhomocysteine (AdoHcy or SAH) to adenosine (Ado) and L-homocysteine (Hcy), and operates to sustain the flux of methionine sulfur toward cysteine. Thus, it regulates the intracellular SAH concentration thought to be important for transmethylation reactions. This reaction also plays an important role in regulating the addition of methyl groups, consisting of one carbon atom and three hydrogen atoms, to other compounds (methylation). Methylation is important in many cellular processes. These include determining whether the instructions in a particular segment of DNA are carried out, regulating reactions involving proteins and lipids, and controlling the processing of chemicals that relay signals in the nervous system (neurotransmitters).

http://www.ncbi.nlm.nih.gov/gene/191

+ Deficiency in this protein is one of a number of causes of hypermethioninemia.
    - Hypermethioninemia is an excess of a particular protein building block (amino acid), called methionine, in the blood. This condition can occur when methionine is not broken down (metabolized) properly in the body.
    - People with hypermethioninemia often do not show any symptoms. Some individuals with hypermethioninemia exhibit intellectual disability and other neurological problems; delays in motor skills such as standing or walking; sluggishness; muscle weakness; liver problems; unusual facial features; and their breath, sweat, or urine may have a smell resembling boiled cabbage.
    - Hypermethioninemia can occur with other metabolic disorders, such as homocystinuria, tyrosinemia and galactosemia, which also involve the faulty breakdown of particular molecules. It can also result from liver disease or excessive dietary intake of methionine from consuming large amounts of protein or a methionine-enriched infant formula.

http://ghr.nlm.nih.gov/gene/AHCY

http://ghr.nlm.nih.gov/condition/hypermethioninemia

+ Catalytic activity:
- S-adenosyl-L-homocysteine + H2O = L-homocysteine + adenosine

+ Cofactor:
- NAD+

+ Pathway: L-homocysteine biosynthesis
- Adenosine kinase is involved in step one of the subpathway that synthesizes L-homocysteine from S-adensyl-L-homocysteine (SAH).
- This subpathway is part of the L-homocysteine biosynthesis, which is part of amino acid biosynthesis.
- Adenosylhomocysteinase (AHCYL1), Adenosylhomocysteinase (AHCYL2), Adenosylhomocysteinase (AHCY)

+ Molecular function:
- Adenosylhomocysteinase activity
- Adenyl nucleotide binding
- NAD binding

+ Biological process:
- Cellular nitrogen compound metabolic process
- Chronic inflammatory response to antigen stimulus
- Circadian sleep/wake cycle
- Homocysteine biosynthetic process
- Methylation
- Response to hypoxia
- Response to nutrient
- SAH catabolic process
- SAM cycle
- Small molecule metabolic process
- Sulfur amino acid metabolic process
- Xenobiotic metabolic process

+ Subcellular location:
- Cytoplasm
- Melanosome

http://www.uniprot.org/uniprot/P23526

AMT

+ **Overview for AMT** *Aminomethyltransferase* (Glycine Cleavage System Protein T)
- *AMT*, rs1464566 (aka, A5736G), rs4855873 (aka, T5998G)

- The AMT gene provides instructions for making an enzyme called aminomethyltransferase. This enzyme is one of four components (subunits) that make up a large complex called glycine cleavage enzyme. Within cells, this complex is active in mitochondria. Glycine cleavage enzyme processes a molecule called glycine by cutting (cleaving) it into smaller pieces. Glycine is an amino acid, which is a building block of proteins. This molecule also acts as a neurotransmitter, which is a chemical messenger that transmits signals in the brain. The breakdown of excess glycine is necessary for the normal development and function of nerve cells in the brain and spinal cord.

http://www.genecards.org/cgi-bin/carddisp.pl?gene=AMT

+ Mutations in the AMT gene are responsible for ten to fifteen percent of all cases of glycine encephalopathy. More than a dozen mutations have been identified in affected individuals. Most of these genetic changes alter single amino acids in aminomethyltransferase. Other mutations delete genetic material from the AMT gene or disrupt how genetic information from the gene is spliced together to make a blueprint for producing aminomethyltransferase.

+ AMT mutations alter the structure and function of aminomethyltransferase. When an altered version of this enzyme is incorporated into the glycine cleavage enzyme complex, it prevents the complex from breaking down glycine properly. As a result, excess glycine can build up to toxic levels in the body's organs and tissues. Damage caused by harmful amounts of this molecule in the brain and spinal cord is responsible for the intellectual disability, seizures, and breathing difficulties characteristic of glycine encephalopathy.

http://ghr.nlm.nih.gov/gene/AMT

+ Molecular function:
  - Aminomethyltransferase activity

+ Biological process:
  - Glycine catabolic activity

http://www.uniprot.org/uniprot/Q49A62

BHMT

+ **Overview for BHMT** *Betaine Homocysteine Methyltransferase* (aka, Betaine--Homocysteine S-Methyltransferase)
  - *BHMT*-02 rs567754 (aka, C13813T), BHMT-04 rs617219 (aka, A26991C), BHMT-08 rs651852 (aka, C6457T)
  - BHMT rs6875201 (aka, A7961G), rs16876512 (aka, C-448T), rs3733890 (aka, R239Q)

- This gene encodes a cytosolic enzyme that catalyzes the conversion of betaine (trimethylglycine) and homocysteine, to dimethylglycine, and methionine, respectively.
- This reaction is also required for the irreversible oxidation of choline.

http://www.genecards.org/cgi-bin/carddisp.pl?gene=BHMT

- It is sometimes referred to as the "shortcut" pathway in homocysteine to methionine conversion.
- BHMT SNPs are associated with decreased conversion of homocysteine to methionine, and can result in higher glycine levels, and sometime (mostly when person under stress) produce results similar to CBS up-regulation (e.g., high ammonia, lower glutathione and lower vitamin B-6).

+ BHMT-08 appears to increase norepinepherine relative to dopamine; also reflected in behaviors.

- Acute stress → norepinepherine increase → tyrosine hydroxylase increase (but not dompaminergic nuclei) → norepinepherine increase relative to dopamine.

http://dramyyasko.com/wp-content/uploads/2010/06/39-A1-BHMT8.pdf

❖ **NOTE**: Norepinepherine receptors may be inhibited by high sulfur (check CBS C699T, vitamin B-6 deficiency).

– Elevated glycine may be seen in someone with a homozygous BHMT 08 mutation.

+ The activity of the betaine homocysteine methyltransferase enzyme can be negatively influenced by stress (cortisol).

- The second pathway involved in BHMT is the amine and polyamine degradation; betaine degradation pathway.

http://www.grenoble.prabi.fr/obiwarehouse/unipathway/upa?upid=UPA00291&entryac=Q93088

+ Betaine homocysteine methyltransferase requires trimethylglycine (TMG) to perform the conversion of homocysteine to methionine. Administering TMG or phosphatidylcholine may be supportive.

http://www.uniprot.org/uniprot/Q93088

+ One of the pathways involved in BHMT is the L-methionine biosynthesis via de novo pathway. Sulfur-containing amino-acid L-methionine (2-amino-4- (methylthio) butanoic acid) is synthesized de novo by most microorganisms after the initial steps of inorganic sulfate assimilation and synthesis of cysteine or homocysteine. There are two alternative pathways of methionine synthesis in microorganisms. The enterobacterial type trans-sulfuration pathway involves cystathionine as an intermediate and utilizes cysteine as the sulfur source. Then there is the direct sulfhydrylation pathway found in yeast (saccharomyces cerevisiae), spirochete (leptospira meyeri) and actinomycetes (corynebacterium glutamicum) which bypasses cystathionine and uses inorganic sulfur instead. Methionine biosynthesis is a central pathway, as it controls a large number of cellular processes such as translation of mRNA into proteins (not only as a substrate for protein elongation, but also as the initiator of protein synthesis) and transmethylation reactions via the formation of S-adenosylmethionine (SAM) (cf activated methyl cycle pathway).

http://www.grenoble.prabi.fr/obiwarehouse/unipathway/upa?upid=UPA00051&entryac=Q93088

+ BHMT is found in the liver and kidneys and not detectable in other organs.

http://www.sciencedirect.com/science/article/pii/S0003986197902460

+ BHMT catalyzes up to fifty percent of homocysteine metabolism.

http://www.ncbi.nlm.nih.gov/pubmed/21093336?dopt=Abstract

+ It plays a role in choline metabolism in the aetiology of oral-facial clefts.

http://www.ncbi.nlm.nih.gov/pubmed/19737740?dopt=Abstract

+ Dr. Amy Yasko at www.holisticheal.com states that, "The activity of this gene product can be affected by stress, by cortisol levels and may play a role in ADD/ADHD by affecting norepinephrine levels."

+ BHMT is one of many genes related to folate-related genes and risks of spina bifida and conotruncal heart defects.

http://www.ncbi.nlm.nih.gov/pubmed/19493349?dopt=Abstract

+ Catalytic activity:
- Trimethylammonioacetate + L-homocysteine = dimethylglycine + L-methionine

+Cofactor:
- Zinc   Binds one zinc ion per subunit

+ **1st** Pathway: Betaine degradation:
- This protein is involved in step one of the subpathway that synthesizes sarcosine from betaine.
    - Step I - Betaine-homocysteine S-methyltransferase 1 (BHMT)
    - Step II – Dimethylglycine dehydrogenase, mitochondrial (DMGDH)
- This subpathway is part of the pathway betaine degradation, which is part of amine and polyamine degradation.

+ **2nd** Pathway: Betaine degradation:
- This protein is involved in step one of the subpathway that synthesizes L-methionine from L-homocysteine.
    - Betaine-homocysteine S-methyltransferase (BHMT2)

- This subpathway is part of the pathway betaine degradation, which is part of amine and polyamine degradation.

+ Molecular function:
  - Betaine-homocysteine S-methyltransferase activity
  - S-adenosylmethionine-homocysteine S-methyltransferase activity
  - Zinc ion binding

+ Biological process:
  - Amino-acid betaine catabolic process
  - Cellular nitrogen compound metabolic process
  - Protein methylation
  - Response to organonitrogen compound
  - S-methionine cycle
  - Amino-acid betaine metabolic process
  - L-methionine salvage
  - Regulation of homocysteine metabolic process
  - Small molecule metabolic process and
  - Sulfur amino acid metabolic process

+ Subcellular location:
  - Cytoplasm

http://www.uniprot.org/uniprot/Q93088

+ Cellular component:
  - Cytoplasm
  - Cytosol
  - Extracellular exosome

❖ **NOTE:** The following four SNPs are grouped together, as they inter-relate in the transsulfuration pathway:

CBS

+ <u>**Overview for CBS**</u> *Cystathionine-beta-synthase* (aka, Cystathionine-β-synthase)
  - *CBS* rs2851391 (aka, A13637G), **rs1801181 (aka, A360A)**, rs706209 (aka, C*351T), rs4920037 (aka, C19150T), **rs234706 (aka, C699T)**, rs12613 (aka, G*299A), rs706208 (aka, T*330C), encodes the enzyme, Cystathionine-β-synthase.

http://ghr.nlm.nih.gov/gene/CBS

  - CBS catalyzes the first step of the transulfuration pathway, from homocysteine and serine, to cystathionine, and down-stream to glutathione production, ammonia, and sulfites/sulfates, and more. Another enzyme then converts cystathionine to the amino acid cysteine, which is used to build proteins or is broken down and excreted in urine.

+ CBS is the only known pyridoxal phosphate-dependent enzyme that contains heme. It is an important regulator of hydrogen sulfide, especially in the brain, utilizing cysteine instead of serine to catalyze the formation of hydrogen sulfide. Hydrogen sulfide is a gastratransmitter with signaling and cytoprotective effects such as acting as a neuromodulator in the brain to protect neurons against hypoxic injury.

http://www.uniprot.org/uniprot/P35520

- **Our Two Cents:** Homocysteine can be converted to methionine via the BHMT pathway (short-cut) when adequate levels of TMG are available. Similarly, homocysteine can be converted to methionine via the MTR (long-way around) when adequate levels of folate and vitamin B-12 are available. Homocysteine however, is functionally broken down, via the transulfuration pathway (e.g., CBS, CTH, etc). The CBS enzyme is P5P dependent (vitamin B-6). Therefore, if the trans-sulfuration pathway is up-regulating, due to, for example, a CBS C699T homozygous SNP, then vitamin B-6 may be depleted. If vitamin B-6 is low, then there may be an impact on adrenal function and neurotransmitter production, as both are vitamin B-6 dependent. There may also be an impact on levels of magnesium (low), zinc (low), glutathione (low), and evidence of higher ammonia (including low arginine and "brain fog"), taurine and sulfate generation.

- **Our Other Two Cents:** Ongoing stress can deplete vitamin B-6 (adrenals). It is also worth mentioning that digestive breakdown of certain plant anti-nutrients (e.g., high oxalate foods) are vitamin B-6 dependent. These include Alanine-glyoxylate amino transferase (AGT), glyoxylate reductase (GR), and hydroxypyruvic reductase (HPR). If there is a history of kidney stones, those same enzymes may be impaired. When a CBS up-regulation is suspected, testing (e.g., GD NutrEval, OATs, Spectracell) may be warranted to determine its impact, as it can have far-reaching consequences on liver mitochondrial function, immune system function, oxidation and neurotransmitter status.

+ The most common mutation in CBS substitutes the amino acid, threonine, for the amino acid, isoleucine, at position 278 in the enzyme (written as Ile278Thr or I278T). Another common mutation, which is the most frequent cause of homocystinuria in the Irish population, replaces the amino acid, glycine, with the amino acid, serine, at position 307 (written as Gly307Ser or G307S). These mutations disrupt the normal function of cystathionine beta-synthase. As a result, homocysteine and other potentially toxic compounds build up in the blood and homocysteine is excreted in urine. Researchers have not determined how excess homocysteine leads to the signs and symptoms of homocystinuria.

http://ghr.nlm.nih.gov/gene/CBS

+ Catalytic activity:
- L-serine + L-homocysteine = L-cystathionine + H2O

+ Cofactor:
- Pyridoxal 5'-phosphate (bioavailable form of vitamin B-6)

+ Enzyme regulation:
- Allosterically activated by adenosyl-methionine (AdoMet)

+ Pathway L-cysteine biosynthesis:
- This protein is involved in step one of the subpathway that synthesizes L-cysteine from L-homcysteine and L-serine.
- Proteins known to be involved in the two steps of the subpathway in this organism are cystathionine beta-synthase (CBS) and cystathionine gamma-lyase (CTH).

+ Molecular function:
- Carbon monoxide binding
- Cystathionine beta-synthase activity
- Enzyme binding
- Heme binding
- Identical protein binding
- Metal ion binding
- Modified amino acid binding
- Nitric oxide binding
- Nitrate reductase (NO-forming) activity
- Oxygen binding
- Protein homodimerization activity
- Pyridoxal phosphate binding
- SAM binding
- Ubiquitin protein ligase binding

+ Biological process:
- Cellular nitrogen compound metabolic process
- Cysteine biosynthetic process
- Cysteine biosynthetic process from serine
- Cysteine biosynthetic process from cystathione
- DNA protection
- Homocysteine catabolic process
- Homocysteine metabolic process
- L-cysteine catabolic process

- L-serine catabolic process
- L-serine metabolic process
- Oxidation-reduction process
- Small molecule metabolic process
- Sulfur amino acid
- Transulfuration

+ Subcellular location:
- Cytoplasm
- Nucleus

+ Cellular component:
- Cytoplasm
- Cytosol
- Intracellular membrane-bound organelle
- Nucleolus
- Nucleus

http://www.uniprot.org/uniprot/P35520

CSAD

+ **Overview for CSAD** *Cysteine Sulfinic Acid Decarboxylase* (aka, Cysteine-Sulfinate Decarboxylase)
- *CSAD* rs1006959 (aka, C13258T), rs11170453 (aka, C15829T), rs2272306 (aka, C25411T), rs12161793 (aka, T7219C), rs2293429 (aka, T5791G), encodes the enzyme, cysteine-sulfinate decarboxylase.
- CSAD encodes a member of the group 2, decarboxylase family. A similar protein in rodents plays a role in multiple biological processes as the rate-limiting enzyme in taurine biosynthesis, catalyzing the decarboxylation of cysteinesulfinate to hypotaurine.

http://www.genecards.org/cgi-bin/carddisp.pl?gene=CSAD&search=CSAD

❖ **NOTE**: Taurine is a sulfur-containing amino acid; it also functions with glycine and GABA as an inhibitory neurotransmitter. Taurine is found in many areas of our body, including our central nervous system, skeletal muscle, and in even greater concentrations, in our heart, and brain. As a powerful inhibitory neurotransmitter, one of taurine's uses has been that of an anticonvulsant. These anticonvulsant effects come from its ability to stabilize nerve cell membranes, which prevents the erratic firing of nerve cells. Therefore, it is also used to calm excitable tissues such as the heart, skeletal muscles, and central nervous system.

+ *In vivo* and *in vitro* the taurine-synthesizing enzyme in the brain, namely cysteine sulfinic acid decarboxylase (CSAD), is activated when phosphorylated and inhibited when dephosphorylated. Furthermore, protein kinase C and protein phosphatase 2C have been identified as the enzymes responsible for phosphorylation and dephosphorylation of CSAD, respectively.

http://www.jneurosci.org/content/17/18/6947.full

+ Cofactor:
- Pyridoxal 5'-phosphate (bioavailable form of vitamin B-6)

+ Molecular function:
- Carboxy-lyase activity
- Pyridoxal phosphate binding

+ Biological process:
- Carboxylic acid metabolic process

http://www.uniprot.org/uniprot/Q86V02

CTH

+ **Overview for CTH** *Cystathionine gamma-lyase*
- *CTH*, rs1145920 (aka, A11886G), rs515064 (aka, A32114G), rs663649 (aka, G25229T), rs10889869 (aka, G6010A), **rs1021737 (aka, S4031I)**, rs12723350 (aka, T16147C), rs681475 (aka, T8763C). Encodes the enzyme, cystathionine gamma-lyase.
- CTH encodes a cytoplasmic enzyme in the trans-sulfuration pathway that converts cystathione derived from methionine into cysteine. Glutathione synthesis in the liver is dependent upon the availability of cysteine. Mutations in this gene cause cystathioninuria.

http://ghr.nlm.nih.gov/gene/CTH

+ Those with homozygous risk alleles (T:T) in rs1021737 may have significantly higher plasma homocysteine concentrations.

http://www.snpedia.com/index.php/Rs1021737(T;T)

+ It is suggested that certain polymorphisms of the CTH gene may participate in the development of chronic hypertension and preeclampsia.

http://www.researchgate.net/publication/274091176_The_importance_of_rs1021737_and_rs482843_polymorphisms_of_cystathionine_gammalyase_in_the_etiology_of_preeclampsia_in_the_Caucasian_population

+ CTH catalyzes the last step in the trans-sulfuration pathway from methionine to cysteine. It has broad substrate specificity. CTH converts cystathionine to cysteine, ammonia, and 2-

oxobutanoate. It also converts two cysteine molecules to lanthionine and hydrogen sulfide, and can accept homocysteine as substrate. Specificity depends on the levels of the endogenous substrates. CTH generates the endogenous signaling molecule hydrogen sulfide (H2S), and so contributes to the regulation of blood pressure. CTH acts as a cysteine-protein sulfhydrase by mediating sulfhydration of target proteins: sulfhydration consists of converting -SH groups into -SSH on specific cysteine residues of target proteins such as GAPDH, PTPN1 and NF-kappa-B subunit RELA, thereby regulating their function. **(See, FIG 5)**

http://ghr.nlm.nih.gov/gene/CTH

+ Catalytic activity:
    - L-cystathionine + H2O = L-cysteine + NH3 + 2-oxobutanoate

+ Cofactor:
    - Pyridoxal 5'-phosphate (bioavailable form of vitamin B-6)

+ Enzyme regulation:
    - Inhibited by propargylglycine, trifluoroalanine and aminoethoxyvinylglycine.

+ Pathway L-cysteine biosynthesis:
    - This protein is involved in step one of the subpathway that synthesizes L-cysteine from L-homcysteine and L-serine.
    - Proteins known to be involved in the two steps of the subpathway in this organism are cystathionine beta-synthase (CBS) and cystathionine gamma-lyase (CTH)

+ Molecular function:
    - Carbon-sulfur lyase activity
    - Cystathionine gamma-lyase activity
    - Homocysteine desulfhydrase activity
    - L-cysteine desulfhydrase activity
    - L-cystine L-cysteine-lyase (deaminating)
    - Pyridoxal phosphate binding

+ Biological process:
    - Cellular nitrogen compound metabolic process
    - Cysteine biosynthetic process
    - Cysteine metabolic process
    - Endoplasmic reticulum unfolder protein response
    - Hydrogen sulfide biosynthetic process
    - Negative regulation of apoptotic signaling pathway
    - Positive regulation of I-kappaB kinase/NF-kappaB signaling
    - Positive regulation of NF-kappaB transcription factor activity
    - Protein homotetramerization

- Protein-pyridoxal-5-phosphate linkage
- Protein Sulfhydration
- Small molecule metabolic process
- Sulfur amino acid catabolic process
- Sulfur amino acid metabolic process
- Transsulfuration

+ Subcellular location:
- Cytoplasm

+ Cellular component:
- Cytoplasm
- Cytosol
- Extracellular exosome
- Nucleoplasm
- Nucleus

http://www.uniprot.org/uniprot/P32929

COMT

+ **Overview for COMT/TXNRD2** *Catechol-O-methyltransferase* **(See FIG. 9 below)**
- COMT **rs769224 (aka, -61 P199P)**, rs2239393 (aka, A 26166G), **rs6269 (aka, A-1324G)**, rs933271 (aka, A2953G), rs174675 (aka, A309G), rs1544325 (aka, A7406G), rs4646316 (aka, C27870T), rs174696 (aka, C28914T), rs174699, (aka, C30196T), rs9332377 (aka, C31430T), rs8192488 (aka, C438T), rs165599 (aka, G*522A), rs739368 (aka, G14834A), rs165656 (aka, G24601C), rs165774 (aka, G28299A0, **rs4633 (aka, H62H)**, rs5993883 (aka, T13376G), rs4646312 (aka, T24075C), rs740601 (aka, T26501G), **rs4680 (aka, V158M)**.
- COMT/TXNRD2 rs737866 (aka, A4251G), rs2020917 (aka, C4622T), rs737865 (aka, T4239C).
- Catechol-*O*-methyltransferase is encoded by COMT and is one of several enzymes that degrade catecholamines such as dopamine, epinephrine, and norepinephrine.

http://www.ncbi.nlm.nih.gov/pubmed/1572656

- Catechol-*O*-methyltransferase also plays a role in estrogen breakdown.
> **Our (long) Two Cents:** COMT V158M and H62H homozygous SNPs almost always have an impact on quality of health/life at some point. In young women with COMT V158M and H62H homozygous SNPs, you may see that chronic health conditions and/or depression take root during the years of post-puberty (e.g., ages 13 to 18-ish).

Beyond that, other "trigger" time frames are post-pregnancy (e.g., depression, autoimmune), BCP introduction, high stress situations (e.g., job loss, holidays, divorce, etc.); times when estrogen levels/breakdown swing and stress hormone breakdown (epinephrine) compete for limited COMT bandwidth. Another issue may be a tendency for formation of 4-hydroxy estrone intermediary metabolites due to a combo of CYP1B1 SNPs (up-regulation via lifestyle) and COMT V158M/H62H SNPs (down-regulation). Over years, these may cause symptoms associated with estrogen dominance (e.g., breast cysts, PMS symptoms that negatively impact life a week or so before period, estrogen related cancers, etc.). Some options are to support glucuronidation and sulfation detox pathways first and then potentially layer in methylation support, but be mindful of other SNPs such as, CBS C699T. Also, those with COMT V158M/H62H homozygous SNPs typically do not do well with too much direct methyl donor supplementation (e.g., SAMe, methyl-B12), because they may push dopamine and epinephrine levels up too quickly. So it is often more effective to support surrounding pathways (transulfuration, methionine/homocysteine, and Krebs cycle) and ensure good GI health and adrenal function first. COMT is supported by magnesium and most tolerate Mg supplementation. Too much folate supplementation however, can result in an increase of excitatory neurotransmitters in those with COMT V158M/H62H homozygous SNPs as does methyl-B12 and SAM, so a "low and slow" approach is best if/when introducing methylation supplements such as, methyl-B12, folate, and SAMe.

- ❖ **NOTE**: Recall that GABA may be called into action to keep high dopamine levels in-check. As a result, GABA levels may be low in those with COMT V158M/H62H homozygous SNPs. (GABA is our calming neurotransmitter). The sympathetic nervous system may dominate over the parasympathetic nervous system in those with COMT V158M/H62H homozygous SNPs, so stress management techniques (such as, life style and dietary changes to remove extraneous inflammatory influences, jettisoning toxic relationships, Heart Math techniques, yoga, etc.) are helpful. Adrenal support (e.g., glandulars, vitamin B-5 and vitamin B-6, adpathogens, etc.) may also be key to reversing affects of stress/sympathetic nervous system tendency conferred by long-term, poor catecholamine breakdown due to COMT V158M/H62H homozygous SNPs.

+ COMT function, like all "MT's", require SAM as a cofactor (methyl donor). SAMe supplements for those with COMT V158M/H62H homozygous SNPs needs to be carefully considered and titrated-up slowly if selected (e.g., in those with MAT SNPs).

+ In summary, physiological substrates of COMT include catecholamine neurotransmitters and the catechol estrogens, produced by cytochrome P-450-mediated metabolism of E2 and E1. **(See FIGs. 3 and 9)**

+ COMT shortens the biological half-lives of the following neuroactive drugs:
- L-DOPA,
- Alpha-methyl DOPA
- Isoproterenol

+ O-methyltransferase activity which catalyzes the transfer of a methyl group to the oxygen atom of an acceptor molecule, http://www.ebi.ac.uk/QuickGO/GTerm?id=GO:0008171, and magnesium ion binding which interacts selectively and non-covalently with magnesium ions. http://www.ebi.ac.uk/QuickGO/GTerm?id=GO:0000287

+ Variations within the catechol-O-methyltransferase (COMT) gene have been associated with pain severity in temporomandibular disorders (TMDs). Psychological factors, such as, personal conflicts, life stress, and depression, are well known to be associated with onset, severity, and chronicity of pain disorders.

http://www.ncbi.nlm.nih.gov/pubmed/20337865

The effect of catechol-O-methyltransferase polymorphisms on pain is modified by depressive symptoms - ResearchGate. Available from:
http://www.researchgate.net/publication/221835085_The_effect_of_catechol-O-methyltransferase_polymorphisms_on_pain_is_modified_by_depressive_symptoms

+ SNPs in COMT V158M and COMT H62H result in three- to four-fold differences in COMT enzyme activity (down-regulation) and may contribute to the process of mental disorders, such as bipolar disorder and alcoholism.

http://www.omim.org/entry/103780

+ COMT SNPs are related to cisplatin toxicity. Cisplatin is used to treat cancers of the testicles, ovaries, or bladder.

http://www.ncbi.nlm.nih.gov/pmc/articles/PMC3217465/

+ Genetic variants in COMT might be involved in modulation of neurocognitive functions and hence conferring increased risk to schizophrenia; specifically, rs737865 in intron 1, rs4680 in exon 4 (Val158Met) and downstream rs165599.

http://www.ncbi.nlm.nih.gov/pubmed/19077118?dopt=Abstract
http://www.sciencedirect.com/science/article/pii/S0165178196031113

+ Because the regulation of catecholamines is impaired in a number of medical conditions (e.g., Parkinson's disease), several pharmaceutical drugs target COMT to alter its activity and therefore the availability of catecholamines.

http://www.ncbi.nlm.nih.gov/pubmed/11873938

+ Specific reactions catalyzed by COMT include:
- Dopamine → 3-Methoxytyramine

http://www.ncbi.nlm.nih.gov/pmc/articles/PMC2956650/

- DOPAC → HVA (homovanillic acid)

http://en.wikipedia.org/wiki/3,4-Dihydroxyphenylacetic_acid

- Norepinephrine → normetanephrine

http://en.wikipedia.org/wiki/Normetanephrine

- Epinephrine → metanephrine

http://en.wikipedia.org/wiki/Metanephrine

- Dihydroxyphenylethylene glycol (DOPEG) → methoxyhydroxyphenylglycol (MOPEG)

http://en.wikipedia.org/wiki/3-Methoxytyramine

- 3,4- Dihydroxymandelic acid (DOMA) → vanillylmandelic acid (VMA)

http://en.wikipedia.org/wiki/3,4-Dihydroxymandelic_acid

+ The oxidative metabolism of 17β-estradiol (E2) and estrone (E1) to catechol estrogens (2-OHE2, 4-OHE2, 2-OHE1, and 4-OHE1) and estrogen quinones has been postulated to be a factor in mammary carcinogenesis.

+ COMT is polymorphic in the human population. Twenty-five percent of United States Caucasians are homozygous for a V158M polymorphism in the *COMT* gene (46 – 48). This polymorphism results in three- to four-fold less enzyme activity (46, 47) and could, therefore, result in *decreased* detoxification and an increase of 4-hydroxyestrone intermediary metabolites.

+ O-Methylation catalyzed by catechol-*O*-methyltransferase is a phase II metabolic inactivation pathway for catechol estrogens. A polymorphism in the *COMT* gene, which codes for a low activity variant of the COMT enzyme (e.g., V158M, H62H), is associated with an increased risk of developing breast cancer.

http://www.researchgate.net/publication/11744930_The_effects_of_catechol-O-methyltransferase_inhibition_on_estrogen_metabolite_and_oxidative_DNA_damage_levels_in_estradiol-treated_MCF-7_cells

+ There are two types of COMT activity in the body. The long form is called, membrane-bound catechol-O-methyltransferase (MB-COMT). It is mainly produced by nerve cells in the brain. The shorter form of the enzyme is called, soluble catechol-O-methyltransferase (S-COMT). This form of the enzyme helps control the levels of certain hormones. Other tissues, including the liver, kidneys, and blood, produce a shorter form of the enzyme.

+ Two alleles, COMT*1 or COMT*H with Val-158 and COMT*2 or COMT*L with Met-158 are responsible for a three- to four-fold difference in enzymatic activity. Low enzyme activity alleles are associated with genetic susceptibility to alcoholism.

http://www.omim.org/entry/103780

+ Catechol-O-methyltransferase is important in the prefrontal cortex, which organizes and coordinates information from other parts of the brain. This region is involved with personality, planning, inhibition of behaviors, abstract thinking, emotions, and working (short-term) memory. COMT helps the prefrontal lobe function with catecholamines (COMT SNPs "cut both ways").

+ 22q11.2 deletion syndrome is a deletion of a small part of chromosome 22 where COMT resides. People with this deletion are more prone to mental illness such as schizophrenia, panic disorder, anxiety, PTSD, and bipolar disorder.

http://ghr.nlm.nih.gov/gene/COMT

- ❖ **NOTE**: Sterling Hill Erdei from MTHFR Support has spoken with many psychiatrists who have run variant reports and several have reported when a patient is chronically ill and has COMT V158M and H62H <u>green</u> on the report, most of the time these individuals have lower levels of dopamine and epinephrine. When psychiatrists have seen someone <u>yellow</u> for these mutations and the patient is chronically ill, they can be low or high on catacholamines, depending on DRD receptor function. When patients are <u>red</u> for these mutations and are chronically ill, they also present with an elevation in dopamine and epinephrine and estrogen/intermediary metabolites.

+ Repeat - Through some amazing doctors like Richard Deth, PhD and Amy Yasko, PhD, we have learned that methyl vitamin B-12 may not be the best form of vitamin B-12 for people with COMT V158M and H62H homozygous and heterozygous. Too many methyl donors can have a negative impact on these individuals, in the form of increased excitatory neurotransmitters.

+ Catalytic activity:
- S-adenosyl-L-methionine + a catechol = S-adenosyl-L-homocysteine + a guaiacol

+ Cofactor:
- Magnesium   Binds one Mg^{2+} ion per subunit

+ Molecular function:
- Catechol O-methyltransferase activity
- Magnesium ion binding
- O-methyltransferase activity

+ Biological process:
- Cellular response to phosphate starvation
- Dopamine catabolic process
- Female pregnancy
- Methylation
- Negative regulation of dopamine metabolic process
- Negative regulation of smooth muscle cell proliferation
- Neurotransmitter catabolic process

- Regulation of sensory perception of pain
- Response to lipopolysaccharide
- Response to pain
- Small molecule metabolic process
- Xenobiotic metabolic process
- Developmental process
- Estrogen metabolic process
- Learning
- Multicellular organismal reproductive process
- Negative regulation of renal sodium excretion
- Neurotransmitter biosynthetic process
- Positive regulation of homocysteine metabolic process
- Response to drugs
- Response to organic cyclic compound
- Short-term memory
- Synaptic transmission

+ Cellular component:
- Axon
- Cell body
- Cytosol
- Dendritic spine
- Extracellular exosome
- Integral component of membrane
- Mitochondrion
- Plasma membrane
- Postsynaptic membrane

http://www.uniprot.org/uniprot/P21964

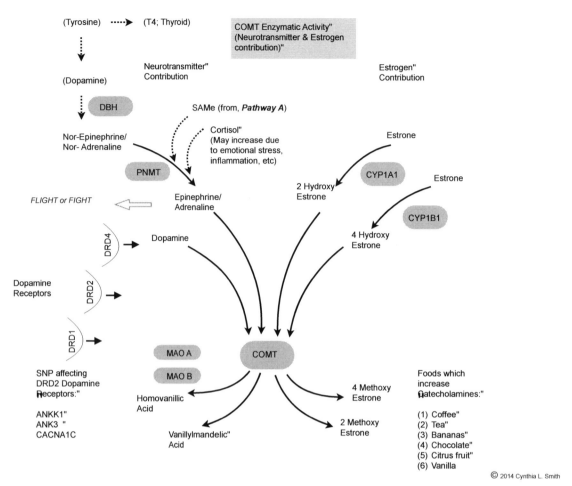

FIGURE 9 – COMT- Neurotransmitter & Estrogen Breakdown

DHFR

+ **Overview for DHFR** *Dihydrofolate Reductase*

- DHFR, rs7387 (aka, A*115T), rs10072026 (aka, A10661G), rs1643649 (aka, A16352G), rs1643659 (aka, A20965G), rs1677693 (aka, C19483A)
- DHFR/MSH, rs1650697 (aka, T-473A)
- The DHFR gene provides instructions for producing the enzyme, dihydrofolate reductase, which converts dihydrofolate into tetrahydrofolate using NADPH (electron donor) as a cofactor. While the functional dihydrofolate reductase gene has been mapped to chromosome 5, multiple intronless processed pseudogenes or dihydrofolate reductase-like genes have been identified on separate chromosomes.
- Recall that tetrahydrofolate is a methyl group shuttle required for the de novo synthesis of purines, thymidylic acid, and certain amino acids.

http://www.genecards.org/cgi-bin/carddisp.pl?gene=DHFR

http://www.ncbi.nlm.nih.gov/gene/1719

+ Mechanism: DHFR catalyzes the transfer of a hydride from NADPH to dihydrofolate to with an accompanying protonation to produce tetrahydrofolate. In the end, dihydrofolate is reduced to tetrahydrofolate and NADPH is oxidized to NADP+. (See FIG 4 on page 99)

- ❖ **NOTE**: SNPs in DHFR (especially in combination with MTHFD1 and MTHFR SNPs) indicate potential issues with subsequent conversion of folic acid into the active bioavailable form of folate. Since 1970's, folic acid has been fortified into many processed foods such as flour, rice, bread, pasta, and cereals, so it is best to avoid them. Natural sources of folate are found in leafy greens, beans, eggs, berries, and more, and require one DHFR step rather than two DHFR steps for folic acid conversion.

+ Folic acid has been found to block L-methylfolate from crossing the blood-brain barrier in individuals with DHFR that is compromised.

+ Dihydrofolate reductase deficiency has been linked to megaloblastic anemia and cerebral folate deficiency.

http://www.cell.com/ajhg/abstract/S0002-9297(11)00008-5

+ DHFR is the target for many anticancer and antibiotic therapies including methotrexate and trimethoprim.

- Because DHFR is associated with levels of tetrahydrofolate, which is needed by rapidly dividing cells to make thymine, the inhibition of DHFR can limit the growth and proliferation of cells that are characteristic of cancer. Methotrexate, a competitive inhibitor of DHFR, is one such anticancer drug that inhibits DHFR. Other drugs include, trimethoprim and pyrimethamine. These three are widely used as antitumor and antimicrobial agents.

http://www.ncbi.nlm.nih.gov/pubmed/10623528

+ Some drugs used to fight cancer and antimalarials can inhibit DHFR:
- Trimethoprim
- Pyrimethamine
- Chloroguanide or Proguanil
- Pentamidine
- Methotrexate
- Trimetrexate

http://www.pharmacorama.com/en/Sections/DNA-RNA-biosynthesis-5.php

+ Catalytic activity:
- $5,6,7,8$-tetrahydrofolate + $NADP^+$ = $7,8$-dihydrofolate + NADPH

+ Pathway; tetrahydrofolate biosynthesis:
- Synthesizes $5,6,7,8$-tetrahydrofolate from $7,8$-dihydrofolate.

+ Molecular function:
- Dihydrofolate reductase activity
- mRNA binding
- Drug binding and
- NADP binding

+ Biological process:
- Folic acid metabolic process
- Glycine biosynthetic process
- Nitric oxide metabolic process
- One-carbon metabolic process
- Regulation of transcription involved in G1/S transition of mitotic cell cycle
- Small molecule metabolic process
- Tetrahydrofolate metabolic process
- Water-soluble vitamin metabolic process
- G1/S transition of mitotic cell cycle
- Mitotic cell cycle
- Nucleotide biosynthetic process
- Regulation of nitric-oxide synthase activity
- Response to methotrexate
- Tetrahydrofolate biosynthetic process
- Vitamin metabolic process

+ Cellular component:
- Cytosol
- Nucleoplasm

http://www.uniprot.org/uniprot/P00374

DMGDH

+ **Overview for DMGDH** *Dimethylglycine Dehydrogenase, mitochondrial* (aka, DMGDHD)
- *DMGDH*, rs479405 (aka, G67591T), rs2253262 (aka, T372G), rs402701 (aka, T39928C), rs532964 (aka, T835C)
- This gene encodes an enzyme involved in the catabolism of choline, catalyzing the oxidative demethylation of dimethylglycine to form sarcosine. Mutations in this gene cause dimethylglycine dehydrogenase deficiency characterized by a fishlike body

odor, chronic muscle fatigue, and elevated levels of the muscle form of creatine kinase in serum.

http://ghr.nlm.nih.gov/gene/DMGDH

+ DMGDH deficiency (DMGDHD): Disorder characterized by fish odor, muscle fatigue with increased serum creatine kinase. Biochemically, it is characterized by an increase of N,N-dimethylglycine (DMG) in serum and urine.
- Treatment for fish odor syndrome is certain dietary restrictions, use of acid lotions and soaps to remove secreted trimethylamine on the skin, use of activated charcoal and copper chlorophyllin, certain antibiotics, laxatives, and riboflavin supplements.

+ Catalytic activity:
- N,N-dimethylglycine + flavoprotein + H2O = sarcosine + formaldehyde + reduced flavoprotein

+ Cofactor:
- FAD

http://www.uniprot.org/uniprot/Q9UI17

FOLR1

+ **Overview for FOLR1** *Folate Receptor 1* [Adult] (aka, Adult Folate-Binding Protein, Folate receptor alpha)
- FOLR1, rs2071010 (aka, G-20A)
- The protein encoded by this gene is a member of the folate receptor family. Members of this gene family bind folic acid and its reduced derivatives and transport 5-methyltetrahydrofolate into cells. This gene product is a secreted protein that either anchors to membranes via a glycosyl-phosphatidylinositol linkage or exists in a soluble form. Mutations in this gene have been associated with neurodegeneration due to cerebral folate transport deficiency. Due to the presence of two promoters, multiple transcription start sites, and alternative splicing, multiple transcript variants encoding the same protein have been found for this gene.

http://www.genecards.org/cgi-bin/carddisp.pl?gene=FOLR1

+ FOLR1 binds to folate and reduced folic acid derivatives and mediates delivery of 5-methyltetrahydrofolate and folate analogs into the interior of cells. Folate receptor alpha has a high affinity for folate and folic acid analogs at neutral pH. Required for normal embryonic development and normal cell proliferation.

http://www.uniprot.org/uniprot/P15328#section_comments

http://www.ncbi.nlm.nih.gov/pubmed/2527252

+ Diseases associated with FOLR1 include acute necrotizing encephalitis and cerebral folate transport deficiency. An important paralog of this gene is FOLR3.

+ Folate receptors (FRα, FRβ and FRγ) are cysteine-rich cell-surface glycoproteins that bind folate with high affinity to mediate cellular uptake of folate. Although expressed at very low levels in most tissues, folate receptors, especially FRα (FOLR1), are expressed at high levels in numerous cancers to meet the folate demand of rapidly dividing cells under low folate conditions. The folate dependency of many tumors has been therapeutically and diagnostically exploited by administration of anti-FRα antibodies, high-affinity antifolates, folate-based imaging agents and folate-conjugated drugs and toxins.

http://www.ncbi.nlm.nih.gov/pubmed/23851396

+ FOLR1 is related to cerebral folate deficiency. Folic acid has been known to prevent/block L-methyfolate from crossing the blood-brain barrier in people with CFD.

http://www.omim.org/entry/136430

+ Molecular function:
- Folic acid binding
- Folic acid transport activity
- Receptor activity

+ Biological process
- Folic acid metabolic process
- Folic acid transport
- Heart looping
- Neural crest cell migration involved in heart formation
- Pharyngeal arch artery morphogenesis
- Receptror mediated endocytosis

http://www.uniprot.org/uniprot/P15328

+ Subcellular location
- Cell membrane; lipid anchor
- Secreted
- Cytoplasmic vesicle
- Endosome
- Apical cell membrane

+ Cellular component
- Anchored component of external side of plasm membrane
- Atypical plasm membrans
- Cell surface
- Clathrin-coated vesicle

- Endosome
- Integral component of plasma membrane
- Nucleus
- Plasma membrane

http://www.uniprot.org/uniprot/P15328

FOLR2

+ **Overview for FOLR2** *Folate Receptor 2* [Fetal] (aka, Folate receptor beta, Folate receptor 2, FBP, and FOLR2)
- *FOLR2*, rs651933 (aka, G-1316A)
- Folate receptor 2 (or beta) is a receptor protein that, in humans, is encoded by the FOLR2 gene.
- The gene's biological process is folic acid binding.

http://en.wikipedia.org/wiki/FOLR2 - cite_note-entrez-3

- The protein encoded by this gene is a member of the folate receptor (FOLR) family. Members of this gene family have a high affinity for folic acid and for several reduced folic acid derivatives, and mediate delivery of 5-methyltetrahydrofolate to the interior of cells. This protein has a sixty-eight percent and seventy-nine percent sequence homology with the FOLR1 and FOLR3 proteins, respectively. The FOLR2 protein was originally thought to exist only in placenta, but is also detected in spleen, bone marrow, and thymus.

http://www.ncbi.nlm.nih.gov/pubmed/2166548
http://www.sinobiological.com/FOLR2-Protein-a-829.html?gclid=Cj0KEQjw-OCqBRDXmlWvveLE3_cBEiQAZWflmf6Slofy7z9Pg1NkNCoZRVrXo1-zHaEoanR1qZVJ2qoaAj7q8P8HAQ

+ FOLR2 may play a role in the transport of methotrexate in synovial macrophages in rheumatoid arthritis patients.

http://www.ncbi.nlm.nih.gov/gene/2350

+ Diseases associated with FOLR2 include rheumatoid arthritis and cerebral folate transport deficiency. An important paralog of this gene is FOLR3.

http://www.genecards.org/cgi-bin/carddisp.pl?gene=FOLR2

+Folate conjugates of therapeutic drugs are a potential immunotherapy tool to target tumor-associated macrophages.

http://www.sinobiological.com/FOLR2-Protein-a-829.html?gclid=Cj0KEQjw-OCqBRDXmlWvveLE3_cBEiQAZWflmf6Slofy7z9Pg1NkNCoZRVrXo1-zHaEoanR1qZVJ2qoaAj7q8P8HAQ

+ Molecular function:
- Folic acid binding
- Folic acid transporter activity

+ Biological process:
- Folic acid transport

+ Subcellular location:
- Cell membrane
- Secreted

+ Cellular component:
- Anchored component of external side of plasma membrane
- Extracellular region
- Membrane

http://www.uniprot.org/uniprot/P14207

FOLR3

+ **Overview for FOLR3** *Folate Receptor 3* (aka, Folate receptor gamma, FR-G; FR-gamma; gamma-hFR)

- *FOLR3*, rs7925545 (aka, A3771G), rs7926875 (aka, C7672A)
- Folate receptor 3 (or gamma) is a receptor protein that, in humans, is encoded by the FOLR3 gene.
- Folate receptor, gamma, binds to folate and reduced folic acid derivatives and mediates delivery of 5-methyltetrahydrofolate to the interior of cells.

http://www.uniprot.org/uniprot/P41439http://en.wikipedia.org/wiki/FOLR2 - cite_note-entrez-3

- This gene encodes a member of the folate receptor (FOLR) family, members of which have a high affinity for folic acid and for several reduced folic acid derivatives, and mediate delivery of 5-methyltetrahydrofolate to the interior of cells. This gene includes two polymorphic variants; the shorter one has two base deletions in the CDS, resulting in a truncated polypeptide, compared to the longer one. Both protein products are constitutively secreted in hematopoietic tissues and are potential serum marker for certain hematopoietic malignancies. The longer protein has a seventy-one percent and seventy-nine percent sequence homology with the FOLR1 and FOLR2 proteins, respectively. Recall that hematopoietic stem cells reside in the bone marrow and are responsible for replenishing blood and immune-system cells.

http://www.genecards.org/cgi-bin/carddisp.pl?gene=FOLR3

+ Evidence that polymorphic variants across the folate receptor genes (FOLR1, FOLR2, FOLR3) and the folate carrier genes (SLC19A1), appear to be statistically significant for association to meningomyelocele in the patient population that was tested. FOLR2 gene (rs13908), three linked variants in the FOLR3 gene (rs7925545, rs7926875, rs7926987), and two variants in the SLC19A1 gene (rs1888530 and rs3788200) were statistically significant.
http://www.ncbi.nlm.nih.gov/pubmed/20683905/

+ FOLR3 is expressed by cells of the myelocyte and B lymphocyte lineage, as well as, by various carcinomas. FOLR3 is more highly expressed in ovarian carcinomas than in breast carcinomas or mesotheliomas. Unlike other folate receptors, FOLR3 does not exhibit stereoselectivity in the binding of folates.
http://www.rndsystems.com/product_results.aspx?m=4171

+ This gene is a 32 kDa protein that binds folic acid and reduced folates.

+ Dietary folates are required for many key metabolic processes including:
    - Nucleotide synthesis
    - Methionine synthesis
    - Interconversion of glycine
    - Interconversion of serine
    - Histidine breakdown

+ Molecular function:
    - Folic acid binding

+ Biological process:
    - Folic acid transport

+ Subcellular location:
    - Secreted

+ Cellular component
    - Extrinsic component of membrane
    - Extracellular region
    - Membrane

http://www.uniprot.org/uniprot/P41439

GAD1

+ **Overview for GAD1** *Glutamate decarboxylase 1 (brain, 67kDa) (GAD67)*
    - GAD, rs2241164 (aka, GAD1), rs769395 (aka, A48604A), rs2241165 (aka, C10180T), rs3828275 (aka, C14541T), rs12185692 (aka, C2627A), rs701492 (aka, C34281T), rs769407 (aka, G25509C), rs3791850 (aka, G39901A),

- rs3791878 (aka, G3992T), rs3749034 (aka, G5276A), rs2058725 (aka, T21922C), rs3791851 (aka, T30473C)
- GAD2, rs1805398 (aka, G264744809T) *Glutamate decarboxylase 2*
- Catalyzes the production of GABA, our calming neurotransmitter.
- GAD67 antibodies are also implicated in pancreas function, via autoimmune and autoreactive T-cell target in insulin-dependent diabetes.

http://www.ncbi.nlm.nih.gov/pubmed/1339255

- **Cyrex Labs** Array 5 can detect antibodies to the GAD1 enzyme as well as many more body tissues and enzymes. Arrays 3, 4 and 10 can detect food antigens.

+ This gene may also play a role in Stiff Man Syndrome.

http://ghr.nlm.nih.gov/gene/GAD1

+ Cerebral palsy, spastic quadriplegic 1 (CPSQ1): A non-progressive disorder of movement and/or posture resulting from defects in the developing central nervous system. Affected individuals manifest symmetrical, non-progressive spasticity and no adverse perinatal history or obvious underlying alternative diagnosis. Developmental delay, mental retardation and sometimes epilepsy can be part of the clinical picture. The disease is caused by mutations affecting the gene.

http://ghr.nlm.nih.gov/condition/pyridoxine-dependent-epilepsy

+ Deficiency of GAD1 enzyme has been shown to lead to pyridoxine dependency (vitamin B-6) seizures (a pyridoxine-dependent epilepsy that requires high levels of vitamin B-6 to mitigate, where standard anticonvulsant drugs are ineffective). Mutations in the ALDH7A1 gene may also cause pyridoxine-dependent epilepsy. ALDH7A1 is also another cause of pyridoxine-dependent epilepsy and is involved in the breakdown of lysine in the brain.

- Reduce foods that deplete vitamin B-6, such as high oxalate foods.
- Check for CBS C699T SNPs where upregulation depletes vitamin B-6. High ammonia, high sulfates, issues with urea cycle, and low arginine are easy-to-measure markers to detect CBS C699T upregulation.
    - High urine taurine is another marker, but excreted levels may also be high due to COMT, BHMT, PEMT and SULT2A1 SNPs where bile recycling is poor and taurine goes unused and is spilled into urine.
    - "Estrogen dominance" can contribute to poor bile recycling via CYP1B1 and COMT SNPs as well. **Precision Analytical** Comprehensive DUTCH test, and **Genova Diagnostics** Complete Hormones, can measure estrogen and their breakdown metabolites.

mnewman@precisionhormones.com

- **Genova Diagnostics** NutrEval can measure CBS markers/analytes.

- Neurotransmitters may be also unbalanced due to lack of vitamin B-6.

http://ghr.nlm.nih.gov/condition/pyridoxine-dependent-epilepsy

+ Alternative splicing of this gene results in two products; the predominant 67-kD form and a less-frequent 25-kD form.

+ GABA SNPs -> impaired GABA production and higher glutamate (brain stimulating). Reduce any foods that increase/stimulate glutamate/receptor reponse. www.unblindmymind.org

- The only true calming neurotransmitter is GABA. Serotonin, however, cuts both ways. Often, supporting GABA and/or serotonin assists in calming the sympathetic nervous system in favor or parasympathetic nervous system, and melatonin production/sleep.
    - Check thyroid markers, including autoimmune thyroid markers.

Our Two Cents: Wrt children on the spectrum, neurotransmitter testing may show higher GABA production in an attempt to "keep up with" high glutamate, NMDA receptor stimulation and high dopamine. The neurotransmitter biomarkers trend towards a sympathetic nervous system (flight/fight) and not parasympathetic (rest/digest). In addition to reducing inflammatory gut foods (permanent GFDF diet), as a first step, 4-amino-3-phenylbutyric acid GABA boosting supplements may be helpful. Supporting mitochondrial health, GI/immune health, and maintaining steady insulin levels are helpful as well.

http://www.ncbi.nlm.nih.gov/pmc/articles/PMC3729335/

- Reducing inflammatory/GMO foods includes removing grains, legumes, dairy, soy, yeast, and eggs. **Cyrex** array 3, 4 and 5 testing may be helpful. A few months may be required to see changes in children's behaviors, but often less time if strict adherence.
- Inflammatory foods and inflammation in general, can stimulate an enzyme, called Indoleamine-pyrrole 2,3-dioxygenase (IDO); that in turn stimulates NMDA receptors via quinolinic acid production due to inflammatory cytokines ("anti-calming"). They affect the gut, immune, neurotransmitter axis. Although not directly affecting GABA, it synergistically, via tryptophan depletion, contributes to upregulation of sympathetic nervous system.
- For adults, in addition to dietary changes that remove inflammatory/GMO grains and animals that eat them, consider using 4-amino-3-phenylbutyric acid GABA boosting supplements as a temporary step, and **Hearth Math** techniques/meditation ifor balancing sympathetic/parasympathetic nervous system.

http://www.heartmath.com

+ Catalytic activity:

- L-glutamate = 4-aminobutanoate + CO_2

+ Cofactor:

- Pyridoxal 5'-phosphate (active form of vitamin B6)

+ Molecular function (GAD1 & GAD2):
- Glutamate binding
- Pyridoxal phosphate binding
- Glutamate decarboxylase activity

+ Biological process (GAD1 & GAD2):
- Gamma-aminobutyric acid biosynthesis
- Glutamate decarboxylation to succinate
- Neurotransmitter secretion
- Response to drugs
- Glutamate catabolic process
- Neurotransmitter biosynthesis process
- Protein P5P linkage
- Synaptic transmission

+ Cellular component:
- Clathrin-sculpted gamma-aminobutyric acid transmport vesicle membrane
- Intracellular
- Plasma membrane
- Vesicle membrane

http://www.uniprot.org/uniprot/Q99259

GAMT

+ **Overview for GAMT** *Guanidinoacetate N-methyltransferase*
- GAMT, rs17851582 (aka, C9110T), rs55776826 (aka, G7497A)
- The GAMT gene requires SAMe, and provides instructions for making the enzyme guanidinoacetate methyltransferase, which is active (expressed) mainly in the liver. This enzyme participates in the two-step production (synthesis) of the compound creatine from the protein building blocks (amino acids) glycine, arginine, and methionine. Specifically, guanidinoacetate methyltransferase controls the second step of this process. In this step, creatine is produced from another compound called guanidinoacetate.

http://ghr.nlm.nih.gov/gene/GAMT

- **Our Two Cents:** Creatine is needed to store and use energy properly. It is involved in providing energy for muscle bulding and contraction and is also important in nervous system functioning. Supplementation with creatine may be recommended, especially if MAT (to free up SAMe) and/or COMT SNPs as well.

+ In addition to its role in creatine synthesis, the guanidinoacetate methyltransferase enzyme is thought to help activate a process called, "fatty acid oxidation". This process encourages fatty acid mobilization as an energy source for cells during times of stress when their easy fuel, glucose, is scarce. Creatine powder in a smoothie may be helpful.

+ At least 15 mutations in the GAMT gene cause severe guanidinoacetate methyltransferase deficiency, a disorder that involves intellectual disability and seizures. Most affected individuals of Portuguese ancestry have a particular mutation in which the amino acid tryptophan is replaced by the amino acid serine at position 20 in the enzyme (written as Trp20Ser or W20S).

+ GAMT gene mutations impair the ability of the guanidinoacetate methyltransferase enzyme to participate in creatine synthesis, resulting in a shortage of creatine. The effects of guanidinoacetate methyltransferase deficiency are most severe in organs and tissues that require large amounts of energy, especially the brain and muscles.

+ Guanidinoacetate methyltransferase deficiency is an inherited disorder that primarily affects the brain and muscles. People with this disorder have intellectual disability that is usually severe, with speech development limited to a few words. Almost all individuals with guanidinoacetate methyltransferase deficiency experience recurrent seizures (epilepsy). Most develop autistic behaviors that affect communication and social interaction; some affected individuals also exhibit self-injurious behaviors such as head banging. Certain involuntary movements (extrapyramidal dysfunction) such as tremors or facial tics occur in about half of affected individuals.

People with guanidinoacetate methyltransferase deficiency may have weak muscle tone and delayed development of motor skills such as sitting or walking. In severe cases they may lose previously acquired skills such as the ability to support their head or to sit unsupported. There have only been eighty cases reported worldwide.

http://ghr.nlm.nih.gov/condition/guanidinoacetate-methyltransferase-deficiency

+ Some defects in this gene have been implicated in neurologic syndromes and muscular hypotonia, probably due to creatine deficiency and accumulation of guanidinoacetate in the brain of affected individuals.

http://www.genecards.org/cgi-bin/carddisp.pl?gene=GAMT

+ Catalytic activity:

    S-adenosyl-L-methionine + guanidinoacetate = S-adenosyl-L-homocysteine + creatine

- ❖ **NOTE**: This protein is involved in step two of the subpathway that synthesizes creatine from L-arginine and glycine.

   Proteins known to be involved in the 2 steps of the subpathway are:
   - Glycine amidinotransferase, mitochondrial (GATM)
   - Guanidinoacetate N-methyltransferase (GAMT)

+ Molecular function:
- Guanidinoacetate N-methyltransferase activity
- Methyltransferase activity

+ Biological process:
- Cellular nitrogen compound metabolic process
- Creatine biosynthetic process
- Creatine metabolic process
- Embryonic liver development
- Muscle contraction
- Organ morphogenesis
- Regulation of multicellular organism growth
- SAH metabolic process
- SAM metabolic process
- Small molecule metabolic process
- Spermatogenesis

+ Cellular component
- Cytosol
- Extracellular exosome

http://www.uniprot.org/uniprot/Q14353

GCSH

+ **Overview for GCSH** Glycine Cleavage System Protein H (Aminomethyl Carrier) (aka, Glycine Cleavage System H Protein, Mitochondrial, Lipoic Acid-Containing Protein)
- *GCSH*, rs8177876 (aka, C10706T)
- Degradation of glycine is brought about by the glycine cleavage system, which is composed of four mitochondrial protein components: P protein (a pyridoxal phosphate-dependent glycine decarboxylase), H protein (a lipoic acid-containing protein), T protein (a tetrahydrofolate-requiring enzyme), and L protein (a lipoamide dehydrogenase). The H protein shuttles the methylamine group of glycine from the P protein to the T protein.
    - Glycine is an inhibitory neurotransmitter in the CNS in addition to its role in a variety of essential cellular processes, e.g., one-carbon metabolism.
    - Other glycine degradation enzymes: AMT, DLD, and GLDC.

+ The protein encoded by this gene is the H protein, which transfers the methylamine group of glycine from the P protein to the T protein.

+ Defects in this gene are a cause of nonketotic hyperglycinemia (NKH), atypical glycine encephalopathy, and neonatal glycine encephalopathy.

http://www.genecards.org/cgi-bin/carddisp.pl?gene=GCSH

http://onlinelibrary.wiley.com/doi/10.1002/humu.20293/abstract;jsessionid=99DF9DDE6D2CDCE52E05AD4802C81A3B.f02t04

+ Glycine and SSRI's: major depressive disorder (MDD) is a common psychiatric disease. Selective serotonin reuptake inhibitors (SSRIs) are an important class of drugs used to treat MDD. However, many patients do not respond adequately to SSRI therapy. Results highlight both a possible role for glycine in SSRI response and the use of pharmacometabolomics to "inform" pharmacogenomics.

http://www.ncbi.nlm.nih.gov/pmc/articles/PMC3034442/

http://europepmc.org/articles/PMC3034442

+ Cofactor:
- (R)-lipoate

+ Molecular function:
- Aminomethyltransferase

+ Biological process:
- Glycine catabolic process
- Glycine decarboxylation via glycine cleavage system
- Methylation

+ Subcellular location:
- Mitochondrian

+ Cellular component:
- Glycine cleavage complex
- Mitochondrian

http://www.uniprot.org/uniprot/P23434

GGH

+ **Overview for GGH** *Gamma-glutamyl hydrolase*
- *GGH*, rs3780127 (aka, C15472T), rs11545078 (aka, C17847T), rs1031552 (aka, C2321T), rs3780126, (aka, C6699T), rs4617146 (aka, G13894A), rs11545077 (aka, G91A).
- Also known as, conjugase, folate conjugase, lysosomal gamma-glutamyl carboxypeptidase, gamma-Glu-X carboxypeptidase, pteroyl-poly-gamma-glutamate hydrolase, carboxypeptidase G, folic acid conjugase, poly (gamma-

glutamic acid) endohydrolase, polyglutamate hydrolase, poly (glutamic acid) hydrolase II, and pteroylpoly-gamma-glutamyl hydrolase.

http://en.wikipedia.org/wiki/Gamma-glutamyl_hydrolase

- GGH encodes an enzyme that catalyzes the hydrolysis of a gamma-glutamyl bond (catalyzes the hydrolysis of folylpoly-gamma-glutamates and antifolylpoly-gamma-glutamates by the removal of gamma-linked polyglutamates and glutamate.)

http://www.ncbi.nlm.nih.gov/gene/8836

- Its cellular location is lysosomal with large amounts of the enzyme constitutively secreted. The highest levels of glutamyl hydrolase mRNA in humans is found in the liver and kidney.

http://www.ncbi.nlm.nih.gov/pubmed/10598552

- Gamma-glutamyl hydrolase is a key enzyme in the metabolism of folic acid and in the pharmacology of many antifolate drugs. Gamma-glutamyl hydrolase catalyzes removal of the poly-gamma-glutamate chains of intracellular folic acid and antifolates.

http://www.ncbi.nlm.nih.gov/pubmed/16945597

+ Diseases associated with polymorphisms in GGH are:
- Tropical sprue
- Pulmonary neuroendocrine tumor

+ GGH is most active at acidic PH.

http://en.wikipedia.org/wiki/Gamma-glutamyl_hydrolase

+ Human GGH showed higher activity toward the pentaglutamate derivative of methotrexate and had little activity against the diglutamate derivative.

http://www.omim.org/entry/601509

+ Expressions of GGH are high in the tissue of the liver, kidney, and placenta. Expressions are low in the spleen, small intestine, and peripheral blood leukocytes.

http://atlasgeneticsoncology.org/Genes/GGHID44358ch8q12.html

+ GGH is significantly higher in people with acromegaly and anorexia nervosa. It plays a role in human development. GH is secreted by vigorous physical activity and immobilization reduces its secretion.

https://www.wikigenes.org/e/gene/e/8836.html

+ Catalytic activity:
- Hydrolysis of a gamma-glutamyl bond

+ Molecular function:
- Exopeptidase activity

- Gamma-glutamyl-peptidase activity
- Omega peptidase activity

+ Biological process:
- Glutamine metabolic process
- Proteolysis
- Response to drug
- Response to ethanol
- Response to insulin
- Response to zince ion

+ Subcellular location:
- Secreted; extracellular space
- Lysosome
- Melanosome

+ Cellular component:
- Cytosol
- Extracellular exosome
- Extracellular space
- Lysosome
- Melanosome
- Nucleus

http://www.uniprot.org/uniprot/Q92820

MAT1A

+ **Overview for MAT1** *Methionine adenosyltransferase I, alpha*
- *MAT1*, rs10788546 (aka, A19581G), rs2993763 (aka, C1131T), rs4934028 (aka, C15656T), rs72558181 (aka, G19502A), rs1985908 (aka, T*1297C),
- The *MAT1A* gene provides instructions for producing the enzyme, methionine adenosyltransferase. The enzyme is produced from the *MAT1A* gene in two forms, designated alpha and beta **(see below)**. The alpha form, called a homotetramer, is made up of four identical protein subunits.
- Both the alpha and beta forms of methionine adenosyltransferase help break down a protein building block (amino acid) called, methionine.
- The enzyme starts the reaction that converts methionine to S-adenosylmethionine, also called AdoMet or SAMe. AdoMet is involved in transferring methyl groups, consisting of a carbon atom and three hydrogen atoms, to other compounds, a process called transmethylation.

- Recall that all enzymes that end with "MT" require SAMe donation of a methyl group in order to carry out their enzymatic function.
- These "MT" enzymes include; determining whether the instructions in a particular segment of DNA are carried out, regulating reactions involving proteins and lipids, and controlling the processing of chemicals that relay signals in the nervous system (neurotransmitters).

+ Mutations in the MAT1A gene have been found to reduce the activity of the methionine adenosyltransferase enzyme. Most of these mutations substitute one amino acid for another amino acid in the enzyme, causing it to process methionine less efficiently → methionine adenosyltransferase deficiency.

http://www.ncbi.nlm.nih.gov/gene/4143

+ Other mutations introduce a premature stop signal in the instructions for making the methionine adenosyltransferase enzyme. As a result, a shortened, nonfunctional enzyme is produced. A reduction in methionine adenosyltransferase function results in a buildup of methionine in the body and less efficient AdoMet production, and in severe cases can cause neurological problems.

http://ghr.nlm.nih.gov/gene/MAT1A
http://onlinelibrary.wiley.com/doi/10.1093/emboj/16.7.1638/full
http://www.sciencedirect.com/science/article/pii/0092867481904992

+ Methionine adenosyltransferase deficiency (MATD) is related to hypermethioninemia. Some neurologic symptoms may be present in rare cases with severe loss of methionine adenosyltransferase activity.

http://www.uniprot.org/uniprot/Q00266

+ Catalytic activity:
- ATP + L-methionine + H_2O = phosphate + diphosphate + S-adenosyl-L-methionine.
❖ **NOTE**: This protein is involved in step one of the subpathway that synthesizes S-adenosyl-L-methionine from L-methionine.

+ Proteins known to be involved in this subpathway are:
- MAT2B
- MAT1A
- MAT2A

+ Cofactor:
- Magnesium
- Potassium

+ Molecular function:
- ATP binding

- Methionine adenosyltransferase activity
- Metal ion binding

+ Biological process:
    - Cellular amino acid metabolic process
    - Methylation
    - S-adenosylmethionine biosynthetic process
    - Sulfur amino acid metabolic process
    - Cellular nitrogen compound metabolic process
    - One-carbo metabolic process
    - Small molecule metabolic process
    - Xenobiotic metabolic process

+ Cellular component:
    - Cytosol

http://www.uniprot.org/uniprot/Q00266

+ Associated disease:
    - Liver cancer
    - Cirrhosis
    - Brain demyelination
    - Alcoholic liver disease
    - Senile dementia

https://www.wikigenes.org/e/gene/e/4143.html

MAT2A

+ **Overview for MAT2A** Methionine Adenosyltransferase II, Alpha (aka, Methionine Adenosyltransferase 2, AdoMet Synthase 2)
    - MAT2A, rs2028900 (aka, C6635T)
    - MAT2A catalyzes the formation of S-adenosylmethionine (aka, SAM or SAMe) from methionine and ATP.

+ Diseases associated with MAT2A are liver cancer and glycine n-methyltransferase deficiency

+ MAT2A is expressed in non-hepatic tissues, whereas MAT1A is expressed in the liver. A third gene, MAT2B, encodes a MAT2A regulatory protein.

http://www.genecards.org/cgi-bin/carddisp.pl?gene=MAT2B

+ For MAT2A, resequencing identified seventy-four polymorphisms, including two nonsynonymous (ns) SNPs. Functional genomic studies of wild type and the two MAT2A variant allozymes (Val11 and Val205), showed that the Val11 allozyme had approximately forty percent decreases in levels of enzyme activity and immunoreactive protein after COS-1 cell transfection.

http://www.ncbi.nlm.nih.gov/pubmed/21813468

http://www.ncbi.nlm.nih.gov/pmc/articles/PMC3376917/

+ Catalytic activity:
- ATP + L-methionine + H_2O = phosphate + diphosphate + S-adenosyl-L-methionine.

+ Cofactor:
- Magnesium
- Potassium
- Cobalt

+ The pathways for s-adenosylmethionine synthase isoform type-s:
- Amino-acid biosynthesis
- S-adenosyl-L-methionine biosynthesis
- S-adenosyl-L-methionine from L-methionine

+ Molecular function:
- ATP binding
- Metal ion binding
- Methionine adensyltransferase activity

+ Biological process:
- Methylation
- One-carbon metabolic process
- S-adenosylmethionine biosynthetic process
- Small molecule metabolic process
- Xenobiotic metabolic process

+ Cellular component:
- Cytosol
- Methionine adenosyltransferase

http://www.uniprot.org/uniprot/P31153

MAT2B

+ **Overview for MAT2B** *Methionine Adenosyltransferase II, Beta* (aka, Methionine adenosyltransferase II beta)

- *MAT2B*, rs4869089 (aka, A7755681G), rs6882306 (aka, C7745233T)
- The non-catalytic regulatory subunit of S-adenosylmethionine synthetase 2 (MAT2A) is an enzyme that catalyzes the formation of S-adenosylmethionine from methionine and ATP. It regulates the activity of S-adenosylmethionine

synthetase 2 by changing its kinetic properties, rendering the enzyme more susceptible to S-adenosylmethionine inhibition.

http://www.ncbi.nlm.nih.gov/gene/27430

+ MAT2A is expressed in non-hepatic tissues, whereas MAT1A is expressed in the liver. A third gene, MAT2B, encodes a MAT2A regulatory protein.

http://www.genecards.org/cgi-bin/carddisp.pl?gene=MAT2B

+ MAT2B encodes for two variant proteins (V1 and V2) that promote cell growth. MAT2B and GIT1 (G protein-coupled receptor kinase interacting ArfGAP 1) form a scaffold, which recruits and activates MEK (mitogen-activated protein kinase 1) and ERK (extracellular signal-regulated kinase) to promote growth and tumorigenesis. This novel MAT2B/GIT1 complex may provide a potential therapeutic gateway in human liver and colon cancer.

http://www.ncbi.nlm.nih.gov/pubmed/23325601

+ Methionine adenosyltransferase 2 subunit betas pathway:
    - Amino-acid biosynthesis
    - S-adenosyl-L-methionine biosynthesis
    - S-adenosyl-L-methionine from L-methionine

+ Molecular function:
    - Enzyme binding
    - Methionine adensyltransferase activity

+ Biological process:
    - Methylation
    - One-carbon metabolic process
    - Regulation of catalytic activity
    - S-adenosylmethionine biosynthetic process
    - Small molecule metabolic process
    - Xenobiotic metabolic process

+ Cellular component:
    - Cytosol
    - Extracellular exosome
    - Intracellular
    - Methionine adenosyltransferase complex
    - Mitochondria
    - Nucleus

http://www.uniprot.org/uniprot/Q9NZL9

MAOA

- **Overview for MAOA** Monomine oxidase A (aka, Amine oxidase [flavin-containing] A, MAOA)
    - MAOA, rs5906883 (aka, A16535C), rs5906957 (aka, A36902G), rs909525 (aka, C42794T), rs5953210 (aka, C42794T), rs5953210 (aka, G3638A), rs6323 (aka, R297R/G492T/T941G), rs2072743 (aka, T89113C) encodes for the enzyme, monomine oxidase A.
    - Monoamine oxidase A is an isozyme of monoamine oxidase. It preferentially deaminates (assists in the breakdown) of norepinephrine (noradrenaline), epinephrine (adrenaline), serotonin, and dopamine (which is equally deaminated by MAOA and MAOB).
    - Catalyzes the oxidative deamination of biogenic and xenobiotic amines and functions in the metabolism of neuroactive and vasoactive amines in the central nervous system and peripheral tissues. MAOA preferentially oxidizes biogenic amines such as 5-hydroxytryptamine (5-HT), norepinephrine and epinephrine.
    - The protein localizes to the outer mitochondrial membrane. Its encoding gene is adjacent to MAOB on the opposite strand of the X chromosome.
    - Monoamine oxidase A is inhibited by clorgyline and befloxatone. Inhibition of both MAOA and MAOB using a MAO inhibitor is used in the treatment of clinical depression, ED, and anxiety.
- **Our Two Cents:** In the case of inhibiting MAOA activity, clorgyline and befloxatone are used to treat depression, ED, and anxiety. This has an effect of slowing the breakdown of nor-epi, epi, serotonin, and dopamine. MAOB and COMT are also part of the picture. In the case of COMT, no SNPs (e.g., green on variant report) indicate maximum/fastest breakdown of epinepherine and dopamine. On the other hand, homozygous SNPs (e.g., red in the variant report) in COMT indicate the slowest breakdown of epinepherine and dopamine. Vitamin D is also in play wrt dopamine breakdown, so consider VDR SNP status.

+ A version of the monoamine oxidase-A gene has been popularly referred to as the *warrior gene*.
https://www.ncbi.nlm.nih.gov/pubmed/17339897
+ Studies have linked methylation of the MAOA gene with nicotine and alcohol dependence in women.
https://www.ncbi.nlm.nih.gov/pubmed/18454435
+ MAOA is involved in the metabolism of tyramine; inhibition, in particular irreversible inhibition of MAOA can result in a dangerous pressor effect when foods high in tyramine are

consumed, such as, cheeses. MAOA is involved in the metabolism of serotonin, noradrenaline, and dopamine, whereas MAOB metabolizes the dopamine neurotransmitter.

+ Monoamine oxidase A inhibitors have been typically used in the treatment of depression.

https://www.ncbi.nlm.nih.gov/pubmed/8313400

+ Nonspecific (i.e. MAOA/B combined) inhibitors can pose problems when taken concomitantly with tyramine-containing foods such as cheese, because the drug's inhibition of MAOA causes a dangerous elevation of serum tyramine levels, which can lead to hypertensive symptoms.

+ Catalytic Activity:

- RCH2NHR' + H2O + O2 = RCHO + R'NH2 + H2O2

+ Cofactor:
- FAD

+ Molecular function:
- Flavin adenine dinucleotide binding
- Primary amine oxidase activity
- Serotonin binding

+ Biological process:
- Cellular biogenic amine metabolic process
- Dopamine catabolic process
- Neurotransmitter biosynthetic process
- Neurotransmitter catabolic process
- Neurotransmitter secretion
- Phenylethylamine metabolic process
- Serotonin metabolic process
- Small molecule metabolic process
- Synaptic transmitssion
- Xenobiotic metabolic process

+ Subcellular location:
- Mitochondrion outer membrane
- Single pass type IV membrane protein
- Cytoplasmic side

http://www.uniprot.org/uniprot/P21397

+ Diseases associated with MAOA:

Brunner syndrom – This is a form of X-linked non-dysmorphic mild mental retardation. Male patients are affected by borderline mental retardation and exhibit abnormal behavior, including disturbed regulation of impulsive aggression. Obligate female carriers have normal intelligence and behavior.

http://www.ncbi.nlm.nih.gov/pubmed/8211186

MAOB

+ <u>**Overview for MAOB**</u> *Monomine oxidase B* (aka, Amine oxidase [flavin-containing] B, MAOB)
- MAOB, **rs1799836 (aka, A118723G)**, rs10521432 (aka, C112982T), rs6651806 (aka, T57758G), encodes for the enzyme monomine oxidase B.
- Monoamine oxidase B is an isozyme of monoamine oxidase. It catalyzes the oxidative deamination of biogenic and xenobiotic amines and has important functions in the metabolism of neuroactive and vasoactive amines in the central nervous system and peripheral tissues. MAOB preferentially degrades benzylamine and phenylethylamin.
- In humans, MAOA preferentially oxidizes serotonin and noradrenaline, whereas MAOB oxidizes/breaks down dopamine.
- **Our Two Cents**: MAOB with COMT, GAD and MAOA SNPs confer susceptibility to dopamine/GABA swings. Like insulin receptors, DRD receptors can become insensitive and cravings can ensue. Alcoholism and addictive behaviors can result.
- Monoamine oxidase B inhibitors are typically used in the treatment of Parkinson's disease. Look at COMT SNPs and Neurotransmitter drawing **(FIG 9)**.

https://www.ncbi.nlm.nih.gov/pubmed/22110357

- Inhibition of MAOB in rats has been shown to prevent many age-related biological changes such as, optic nerve degeneration, and extend average lifespan by up to thirty-nine percent.

https://www.ncbi.nlm.nih.gov/pubmed/23082958

+ Homovanillic acid (HVA), 5-hydroxyindoleacetic acid (5-HIAA), and 3-methoxy-4-hydroxyphenylglycol (MHPG), are the major degradation products of the monoamines dopamine, serotonin, and noradrenaline, respectively. Schizophrenia has been associated with monoamine metabolite concentrations, mainly HVA. HVA concentrations have been reported to be significantly lower in drug-free schizophrenic patients compared to controls. Rs1799836 has been associated with schizophrenia in women.

http://www.behavioralandbrainfunctions.com/content/10/1/26#B9

+ Alzheimer's disease and Parkinson's disease are both associated with elevated levels of MAOB in the brain. The normal activity of MAOB creates reactive oxygen species, which directly damage cells.

https://www.ncbi.nlm.nih.gov/pubmed/17447416

+ MAOB levels have been found to increase with age, suggesting a role in age-related cognitive decline and the increased likelihood of developing neurological diseases later in life.
https://www.ncbi.nlm.nih.gov/pubmed/15247489

+ Catalytic activity:
  - RCH2NHR' + H2O + O2 = RCHO + R'NH2 + H2O2

+ Cofactor:
  - FAD

+ Molecular function:
  - Electron carrier activity
  - Flavin adenine dinucleotide binding
  - Primary amine oxidase activity

+ Biological process:
  - Dopamine catabolic process
  - Hydrogen peroxide biosynthetic process
  - Negative regulation of serotonin secretion
  - Positive regulation of dopamine metabolic process
  - Response to aluminum ion
  - Response to corticosterone
  - Response to drug
  - Response to ethanol
  - Response to lipopolysaccharides
  - Response to selenium ion
  - Small molecule metabolic process
  - Substantia nigra development
  - Xenobiotic metabolic process

+ Subcellular location:
  - Mitochondrion outer membrane
  - Single pass type IV membrane protein
  - Cytoplasmic side

+ Cellular component:
  - Extracellular exosome
  - Integral component of membrane
  - Mitochondrial envelope
  - Mitochindrial inner membrane
  - Mitochindrial outer membrane

- Mitochondrian

http://www.uniprot.org/uniprot/P27338

MMAB

+ **Overview for MMAB** *Cob(I)yrinic acid a,c-diamide adenosyltransferase, mitochondrial*
  (aka, methylmalonic aciduria type B protein)
  - *MMAB*, rs11836136 (aka, A13G), rs7134594 (aka, G16110A), rs11067231 (aka, MMAB/MVK A818G).
  - This gene encodes a protein that catalyzes the final step in the conversion of vitamin B-12 into adenosylcobalamin (AdoCbl), a vitamin B-12-containing coenzyme for methylmalonyl-CoA mutase. Mutations in the gene are the cause of vitamin B-12-dependent methylmalonic aciduria linked to the cblB complementation group.

http://www.genecards.org/cgi-bin/carddisp.pl?gene=MMAB

  - Methylmalonic aciduria is a disorder of methylmalonate and cobalamin metabolism due to defective synthesis of adenosylcobalamin.

http://www.uniprot.org/uniprot/Q96EY8

+ Methylmalonic acidemia is a condition characterized by feeding difficulties in babies, developmental delay, and long-term health problems. Some of these genetic changes delete or duplicate a small amount of genetic material in the MMAB gene. Other mutations change a single protein building block (amino acid) used to make the MMAB enzyme. Researchers believe that many of these mutations lead to the production of a nonfunctional version of the enzyme. This causes adenoslyl B12 to be made improperly. A lack of adenosyl cobalimin impairs the function of methylmalonyl CoA mutase, which results in the incomplete breakdown of certain proteins and lipids. This defect allows toxic compounds to build up in the body's organs and tissues, causing the signs and symptoms of methylmalonic acidemia.

http://ghr.nlm.nih.gov/gene/MMAB

+ The *KCTD10* (V206VT→C and i5642G→C) and *MMAB*_3U3527G→C variants may contribute to the variation in HDL-cholesterol concentrations (e.g., low HDL), particularly in subjects with high carbohydrate intakes.

http://www.ncbi.nlm.nih.gov/pmc/articles/PMC2728650/
http://www.ncbi.nlm.nih.gov/pmc/articles/PMC2860891/

+ Catalytic activity:
  - ATP + cob(I)yrinic acid a, c-diamide = triphosphate + adenosylcob(III)yrinic acid a, c-diamide.
  - ATP + cobinamide = triphosphate + adenosylcobinamide

+ Pathway: adenosylcobalamin biosynthesis:
- Cofactor biosynthesis;
- Adenosylcobalamin biosynthesis
- Adenosylcobalamin from cob(II)yrinate a,c-diamide

+ Molecular function:
- ATP binding
- Cob(I)yrinic acid a,c-diamide adenosyltransferase activity

+ Biological process:

Cobalamin biosynthetic process
- Cobalamin metabolic process
- Small molecule metabolic process
- Vitamin metabolic process
- Water-soluble vitamin metabolic process

+ Subcellular location:
- Mitochondrion

+ Cellular component:
- Mitochondrial matrix

http://www.uniprot.org/uniprot/Q96EY8

MTHFD1

+ **Overview for MTHFD1** *Methylenetetrahydrofolate Dehydrogenase (NADP+ Dependent) 1, Methenyltetrahydrofolate* (aka, C-1-tetrahydrofolate synthase, cytoplasmic) *MTHFD1*, rs1076991 (aka, C105T), rs2236225 (aka, G1958A).

- This gene encodes a protein that possesses three distinct enzymatic activities/steps; 5,10-methylenetetrahydrofolate dehydrogenase, 5,10-methenyltetrahydrofolate cyclohydrolase, and 10-formyltetrahydrofolate synthetase.
- Each of these steps catalyzes one of three sequential reactions in the interconversion of 1-carbon derivatives of tetrahydrofolate, which are substrates for methionine, thymidylate, and de novo purine syntheses. **(See FIG. 4)**
- The tri-functional enzymatic activities are conferred by two major domains. DHFR preceeds MTHFD1. (One or two steps, depending on whether foic acid or folate input.) MTHFR follows.

http://www.genecards.org/cgi-bin/carddisp.pl?gene=MTHFD1

+ Diseases associated with MTHFD1 include:

- Upper thoracic spina bifida cystica and cervicothoracic spina bifida cystica.

- Colorectal cancer; genetic alterations are often associated with progression from premalignant lesion (adenoma) to invasive adenocarcinoma. Risk factors for cancer of the colon and rectum include colon polyps, long-standing ulcerative colitis, and genetic family history.

http://ghr.nlm.nih.gov/gene/MTHFD1

+ The most common diseases related to MTHFD1 are:

- NTDs (neural tube defects)
- Open spina bifida (myelomeningocele) and anencephaly

http://www.uniprot.org/uniprot/P11586

+ Women who are MTHFD1 1958AA (i.e., MTHFD1 1958G→A) homozygous (rs2236225) have a 1.64-fold increased risk of having an unexplained second trimester loss compared to women who are MTHFD1 1958AG or 1958GG.

http://www.ncbi.nlm.nih.gov/pubmed/16123074

+ Many people who have dysfunctional MTHFD1 SNPs and a poor diet of folate rich foods can get a buildup of carcenogenic lesions on the colon.

http://onlinelibrary.wiley.com/doi/10.1002/ijc.20148/full

+ The role of folate and MTHFD1 functioning is important in preventing congenital heart defects.

http://onlinelibrary.wiley.com/doi/10.1002/humu.20830/abstract

+ Dysfunctional MTHFD1 is related to DNA damage in Alzheimer's and Parkinson's disease.

http://www.zla.ane.pl/pdf/6713.pdf

+ MTHFD1, an enzyme that generates methylenetetrahydrofolate from formate, ATP and NADPH, functions in the nucleus to support de novo thymidylate biosynthesis.

Nuclear localization of MTHFD1 protects DNA by limiting uracil misincorporation into DNA.

http://www.jbc.org/content/early/2014/09/11/jbc.M114.599589

+ Catalytic activity:

- 5,10-methylenetetrahydrofolate + NADP+ = 5,10-methenyltetrahydrofolate + NADPH.
- 5,10-methenyltetrahydrofolate + H_2O = 10-formyltetrahydrofolate.
- ATP + formate + tetrahydrofolate = ADP + phosphate + 10-formyltetrahydrofolate

+ Molecular function:

- ATP binding
- Formate-tetarhydrofolate ligase activity

- Methylenetetrahydrofolate dehydrogenase (NAD) activity
- Methylenetetrahydrofolate dehydrogenase (NADP+) activity
- Methylenetetrahydrofolate dehydrogenase [NAD(P)+] activity

+ Biological process:

- 10-formyltetrahydrofolate biosynthetic process
- Embryonic neurocranium morphogenesis
- Embryonic viscerocranium morphogenesis
- Folic acid metabolic process
- Heart development
- Methionine biosynthetic process
- Methionine metabolic process
- Neural tube closure
- One-carbon metabolic process
- Purine nucleotide biosynthetic process
- Serine family amino acid biosynthetic process
- Serine family amino acid metabolic process
- Small molecule metabolic process
- Somite development
- Tetrahydrofolate interconversion
- Vitamin metabolic process
- Water-soluble vitamin metabolic process

+ Subcellular location:

- Cytoplasm

+ Cellular component:

- Cytosol
- Extracellular exosome
- Membrane
- Mitochondria

http://www.uniprot.org/uniprot/P11586

MTHFD1L

+ **Overview for MTHFD1L** *Methylenetetrahydrofolate Dehydrogenase (NADP+ Dependent) 1-Like* (aka, Monofunctional C1-tetrahydrofolate synthase, mitochondrial)

- *MTHFD1L*, rs803422 (aka, A33780G), rs11754661 (aka, G25264A), rs6922269 (aka, G71171A), rs17349743 (aka, T31397C).

- MTHFD1L encodes the enzyme, monofunctional C1-tetrahydrofolate synthase, mitochondrial, also known as, formyltetrahydrofolate synthetase, formyltetrahydrofolate synthetase domain containing 1, monofunctional C1-tetrahydrofolate synthase, mitochondrial, 10-Formyl-THF synthetase, mitochondrial C1-tetrahydrofolate synthase, and formyltetrahydrofolate synthetase.
- MTHFD1L is an enzyme involved in THF synthesis in mitochondria.

http://www.ncbi.nlm.nih.gov/gene?Db=gene&Cmd=ShowDetailView&TermToSearch=25902

- In contrast to MTHFD1 that has trifunctional enzymatic activities, MTHFD1L only has formyltetrahydrofolate synthetase activity.

https://www.ncbi.nlm.nih.gov/pubmed/15611115

- The protein encoded by this gene is involved in the synthesis of tetrahydrofolate (THF) in the mitochondrion. THF is important in the de novo synthesis of purines and thymidylate and in the regeneration of methionine from homocysteine. Several transcript variants encoding different isoforms have been found for this gene.

http://www.genecards.org/cgi-bin/carddisp.pl?gene=MTHFD1L

+ MTHFD1L is related to neural tube defects.

https://www.ncbi.nlm.nih.gov/pubmed/19777576

+ MTHFD1L may provide the missing metabolic reaction required to link the mitochondria and the cytoplasm in the mammalian model of one-carbon folate metabolism in embryonic and transformed cells complementing thus, the enzymatic activities of MTHFD2.

http://www.uniprot.org/uniprot/Q6UB35

+ MTHFD1L is detected in most tissues, highest expression found in placenta, thymus, and brain. Low expression is found in liver and skeletal muscle. Up-regulated in colon adenocarcinoma.

http://www.uniprot.org/uniprot/Q6UB35

+ Controversy regarding MTHFD1L rs 6922269 and cardiovascular risk:

MTHFD1L rs6922269 genotype is associated with active vitamin B-12 levels at baseline and may be a marker of prognostic risk in patients with established coronary heart disease.

http://www.ncbi.nlm.nih.gov/pubmed/24618918
http://www.ncbi.nlm.nih.gov/pubmed/25809277
http://www.ncbi.nlm.nih.gov/pubmed/22216278

+ Catalytic activity:
- ATP + formate + tetrahydrofolate = ADP + phosphate + 10-formyltetrahydrofolate

+ Kinetic:
- THF (tetrahydrofolate) monoglutamate

- THF (tetrahydrofolate) triglutamate
- THF (tetrahydrofolate) pentaglutamate

+ The molecular functions for MTHFD1L are:
- ATP binding
- Formate-tetrahydrofolate ligase activity
- Protein homodimerization activity

+ MTHFD1L biological process:
- Embryonic neurocranium morphogenesis
- Embryonic viscerocranium morphogenesis
- Folic acid-containing compound biosynthetic process
- Folic acid-containing compound metabolic process
- Formate metabolic process
- Neural tube closure
- One carbon metabolic process
- Oxidation-reduction process
- Tetrahydrofolate interconversion
- Tetrahydrofolate metabolic process

+ Subcellular location:
- Mitochondrian

+ Cellular component:
- Membrane
- Mitochondrian

http://www.uniprot.org/uniprot/Q6UB35

MTHFD2

+ **Overview for MTHFD2** *Bifunctional methylenetetrahydrofolate dehydrogenase/cyclohydrolase, mitochondria* MTHFD2, rs1667627 (aka, C8503T).

- The MTHFD2 gene encodes a nuclear-encoded mitochondrial bi-functional enzyme with methylenetetrahydrofolate dehydrogenase and methenyltetrahydrofolate cyclohydrolase activities.
- The enzyme functions as a homodimer and is unique in its absolute requirement for **magnesium** and inorganic **phosphate**. Formation of the enzyme-magnesium complex allows binding of NAD.

http://www.ncbi.nlm.nih.gov/gene?Db=gene&Cmd=ShowDetailView&TermToSearch=10797

+ It has been proposed that a key enzyme, MTHFD2, up-regulated in rapidly proliferating tumors but not in normal adult cells, is the mitochondrial enzyme. The development of selective inhibitors of mitochondrial methylene tetrahydrofolate dehydrogenase may have substantial anticancer activity.

http://www.ncbi.nlm.nih.gov/pubmed/26101208

+ Catalytic Activity:

- 5,10-methylenetetrahydrofolate + NAD+ = 5,10-methenyltetrahydrofolate + NADH.
- 5,10-methenyltetrahydrofolate + H2O = 10-formyltetrahydrofolate.

+ Cofactor:

- Magnesium

+ Molecular function:

- Magnesium iron binding
- Methenyltetrahydrofolate cyclohydrolase activity
- Methenyltetrahydrofolate dehydrogenase (NAD+) activity
- Methenyltetrahydrofolate dehydrogenase (NADP+) activity

+ Biological process:

- Folic acid-containing compound biosynthetic process
- Onc carbon metabolic process
- Tetrahydrofolate metabolic process

+ Subcellular location:

- Mitochondrian

+ Cellular component:

- Extracellular space
- Mitochondrian

http://www.uniprot.org/uniprot/P13995

MTHFR

+ **Overview for MTHFR** *Methylenetetrahydrofolate reductase (NAD(P)H)*

MTHFR, rs2066470 (aka, 03 P39P), rs4846049 (aka A*372C), **rs1801131 (aka, A1298C)**, rs17367504 (aka, A1572G), rs3737964 (aka, A4117C), rs13306561 (aka, A4598G), rs13306560 (C-137T), rs17037390 (aka, C10318T), rs4846048 (aka, C24909T), **rs1801133 (aka, C677T)**, rs17037396 (aka, C841T), rs12121543 (aka, G16490T), rs2274976 (G1793A or R594Q), rs1476413, (aka, G18861A), encodes for the enzyme methylenetetrahydrofolate reductase.

- Methylenetetrahydrofolate reductase is the rate-limiting enzyme in the methyl cycle, and is encoded by the MTHFR gene. Methylenetetrahydrofolate reductase catalyzes the conversion of 5,10-methylenetetrahydrofolate to 5-methylenetetrahydrofolate, a co-substrate for homocysteine remethylation to methionine.

- Genetic variations in this gene may influence susceptibility to occlusive vascular disease, neural tube defects, Alzheimer's disease, colon cancer, and acute myeloid leukemia because mutations in this gene are associated with methylene tetrahydrofolate reductase deficiency.

+ MTHFR C677T - A homozygosity reduces the risk for colorectal cancer in individuals with adequate folate status; decreased risk for adult acute leukemia; increased risk for NTDFS; thermolabile; fifty percent reduced activity.

http://www.ncbi.nlm.nih.gov/pubmed/10536004

+ Medications that deplete vitamin B-9 (folate):

- **Birth Control pills**
- **Antacids**
- Sulfasalazine (anti-inflammatory)
- Beclomethasone (anti-inflammatory)
- Budesonide (anti-inflammatory)
- Dexamethasone (anti-inflammatory)
- Fluticasone (anti-inflammatory)
- Hydrocortisone (anti-inflammatory)
- Methylaprednisolone (anti-inflammatory)
- Mometasone Furoate (anti-inflammatory)
- Prednisone (anti-inflammatory)
- Triamcinolone (anti-inflammatory)
- Many **NSAIDs**, including Ibuprofen and Naproxen
- **Aspirin**
- Co-Trimoxazole (antibiotic)
- Trimethoprim (antibiotic)
- Some cephalosporins
- Some macrolides
- Penicilin derivatives, including Amoxicillin and penicillin V potassium
- Many **Quinolones** (antibiotic) including Ciprofloxacin and Levofloxacin

➤ **Our Two Cents:** Folks with SNPs related to **Ehlers-Danlos Syndrome**, which can lead to varicose veins, easy bruising, joint hypermobility (loose joints), skin that stretches easily (skin hyperelasticity or laxity), and repeated connective tissue sports injuries due to weakness of tissues, need to be particularly vigilant when taking fluoroquinolone meds. A suspected UTI does not warrent a fluoroquinolone "machine gun" and the long-term risks they pose, when other options (e.g., cranberry extract, D-mannose, and a good pre- and probiotic), may be able to clear it. It is suspected that fluoroquinolones damage our mitochondrial DNA, which is derived from a particular bacterial DNA, way back in our species genetic evolution. Currently EDS SNPs are not on the variant report, but if you would like the rs number list, please contact me and I will email it to you. They will be listed and discussed in Compedium II. The rs number list can be used to check your raw data and see what risk alleles you may have.

- Some tetracycline derivatives
- Some anticonvulsants including phenobarbital, phenytoin, valproic acid (and derivatives) and carbamazepine
- Metformin
- Cholstyramine (cholesterol)
- Colestipol (cholesterol)
- Many potassium sparing drugs (diuretics) including amiloride, spirolactone
- Many ulcer medications including cimetidine, ranitidine

http://umm.edu/health/medical/altmed/supplement-depletion-links/drugs-that-deplete-vitamin-b9-folic-acid

+ Catalytic activity:
    - 5-methyltetrahydrofolate + NAD(P)+ = 5,10-methylenetetrahydrofolate + NAD(P)H
+ Cofactor:
  - FAD (flavin adenine dinucleotide, derived from vitamin B-2)
+ Enzyme regulation:
  - Allosterically regulated by S-adenosylmethionine
+ Molecular function:
  - Flavin adenine dinucleotide binding
  - Methylenetetrahydrofolate reductase (NAD(P)H) activity
  - Modified amino acid binding
  - NADP binding
  - Protein complex binding
+ Biological process:
  - Blood circulation

- Cellular amino acid metabolic process
- Folic acid metabolic process
- Heterochromatin maintenance
- Homocysteine metabolic process
- Methionine biosynthetic process
- Methionine metabolic process
- Regulation of histone methylation
- Response to drug
- Response to folic acid
- Response to hypoxia
- Response to interleukin-1
- Response to vitamin B-2
- S-adenosylmethionine metabolic process
- Small molecule metabolic process
- Tetrahydrofolate interconversion
- Vitamin metabolic process
- Water-soluble vitamin metabolic process

+ Cellular component:
- Cytosol
- Neuron projection

http://www.uniprot.org/uniprot/P42898

+ Diseases associated with MTHFR:
- Methylenetetrahydrofolate reductase deficiency - Autosomal recessive disorder with a wide range of features including, homocysteinuria and homocysteinemia. Also, developmental delay, severe mental retardation, perinatal death, psychiatric disturbances, and later-onset neurodegenerative disorder.

http://www.ncbi.nlm.nih.gov/pubmed/7726158
http://www.ncbi.nlm.nih.gov/pubmed/8940272
http://www.ncbi.nlm.nih.gov/pubmed/9781030
http://www.ncbi.nlm.nih.gov/pubmed/10679944

- Ischemic stroke – A stroke is an acute neurologic event leading to death of neural tissue of the brain and resulting in loss of motor, sensory, and/or cognitive function. Ischemic strokes, resulting from vascular occlusion, are considered to be a highly complex disease consisting of a group of heterogeneous disorders with multiple genetic and environmental risk factors.

http://www.ncbi.nlm.nih.gov/pubmed/15534175
- Neural tube defect - The most common NTDs are open spina bifida (myelomeningocele) and anencephaly.

http://www.ncbi.nlm.nih.gov/pubmed/7564788

http://www.ncbi.nlm.nih.gov/pubmed/8826441

http://www.ncbi.nlm.nih.gov/pubmed/10323741

The following is a list of commonly asked MTHFR questions, with answers from Sterling:

❖ You've been "diagnosed" with MTHFR, now what is the next step?

Find an on-line support system. Also, finding a doctor or nutritionist that understands MTHFR and methylation is very important. As with most SNPs, because you have an MTHFR SNP does not mean it is expressing. Health history is important.

❖ Many people have MTHFR but who needs supplemental L-Methylfolate?

If folic acid levels are high, this may be an indication that MTHFR function is compromised. People who have this gene compromised will have trouble converting folic into the more active bioavailable form of folate, so in turn, you will see folate low if they are not getting folate rich foods like eggs, leafy greens, beans, and berries. The next step would be testing whole serum folate levels. If you are eating a diet rich in natural folate such as leafy greens, and berries and your folate is still low, then your doctor/nutrionist will want to consider giving you a more active bioavailable form of folate such as 5 MTHF, after addressing surrounding pathways.

❖ Many doctors are giving high doses of folate supplementation. When should they consider lower dosages?

When serum folate levels are not extremely low. Many people have done well on just 400mcg-800mcg of folate every few days, along with a folate (not folic) rich diet. Unmetabolized folic acid is one of the risk factors for colorectal cancer. High levels of L-methylfolate may be contraindicated in the case of COMT V158M and H62H homozygous SNPs as breakdown of catecholamines such as dopamine, norepinephrine, and epinephrine are compromised. Increased anxiety and/or panic attacks can result.

- ❖ If folate levels are low what should I be concerned about?

    You should be concerned about autoimmune diseases because folate plays a role in the immune system. Many people with MTHFR SNPs have been diagnosed with Hashimoto's thyroiditis. In that case, TSH (thyroid stimulating hormone) alone is not adequate. T3, T4, reverse T3/ T4, TG (thyroglobulin), TGAF (thyroblobulin antibody), and TPO (thyroid peroxidase) levels should also be tested.

- ❖ What do I do if my doctor will not run these tests or just wants to give me folic acid?

    Find another doctor. We have a list started at www.MTHFRSupport.com.

- ❖ What do I do if my doctor tells me not to worry about MTHFR?

    Again, if you have a concern, please find a doctor who will listen and run the proper tests before they say that there is nothing to worry about.

- ❖ My doctor says that my homocysteine is fine so I have nothing to worry about. Is this true?

    What is your homocysteine? Many doctors and nutritionists that understand methylation and MTHFR believe that a homocysteine level between six and eight is optimal and others are believe that a homocysteine level between seven and nine is optimal. If a homocysteine level is over nine, or under six, MTHFR or MTR/MTRR enzymatic activity could be compromised.

- ❖ What form of vitamin B-12 should I be taking with my L-methylfolate, and how much?

    Methylcobalamin is the most active form of vitamin B-12 and the one that most doctors who are familiar with methylation recommend. Individuals with COMT V158M and H62H homozygous SNPs, typically do better with hydroxy and/or adenosyl B-12 (check MMAB status). Methylcobalamin can do more oxidative damage to people with COMT compromised.

- I have psoriasis and when I take L-methylfolate my psoriasis gets worse, but I have been diagnosed with MTHFR. What can I do?

    Many who have psoriasis have experienced flare-ups when taking L-Methylfolate. Increase leafy greens and support surrounding pathways.

- If MTHFR is compromised how does this relate to glutathione?

    When folate is low, glutathione may be low as glutathione production is one of the end products of the transulfuration pathway.

- I'm trying to conceive and have been unable to or I have a history of miscarriage and have been diagnosed with MTHFR. Is this important to address?

    Yes it is. Folate deficiency, infertility, and miscarriage is directly linked to MTHFR. Your OB/GYN should know the difference between folic acid and folate. Folic acid is not recommended.

- My doctor wants to put me on oral birth control pills and I have been diagnosed with MTHFR. Should I be concerned?

    Yes. Oral birth control pills reduce folate.

- I have elevated oxalates. How does this affect someone with MTHFR?

    When oxalates are elevated, oxalic acid can impair the folate cycle. Also, vitamin B6 and C may be depleted. If gut yeast markers on testing, address with a proper botanical supplement. **Please see CBS write-up on page 122**.

MTHFS

+ **Overview for MTHFS** *5,10-methenyltetrahydrofolate synthetase (5-formyltetrahydrofolate cyclo-ligase)* MTHFS, rs6495446 (aka, ST20 MTHFS G39646A), rs2733103 (aka, ST20 *MTHFS* G56057A), encodes for the enzyme 5,10-methenyltetrahydrofolate synthetase.

- Methenyltetrahydrofolate synthetase (MTHFS) catalyses the obligatory initial metabolic step in the intracellular conversion of 5-formyltetrahydrofolate to other reduced folates.

http://www.ncbi.nlm.nih.gov/pubmed/8522195

- Helps regulate carbon flow through the folate-dependent one-carbon metabolic network that supplies carbon for the biosynthesis of purines, thymidine, and amino acids.

http://www.uniprot.org/uniprot/P49914

http://www.genecards.org/cgi-bin/carddisp.pl?gene=MTHFS

+ An increased activity of the encoded protein may result in an increased folate turnover-rate and associated folate depletion.

http://www.ncbi.nlm.nih.gov/gene/10588

+ People who have an MTHFS defect can have a problem metabolizing folinic acid. One popular drug called leucovorin contains folinic acid. Also, be mindful of prenatal vitamins.

http://www.jbc.org/content/286/17/15377.full.pdf

http://onlinelibrary.wiley.com/doi/10.1002/stem.140033/pdf

+ MTHFS SNP rs6495446 in the gene was significantly associated with chronic kidney disease.

http://www.ncbi.nlm.nih.gov/pubmed/18522750?dopt=Abstract

+ Catalytic activity:

- ATP + 5-formyltetrahydrofolate = ADP + phosphate + 5,10-methenyltetrahydrofolate

+ Cofactor:
- Magnesium

+ Molecular function:
- 5-formyltetrahydrofolate cyclo-ligase
- ATP binding
- Folic acid binding
- Metal ion binding

+ Biological process:
- Formate metabolic process
- Tetrahydrofolate metabolic process

+ Cellular component:
- Cytoplasm

http://www.uniprot.org/uniprot/P49914

MTR

+ **Overview for MTR** *Methionine synthase* (aka, MS, MeSe, MetH)

MTR, rs2853522 (aka, A*112C), rs2853523 (aka, A*1254C), rs1050993 (aka, A*1361G), rs11799670 (aka, A*153G), **rs1805087 (aka, A2765G)**, rs2789352 (aka, A50417C), rs10925250 (aka, A68550G), rs10925257 (aka, A92580G), rs7526063 (aka, C18418T), rs2275568 (aka, C62048T), rs3820571 (aka, G106853T), rs12749581 (aka, G155A), rs12060264 (aka, G34783A), rs12060570 (aka, G35489C), rs3768142 (aka, G74984T), rs4659736 (aka, G81204T), rs2275566 (aka, G94982A), rs2275565 (aka, G95096T), rs1770449 (aka, T84581C), rs10925235 (aka, T9195C), encodes for the enzyme methionine synthase.

- Catalyzes the transfer of a methyl group from methyl-cobalamin to homocysteine, yielding enzyme-bound cob(I)alamin and methionine. Subsequently, remethylates the cofactor using methyltetrahydrofolate.
- Methionine synthase is responsible for the regeneration of methionine from homocysteine (the "long pathway" vs BHTM, the "short pathway").
- This gene encodes the 5-methyltetrahydrofolate-homocysteine methyltransferase. This enzyme, also known as cobalamin-dependent methionine synthase, catalyzes the final step in methionine biosynthesis. Mutations in MTR have been identified as the underlying cause of methylcobalamin deficiency complementation group G. Alternatively spliced transcript variants encoding distinct isoforms have been found for this gene.

http://www.genecards.org/cgi-bin/carddisp.pl?gene=MTR

+ Methionine synthase forms part of the SAMe biosynthesis and regeneration cycle. This enzyme requires vitamin B-12 as a cofactor.

https://www.ncbi.nlm.nih.gov/pubmed/2407589

+ Catalytic activity:

- 5-methyltetrahydrofolate + L-homocysteine = tetrahydrofolate + L-methionine

+ Cofactor:
- Zinc
- Methyl(III)cobalamin

+ Molecular function:

- Cobalamin binding
- Methionine synthase activity
- S-adenosylmethionine-homocysteine S-methyltransferase activity
- Zinc ion binding

+ Biological process:
- Cellular nitrogen compound metabolic process
- Cobalamin metabolic process
- Methionine biosynthetic process
- Methylation
- Nervous system development
- Pteridine-containing compound metabolic process
- Small molecule metabolic process
- Sulfur amino acid metabolic process
- Vitamin metabolic process
- Water-soluble vitamin metabolic process
- Xenobiotic metabolic process

+ Cellular component:
- Cytoplasm
- Cytosol

http://www.uniprot.org/uniprot/Q99707

+ Diseases associated with MTR:

Homocystinuria-megaloblastic anemia - An autosomal recessive inborn error of metabolism resulting from defects in the cobalamin-dependent pathway that converts homocysteine to methionine. It causes delayed psychomotor development, megaloblastic anemia, homocystinuria, and hypomethioninemia.

http://www.ncbi.nlm.nih.gov/pubmed/8968737

Neural tube defects, folate-sensitive - The most common NTDs are open spina bifida (myelomeningocele) and anencephaly.

http://www.ncbi.nlm.nih.gov/pubmed/12375236

MTRR

+ **Overview for MTRR** *5-methyltetrahydrofolate-homocysteine methyltransferase reductase* (aka, methionine synthase reductase) *MTRR*, rs1802059 (aka, -11 A664A), rs3815743 (aka, A22893G), **rs1801394 (aka, A66G)**, rs10064631 (aka, C1078G), rs3776455 (aka, C32295T), rs1532268 (aka, C524T), rs9332 (aka, G*541A), rs326120 (aka, G10631A), rs2287779 (aka,

G1155A), rs3776467 (aka, G12099A), rs7703033 (aka, G15734A), rs162049 (aka, G28905A), **rs10380 (aka, H595Y), rs162036 (aka, K350A)**, rs2287780 (aka, R415T), rs10520873 (aka, T*1059C), rs8659 (aka, T*662A), rs326121 (aka, T12072C), rs162031 (aka, T16071C), encodes for the enzyme methionine synthase reductase.

- Methionine synthase reductase is involved in the reductive regeneration of cob(I)alamin (vitamin B-12) cofactor required for the maintenance of methionine synthase in a functional state. It is necessary for utilization of methyl groups from the folate cycle, thereby affecting transgenerational epigenetic inheritance. Folate pathway donates methyl groups necessary for cellular methylation and affects different pathways such as DNA methylation, possibly explaining the transgenerational epigenetic inheritance effects.

+ Methionine synthase reductase regenerates a functional methionine synthase via reductive methylation. It is a member of the ferredoxin-NADP(+) reductase (FNR) family of electron transferases.

http://www.ncbi.nlm.nih.gov/gene?Db=gene&Cmd=ShowDetailView&TermToSearch=4552

+ Medications that deplete vitamin B-12:

- Many anti-inflammatory medications including hydrocortisone and prednisone
  - Genatamicin (antibiotic)
  - Neomycin (antibiotic)
  - Tobramycin (antibiotic)
  - Some Sulfa drug antibiotics including Co-Trimoxazole and Trimethoprim
  - Some Cephalosporins including Cefprozil and Loracarbef
  - Some Macrolides including Azithromycin and Erythromycin
  - Penicillin dervatives including AMoxicillian and Penicillin V Potassium
- Quinolones **(See MTHFR write-up above)**
- Phenobarbital (anti-convulsant)
  - Metformin (anti-diabetic)
  - Birth Control pills
  - Potassium chloride (cardiovascular)
- Some cholesterol lowering medications including Cholestyramine and Colestipol
  - Colchicine (gout)
  - Many Ulcer medications including Cimetidine and Ranitidine

- **Proton Pump Inhibitors (PPIs)** including Lansoprazole and Opeprazole

➤ **Our Two Cents:** PPIs have their place in assisting with gastroesophageal reflux disease. In addition to causing decreased mineral absorption however, PPIs taken long-term, eventually impact parietal cell function. Parietal cells line the stomach and have two primary jobs. Their first job is to make somach acid, needed to begin the process of protein and subsequent amino acid assimilation from chewed food. The panceas further assists by releasing its enzymes, with its function partially triggered by the robustness of the acidity of the food/HCl moving from the stomach into the small intestine. PPIs = "low functioning stomach acid" (i.e., the pH of stomach acid is too high); exactly the wrong thing needed to keep the valve between the stomach and the esophagus (LES) closed to prevent heartburn.

(See references in Chapter 5 for 2nd Brain book)

PPI's operate to damp down the acidity of stomach contents so that the sensation of burning is minimized when the LES valve opens, but they do nothing to address the underlying issues. The underlying issue is actually low-functioning stomach acid (higher pH). Simple aging and poor diet contribute to poor HCl production.

The bottom line is that wimpy HCl leads to wimpy pancreas response, and potentially undigested food in stool and poor amino acid assimiliation. (Gallbladder function and bile production are in play as well, but that will be discussed in Compendium 2).

The amino acids subsequently derived from robust digestion provide the building blocks of neurotransmitter production and much more, including liver detoxification. So, when amino acid assimilation is impaired by PPI's, the domino effect may be wide spread in body's biochemical pathways.

The second job of the parietal cells is to make a glycoprotein referred to as, "intrinsic factor". Intrinsic factor "escorts" vitamin B-12, derived from specific foods such as eggs and beef, to the distal (lower) end of our small intestine, where it is absorbed into our blood stream. Once in the bloodstream, its second escorts, TCN 1 and 2 pick up vitamin B-12, where it is subsequently ferried into our cells. Without intrinsic factor much of vitamin B-12 from foods or oral supplements is lost and the SO IMPORTANT folate and vitamin B-12 methyl-swap, required for methylation, may be compromised. Vegetarians are also at risk as vitamin B-12 is typically source from animal protein.

If you are reading this this, you likely have an MTHFR SNP. Remember, addressing folate deficiency via 5MTHF supplementation will not be effective without adequate vitamin B-12, as they work hand in glove to run the biochemical pathways of a healthy body.

Much of the time, supporting methylation with the proper form of vitamin B-12, may reduce the need for daily 5MTHF supplementation. Too much 5MTHF may cause excitatory neurotransmitters to ramp up, especially in those with COMT SNPs and/or high dopamine and/or epinephrine for other reasons. It is also worth noting that supporting vitamin B-12 transport proteins, TCN 1 and 2 with lithium orotate a few days per week, is often helpful in those with TCN1 and 2 SNPs.

+ Catalytic activity:

-2 [methionine synthase]-methylcob(I)alamin + 2 S-adenosylhomocysteine + NADP+ = 2 [methionine synthase]-cob(II)alamin + NADPH + 2 S-adenosyl-L-methionine

+ Cofactor:
- FAD
- FMN

+ Molecular function:
- Methionine synthase reductase activity
- Aquacobalamin reductase (NADPH) activity
- FAD binding
- Flavin adenine dinucleotide binding
- FMN binding
- Iron ion binding
- NADP binding
- NADPH binding
- NADPH-hemoprotein reductase activity
- Oxidoreductase activity, acting on paired donors, with incorporation or reduction of molecular oxygen, NAD(P)H as one donor, and incorporation of one atom of oxygen
- Oxidoreductase activity, oxidizing metal ions, NAD or NADP as acceptor

+ Biological process:
- Cellular nitrogen compound metabolic process
- Cobalamin metabolic process
- DNA methylation
- Folic acid metabolic process
- Homocysteine catabolic process
- Methionine biosynthetic process
- Methionine metabolic process
- Methylation
- Negative regulation of cystathionine beta-synthase activity

- Oxidation-reduction process
- S-adenosylmethionine cycle
- Small molecule metabolic process
- Sulfur amino acid metabolic process
- Vitamin metabolic process
- Water-soluble vitamin metabolic process
- Xenobiotic metabolic process

+ Cellular component:
- Cytoplasm
- Cytosol
- Intermediate filament cytoskeleton
- Nucleoplasm

http://www.uniprot.org/uniprot/Q9UBK8

+ Diseases associated with MTRR:
- Homocystinuria-megaloblastic anemia - An autosomal recessive inborn error of metabolism resulting from defects in the cobalamin-dependent pathway that converts homocysteine to methionine. It causes delayed psychomotor development, megaloblastic anemia, homocystinuria, and hypomethioninemia.

http://www.ncbi.nlm.nih.gov/pubmed/8968737

- Neural tube defects, folate-sensitive - The most common NTDs are open spina bifida (myelomeningocele) and anencephaly.

http://www.ncbi.nlm.nih.gov/pubmed/12375236

MUT

+ **Overview for MUT** *Methylmalonyl CoA mutase, mitochondrial*

MUT, rs6458687 (aka, A2011G), rs6458690 (aka, T24234C), which encodes for the enzyme, Methylmalonyl Coenzyme A mutase.

- Methylmalonyl Coenzyme A mutase is an enzyme that catalyzes the isomerization of methylmalonyl-CoA to succinyl-CoA. It requires a vitamin B-12-derived prosthetic group adenosylcobalamine (aka, AdoCbl), to function.
- MUT is active in the mitochondria

+ Methylmalonyl CoA mutase is responsible a step in the breakdown of several amino acids, specifically isoleucine, methionine, threonine, and valine. The enzyme also helps break down certain types of fats (lipids) and cholesterol. First, several chemical reactions convert the amino acids, lipids, or cholesterol to a molecule called methylmalonyl CoA. Then, working with adenosylcobalamin (AdoCbl), methylmalonyl CoA mutase converts methylmalonyl CoA to a compound called succinyl-CoA. Other enzymes break down succinyl-CoA into molecules that are later used for energy production in the Krebs cycle.

http://ghr.nlm.nih.gov/gene/MUT

+ Mutations in MUT may be associated with methylmalonic acidemia; a condition characterized by feeding difficulties, developmental delay, and long-term health problems. These genetic changes prevent the production of functional methylmalonyl CoA mutase, or reduce the activity of the enzyme. As a result, certain proteins and lipids are not broken down properly. This defect allows methylmalonyl CoA and other toxic compounds to build up in the body's organs and tissues, causing the signs and symptoms of methylmalonic academia.

http://ghr.nlm.nih.gov/gene/MUT

https://www.ncbi.nlm.nih.gov/pubmed/19699272

https://en.wikipedia.org/wiki/Methylmalonyl-CoA_mutase

+ Catalytic activity:
- (R)-methylmalonyl-CoA = succinyl-CoA

+ Cofactor:
- Adenosylcob(III)alamin

+ Molecular function:
- Cobalamin binding
- Metal ion binding
- Methylmalonyl-CoA mutase activity
- Modified amino acid binding

+ Biological process:
- Cellular lipid metabolic process
- Cobalamin metabolic process
- Fatty acid beta-oxidation
- Homocysteine metabolic process
- Post-embryonic development
- Short chain fatty acid catabolic process
- Small molecule metabolic process
- Vitamin metabolic process
- Water-soluble vitamin metabolic process

+ Subcellular location:
- Mitochondrian matrix

+ Cellular component:
- Mitochondrial matrix

- Mitochondrian

http://www.uniprot.org/uniprot/P22033

NOS1

+ <u>**Overview for NOS1**</u> *Nitric oxide synthase 1 (neuronal)* (aka, nNOS, Nitric oxide synthase, brain) *NOS1*, rs7298903 (aka, A57373G), rs3782206 (aka, G59494A), rs2293054 (aka, T2202C), encodes for the enzyme, nitric oxide synthase 1.

- Nitric oxide (NO) is a messenger molecule with diverse functions throughout the body. In the brain and peripheral nervous system, NO displays many properties of a neurotransmitter.
- NO is implicated in neurotoxicity associated with stroke and neurodegenerative diseases, <u>neural regulation of smooth muscle</u>, including peristalsis, and penile erection. NO is also responsible for endothelium-derived relaxing factor activity regulating blood pressure.

https://www.ncbi.nlm.nih.gov/pubmed/1379716

- nNOS is one of three isoforms that synthesize nitric oxide, a small gaseous and lipophilic molecule that participates of several biological processes.

https://www.ncbi.nlm.nih.gov/pubmed/20388537

+ In macrophages, NO mediates tumoricidal and bactericidal actions, as evidenced by the fact that NO synthase inhibitors block these effects. Both the neuronal and the macrophage forms are unusual among oxidative enzymes in that they require several electron donors: FAD, flavin, flavin mononucleotide (FMN), NADPH, and tetrahydrobiopterin (BH4).

https://en.wikipedia.org/wiki/NOS1

+ Catalytic activity:

- 2 L-arginine + 3 NADPH + 4 O2 = 2 L-citrulline + 2 nitric oxide + 3 NADP+ + 4 H2O

+ Cofactor:

- Heme
- FMN
- 5,6,7,8-tetrahydrobiopterin

+ Molecular function:

- Arginine binding
- Cadmium ion binding
- Flavin adenine dinucleotide binding
- FMN binding

- Heme binding
- Ion channel binding
- Iron ion binding
- NADP binding
- NADPH-hemoprotein reductase activity
- Nitric-oxide synthase activity
- Scaffold protein binding
- Sodium channel regulator activity
- Tetrahydrobiopterin binding

+ Biological process:

- Aging
- Arginine catabolic process
- Behavioral response to cocaine
- Blood coagulation
- Cellular response to growth factor stimulus
- Cellular response to mechanical stimulus
- Exogenous drug catabolic process
- Female pregnancy
- Interaction with host
- Multicellular response to stress
- Muscle contraction
- Myoblast fusion
- Negative regulation of adrenergic receptor signaling pathway
- Negative regulation of apoptotic process
- Negative regulation of blood pressure
- Negative regulation of calcium ion transport
- Negative regulation of calcium ion transport into cytosol
- Negative regulation of cell proliferation
- Negative regulation of cytosolic calcium ion concentration
- Negative regulation of heart contraction
- Negative regulation of hydrolase activity
- Negative regulation of insulin secretion
- Negative regulation of potassium ion transport
- Negative regulation of serotonin uptake

- Negative regulation of vasoconstriction
- Neurotransmitter biosynthetic process
- Nitric oxide biosynthetic process
- Nitric oxide mediated signal transduction
- Peptidyl-cysteine S-nitrosylation
- Phagosome maturation
- Positive regulation of adrenergic receptor signaling pathway in heart process
- Positive regulation of guanylate cyclase activity
- Positive regulation of of histone acetylation
- Positive regulation of long-term synaptic potentiation
- Positive regulation of neuron death
- Positive regulation of sodium ion transmember transport
- Positive regulation of the force of the heart
- Positive regulation of transcription, DNA-templated
- Positive regulation of transcription from RNA polymerase II promoter
- Positive regulation of vasodilation
- Regulation of cardiac muscle contraction
- Regulation of generation of L-type calcium current
- Regulation of neurogenesis
- Regulation of ryanodine-sensitive calcium-release channel activity
- Regulation of sensory perception of pain
- Regulation of sodium ion transport
- Response to activity
- Response to estrogen
- Response to ethanol
- Response to heat
- Response to hypoxia
- Response to lead ion
- Response to lipopolysaccharide
- Response to nicotine
- Response to nitric oxide

- Response to peptide hormone
- Response to vitamin E
- Striated muscle contraction

+Cellular component:
- Azurophil granule
- Caveola
- Cytoplasm
- Cytoskeleton
- Cytosol
- Dendritic spine
- Membrane raft
- Mitochondrial outer membrane
- Mitochondrion
- Nuclear membrane
- Perinuclear region of cytoplasm
- Photoreceptor inner segment
- Postsynaptic density
- Protein complex
- Sarcoplasmic reticulum membrane
- Synapse
- T-tubule
- Vesical membrane
- Z disc

http://www.uniprot.org/uniprot/P29475

NOS2

+ **Overview for NOS2** *Nitric oxide synthase 2 (inducible)* (aka, Inducible NO synthase - iNOS) NOS2, rs2297518 (aka, C1823T), rs2248814 (aka, T32235C), rs2274894 (aka, T836165G), encodes for the enzyme nitric oxide synthase 2 (NOS2).

- *iNOS* is a <u>reactive free radical</u> that acts as a biologic mediator in several processes, including neurotransmission and antimicrobial and antitumoral activities. It is inducible by a combination of lipopolysaccharides and particular cytokines. In other words, its expression is typically induced in inflammatory diseases.

http://www.uniprot.org/citations/7528267

- ❖ **NOTE**: Lipopolysaccharides are an endotoxin, found in the outer membrane of gram-negative bacteria and released into the surrounding environment (e.g., GI tract), which elicit a strong immune response. Detection of lipopolysaccharide antibodies as well as occluding and zonulin can be measured via **Cyrex Labs**, to determine if leaky gut has occured.

+ NOS2 is regulated by calcium/calmodulin. Aspirin inhibits expression and function of this enzyme and effects may be exerted at the level of translational/post-translational modification and directly on the catalytic activity.

+ Catalytic activity:

  - 2 L-arginine + 3 NADPH + 4 O2 = 2 L-citrulline + 2 nitric oxide + 3 NADP+ + 4 H2O

+ Cofactor:
- Heme
- FAD
- FMN
- 5,6,7,8-tetrahydrobiopterin

+ Molecular function:
- Arginine binding
- Flavin adenine dinucleotide binding
- FMN binding
- Heme binding
- Iron ion binding
- NADP binding
- NADPH-hemoprotein reductase activity
- Nitric oxide synthase activity
- Protein homodimerization activity
- Receptor binding
- Tetrahydrobiopterin binding

+ Biological process:
- Arginine catabolic process
- Blood coagulation
- Cellular response to interferon-gamma
- Cellular response to lipopolysaccharide
- Circadian rhythm
- Defense response to bacterium
- Defense response to gram-negative bacterium

- Inflammatory response
- Innate immune response in mucosa
- Interaction with host
- Negative regulation of blood pressure
- Negative regulation of gene expression
- Negative regulation of protein catabolic process
- Nitric oxide biosynthetic process
- Nitric oxide mediated signal transduction
- Peptidyl-cysteine S-nitrosylation
- Phagosome maturation
- Positive regulation of guanylate cyclase activity
- Positive regulation of killing cells of other organism
- Positive regulation of leukocyte mediated cytotoxicity
- Positive regulation of vasodilation
- Regulation of cardiac muscle contraction
- Regulation of cell proliferation
- Regulation of cellular respiration
- Regulation of insulin secretion
- Response to bacterium
- Response to hypoxia
- Superoxide metabolic process

+Cellular component:

- Cortical cytoskeleton
- Cytoplasm
- Cytosol
- Intracellular
- Nucleus
- Perinuclear region of cytoplasm
- Peroxisome

+ Tissue specificity; expressed in:

- Liver
- Retina
- Bone cells
- Airway epithelial cells of the lungs

http://www.uniprot.org/uniprot/P35228

NOS3

+ **Overview for NOS3** *Nitric oxide synthase 3 (endothelial)* (aka, eNOS, Constitutive NOS) *NOS3*, rs1800783 (aka, A6251T), rs3918188 (aka, C19635T), rs7830 (aka, G10T), rs1800779 (G6797A), rs2070744 (aka, T786C) encodes for the enzyme Nitric oxide synthase 3 (NOS3).

- NOS3 produces nitric oxide (NO) that is implicated in vascular smooth muscle relaxation through a cGMP-mediated signal transduction pathway. NO mediates vascular endothelial growth factor (VEGF)-induced angiogenesis in coronary vessels and promotes blood clotting through the activation of platelets.

+ eNOS is primarily responsible for the generation of NO in the vascular endothelium, a monolayer of flat cells lining the interior surface of blood vessels, at the interface between circulating blood in the lumen and the remainder of the vessel wall. NO produced by eNOS in the vascular endothelium plays crucial roles in regulating vascular tone, cellular proliferation, leukocyte adhesion, and platelet aggregation. Therefore, a functional eNOS is essential for a healthy cardiovascular system.

https://www.ncbi.nlm.nih.gov/pubmed/16416260
https://www.ncbi.nlm.nih.gov/pubmed/12379270
https://www.ncbi.nlm.nih.gov/pubmed/16585403

+ Catalytic activity:
   - 2 L-arginine + 3 NADPH + 4 O2 = 2 L-citrulline + 2 nitric oxide + 3 NADP+ + 4 H2O

+ Cofactor:
   - Heme
   - FAD
   - FMN
   - 5,6,7,8-tetrahydrobiopterin

+ Enzyme regulation:
   - Stimulated by calcium/calmodulin
   - Inhibited by NOSIP and NOSTRIN

+ Molecular function:
   - Actin monomer binding
   - Arginine binding
   - Cadmium ion binding
   - Flavin adenine dinucleotide binding
   - FMN binding

- Heme binding
- Iron ion binding
- NADP binding
- NADPH-hemoprotein reductase activity
- Nitric oxide synthase activity
- Tetrahydrobiopterin binding

+ Biological process:

- Angiogenesis
- Arginine catabolic process
- Blood coagulation
- Blood vessel remodeling
- Endothelial cell migration
- Interaction with host
- In-utero embryonic development
- Lipopolysaccharide-mediating signaling pathway
- Lung development
- Mitochondrion organization
- Negative regulation of blood pressure
- Negative regulation of calcium ion transport
- Negative regulation of cell proliferation
- Negative regulation of extrinsic apoptotic signaling pathway
- Negative pathway of hydrolase activity
- Negative regulation of muscle hyperplasia
- Negative regulation of platelet activation
- Negative regulation of potassium ion transport
- Nitric oxide biosynthetic process
- Nitric oxide mediated signal transduction
- Ovulation from ovarian follicle
- Phagosome maturation
- Positive regulation of angiogenesis
- Positive regulation of guanylate cyclase activity
- Positive regulation of vasodilation
- Regulation of blood pressure
- Regulation of blood vessel size

- Regulation of nitric-oxide synthase activity
- Regulation of sodium ion transport
- Regulation of systemic arterial blood pressure by endothelin
- Regulation of the force of heart contraction by chemical signal
- Response to fluid shear stress
- Response to heat
- Smooth muscle hyperplasia
- Vascular endothelial growth factor receptor signaling pathway

+Cellular component:
- Caveola
- Cytoplam
- Cytoskeleton
- Cytosol
- Endocytic vesicle membrane
- Golgi membrane
- Nucleus
- Plasma membrane

+ Tissue specificity; expressed in:
- Platelets
- Placenta
- Liver
- Kidney

http://www.uniprot.org/uniprot/P29474

PEMT

+ **Overview for PEMT** *Phosphatidylethanolamine N-methyltransferase*

PEMT, rs7946 (aka, G634A), rs4646406 (aka, T17020543A), rs4244593 (aka, T17023592G), encodes for the enzyme, phosphatidylethanolamine N-methyltransferase.

- PEMT is a transferase enzyme that converts phosphatidylethanolamine (PE) to phosphatidylethanolamine (PC) in the liver, via three sequential methylation steps by SAM (i.e., three molecules of SAM).
- Although the CDP-choline pathway accounts for approximately seventy percent of PC biosynthesis in the liver, the PEMT pathway has been shown to play a critical (evolutionary) role in providing PC during times of starvation.

https://www.ncbi.nlm.nih.gov/pubmed/22877991

❖ **NOTE**: The CDP-choline pathway is one where choline is obtained either by dietary consumption (e.g., eggs) or by metabolism of choline-containing lipids is converted to PC.

+ PC made via PEMT plays a wide range of physiological roles, utilized in choline synthesis, hepatocyte membrane structure, bile secretion, and VLDL secretion.

https://www.ncbi.nlm.nih.gov/pubmed/24184426

+ Estrogen has also been shown to be a (positive) regulator of hepatocyte PEMT transcription.

➤ **Our Two Cents:** If PEMT SNPs and menopausal, consider using a PC supplement or lecithin, unless antiphospholipid antibodies or other contraindications are present.

+ A major pathway for hepatic PC utilization is secretion of bile into the intestine.

https://www.ncbi.nlm.nih.gov/pubmed/22877991

+ The enzyme is found in endoplasmic reticulum and mitochondria-associated membranes. It accounts for more than half of cell membrane phospholipids and approximately thirty percent of all cellular lipid content, so is therefore crucial for maintaining membrane integrity.

➤ **Our Other Two Cents:** when methyl donors are needed due to compromised methylation (e.g., low folate, low vitamin B-12, etc), call membranes are often a "back-up" source of methyl groups, to the detriment of the membranes, bile production, etc.

+ PEMT partially modulates levels of blood plasma homcysteine, as PC can be utilized to produce TMG, needed by the BHMT enzyme to reduce homocystein to methionine. **(See FIG. 3)**

+ Catalytic activity:

- S-adenosyl-L-methionine + phosphatidyl-N-methylethanolamine = S-adenosyl-L-homocysteine + phosphatidyl-N-dimethylethanolamine

- S-adenosyl-L-methionine + phosphatidyl-N-dimethylethanolamine = S-adenosyl-L-homocysteine + phosphatidylcholine

- S-adenosyl-L-methionine + phosphatidylethanolamine = S-adenosyl-L-homocysteine + phosphatidyl-N-methylethanolamine

+ Molecular function:

- Phosphatidylethanolamine binding
- Phosphatidylethanolamine N-methylatransferase activity
- Phosphatidyl-N-dimethylethanolamine N-methyltransferase activity
- Phosphatidyl-N-methylethanolamine N-methyltransferase activity

+ Biological process:

- Cell proliferation
- Glycerophospholipid biosynthetic process
- Lipid metabolic process
- Negative regulation of cell proliferation
- Phosphatidylcholine biosynthetic process
- Phospholipid metabolic process
- Positive regulation of lipoprotein metabolic process
- Positive regulation of protein targeting to mitochondria
- Response to amino acids
- Response to drug
- Response to ethanol
- Response to vitamin
- SAH metabolic process
- SAM metabolic process
- Small molecule process

+ Subcellular location:

- Endoplasmic reticulum membrane
- Mitochondrion membrane

+ Cellular component:

- Brush border membrane
- Endoplasmic reticulum membrane
- Integral component of membrane
- Mitochondrial membrane
- Sarcolemma

http://www.uniprot.org/uniprot/Q9UBM1

SHMT1

+ **Overview for SHMT1** *Serine hydroxymethyltransferase* (aka, Glycine hydroxymethyltransferase, Serine methylase) *SHMT1*, rs9909104 (aka, A23836G), rs1979277 (aka, C1420T), encodes for the enzyme, serine hydroxymethyltransferase.

- SHMT1 is a transferase enzyme that plays an important role in cellular one-carbon pathways by catalyzing the reversible, simultaneous conversions of L-serine to glycine and tetrahydrofolate to 5, 10 methylenetetrahydrofolate, requiring SAM.

https://www.ncbi.nlm.nih.gov/pubmed/12686103

- SHMT1 also catalyzes other reactions that may be biologically significant, including the conversion of 5,10-methenyltetrahydrofolate to 10-formyltetrahydrofolate.

https://www.ncbi.nlm.nih.gov/pubmed/2201683

+ Smith-Magenis Syndrome (SMS) is a rare disorder that manifests as a complex set of traits including facial abnormalities, unusual behaviors, and developmental delay. It results from an interstital deletion within chromosome 17p11.2, including the cSHMT gene. A small study showed SHMT activity in SMS patients was ~50% of normal.

+ Reduced SHMT activity may result in less glycine.

https://www.ncbi.nlm.nih.gov/pubmed/8533763

+ Catalytic activity:

- 5,10-methylenetetrahydrofolate + glycine + H2O = tetrahydrofolate + L-serine

+ Cofactor:

- Pyridoxal 5'-phosphate (P5P is the active form of Vitamin B6)

+ Molecular function:
- Amino acid binding
- Glycine hydroxymethyltransferase activity
- L-allo-threonine aldolase activity
- Protein homodimerization activity
- Pyridoxal phosphate binding

+ Biological process:
- Carnitine biosynthetic process
- Cellular nitrogen compound metabolic process
- Folic acid metabolic process
- Glycine biosynthetic process from serine
- L-serine catabolic process
- Protein homotetramerization
- Protein tetramerization
- Purine nucleobase biosynthetic process
- Small molecule metabolic process
- Tetrahydrofolate interconversion
- Vitamin metabolic process
- Water-soluble vitamin metabolic process

+ Subcellular location:
- Cytoplasm

+ Cellular component:
- Cytoplasm
- Cytosol
- Extracellular exosome
- Mitochondrion
- Nucleoplasm
- Nucleus

http://www.uniprot.org/uniprot/P34896

SLC19A1

+ **Overview for SLC19A1** *Solute carrier family 19 (folate transporter), member 1* (aka, folate transporter 1, reduced folate carrier protein). SLC19A1, rs1888530 (aka, G30963A), rs3788200 (aka, T10815C), encodes for the folate transporter solute carrier family 19, member 1.

- The membrane protein encoded by this gene is a **transporter of folate** and is involved in the regulation of intracellular concentrations of folate receptor, the folate transporter, and a V-type H+-pump.

http://www.genecards.org/cgi-bin/carddisp.pl?gene=SLC19A1

+ Diseases associated with SLC19A1 include methotrexate dose selection and thiamine-responsive megloblastic anemia syndrome (related to cone-rod dystrophy).

http://www.malacards.org/card/methotrexate_dose_selection
http://www.malacards.org/card/thiamine_responsive_megaloblastic_anemia_syndrome

+ The uptake of folate in human placental choriocarcinoma cells occurs via a novel mechanism called, potocytosis, which functionally couples three components, namely the folate receptor, the folate transporter, and a V-type H+-pump.

http://www.uniprot.org/uniprot/P41440

+ Molecular function:
- Folic acid binding
- Folic acid transporter activity
- Methotrexate transporter activity

+ Biological process:
- Folic acid metabolic process
- Folic acid transport
- Small molecule metabolic process
- Vitamin metabolic process
- Water-soluble vitamin metabolic process

+ Cellular component:
- Integral component of plasma membrane
- Membrane
- Plasma membrane

http://www.uniprot.org/uniprot/P41440

SPR

+ **Overview for SPR** *Sepiapterin reductase (7,8-dihydrobiopterin:NADP+ oxidoreductase)*. SPR, rs10174540 (aka, 7413A>G)

- The *SPR* gene provides instructions for making the sepiapterin reductase enzyme. This enzyme is involved in the last of three steps in the production of a molecule called tetrahydrobiopterin (BH4). Other enzymes help carry out the first and second steps in this process.
- The sepiapterin reductase enzyme converts a molecule called, 6-pyruvoyl-tetrahydropterin, to tetrahydrobiopterin. Tetrahydrobiopterin helps process several building blocks of proteins (amino acids), and is involved in the production of neurotransmitters (e.g., serotonin, dopamine -> norepinepherine, epinephrine).
- This FAD binding protein forms homodimers and performs two-electron reduction of quinones to hydroquinones.

https://www.ncbi.nlm.nih.gov/pubmed/1657151

+ As SPR is involved in BH4 and subsequent dopamine production, SNPs in SPR are sometimes associated with DOPA-responsive dystonia: In the majority of cases, patients manifest progressive psychomotor retardation, dystonia, and spasticity. Cognitive anomalies are also often present. The disease is due to severe dopamine and serotonin deficiencies in the central nervous system caused by a defect in BH4 synthesis. Dystonia is defined by the presence of sustained involuntary muscle contractions, often leading to abnormal postures.

http://www.uniprot.org/uniprot/P35270

+ Catalytic activity:
- L-erythro-7,8-dihydrobiopterin + NADP+ = sepiapterin + NADPH
- L-erythro-tetrahydrobiopterin + 2 NADP+ = 6-pyruvoyl-5,6,7,8-tetrahydropterin + 2 NADPH

+ Molecular function:
- Aldo-keto reductase (NADP) activity
- NADP binding
- Sepiapterin reductase activity

+ Biological process:
- Cell morphogenesis involved in neuron differentiation
- Death
- Dopamine metabolic process
- L-phenylalanine process
- Nitric oxide biosynthetic process
- Nitric oxide metabolic process
- Norepinepherine metabolic process
- Oxidation-reduction process
- Pteridine metabolic process
- Regulation of multicellular growth
- Regulation of nitric-oxide synthase (NOS) process
- Small molecule metabolic process
- Tetrahydrobiopterin biosynthetic process
- Voluntary musculoskeletal movement

+ Subcellular location:
- Cytoplasm

+ Cellular component:
- Cytoplasm
- Cytosol
- Extracellular exosome
- Mitochondrion
- Nucleoplasm

http://www.uniprot.org/uniprot/P35270

SUOX

+ **Overview for SUOX** *Sulfite oxidase.* SUOX, rs705703 (aka, C5444T), encodes for the enzyme, sulfite oxidase utilizes in sulfur pathway metabolism.

- Sulfite oxidase is a homodimeric protein localized to the intermembrane space of mitochondria. Each subunit contains a heme domain and a molybdopterin-binding domain.
- The enzyme catalyzes the oxidation of sulfite to sulfate, the final reaction in the oxidative degradation of the sulfur amino acids cysteine and methionine.
- Sulfite oxidase deficiency results in neurological abnormalities that are often fatal at an early age.

http://ghr.nlm.nih.gov/gene/SUOX

> **Our Two Cents:** I have never seen a variant report with homozygous SUOX SNPs at rs705703.

+ Sulfite oxidase is an enzyme in the mitochondria. It oxidizes sulfite to sulfate, via cytochrome c, transfers the electrons produced to the electron transport chain, thereby allowing genetation of ATP in oxidative phosphorylation. This is the last step in the metabolism of sulfur-containing compounds (i.e., the trans-sulfuration pathway) and the sulfate is excreted.

https://www.ncbi.nlm.nih.gov/pubmed/16140720

http://www.wikigenes.org/e/gene/e/6821.html

+ Catalytic activity:
- Sulfite + O_2 + H_2O = sulfate + H_2O_2

+ Cofactor:
- Heme b; (iron(II)-protoporphyrin IX) group non-covalently per subunit
- Mo-molybdopterin (Mo-MPT) cofactor per subunit

+ Molecular function:
- Heme binding
- Molybdenum ion binding
- Molybdopterin cofactor binding
- Sulfite oxidase activity

+ Biological process:
- Cellular nitrogen compound metabolic process
- Nitrate assimilation
- Response to nutrient
- Small molecule metabolic process
- Sulfide oxidation, using sulfide: quinone oxidoreductase
- Sulfur amino acid catabolic process
- Sulfur amino acid metabolic process

+ Subcellular location
- Mitochondrion intermembrane space

+ Cellular component:
- Cytosol
- Mitochondrial intermembrane space
- Mitochindrial matrix

http://www.uniprot.org/uniprot/P51687

+ Associated disease:

- Isolated sulfite oxidase deficiency (ISOD) – is characterized by neurological abnormalities including, multicystic leukoencephalopathy with brain atrophy. Patients often suffer from seizures. Often leads to death at an early age.

TCN1

+ **Overview for TCN1** *Transcobalamin I (vitamin B-12 binding protein, R binder family) [Homo sapiens (human)].* TCN1, rs526934 (aka, G4939288A) encodes a member of the vitamin B-12-binding protein family, transcobalamin I.

- This family of proteins, alternatively referred to as R binders, is expressed in various tissues and secretions. This protein is a major constituent of secondary granules in neutrophils and facilitates the transport of cobalamin into cells.

http://www.ncbi.nlm.nih.gov/gene/6947

> **Our Two Cents:** Because TCN1 (as well as other TCNs) are involved in B-12 transport from the blood stream "into" the cells, in addition to folate and B-12 supplementation, it has been suggested that a lithium orotate supplement (4.6 mgs), pulsed, may be helpful when addressing high MMA levels and/or high homocysteine levels. Positive antibodies to intrinsic factor, or ongoing PPI medication (due to heartburn), may contribute to poor B-12 absorption in the GI.

+ Molecular function:
- Cobalamin binding

+ Biological process:
- Cobalamin metabolic process
- Cobalamin transport
- Cobalt ion transport
- Small molecule metabolic process
- Vitamin metabolic process
- Water-soluble vitamin metabolic process

+ Subcellular location:
- Secreted

+ Cellular component:
- Extracellular region

- Extracellular space

http://www.uniprot.org/uniprot/P20061

TCN2

+ Overview for TCN2 *Transcobalamin 2 (vitamin B-12 binding protein, R binder family) [Homo sapiens (human)].* TCN2, rs9606756 (aka, A8700G), rs1801198 (aka, C766G) encodes a member of the vitamin B-12-binding protein family, transcobalamin II.

- This family of proteins, alternatively referred to as R binders, is expressed in various tissues and secretions. This protein is a major constituent of secondary granules in neutrophils and facilitates the transport of cobalamin into cells.

http://www.ncbi.nlm.nih.gov/gene/6947

> **Our Two Cents:** Because TCN2 (as well as other TCNs) are involved in B-12 transport from the blood stream "into" the cells, in addition to folate and B-12 supplementation, it has been suggested that a lithium orotate supplement (4.6 mgs), pulsed, may be helpful when addressing high MMA levels and/or high homocysteine levels. Positive antibodies to intrinsic factor, or ongoing PPI medication (due to heartburn), may contribute to poor B-12 absorption in the GI.

+ TCN2 SNPs have been associated with decreased vitamin B-12 and increased risk of fragility.

http://www.ncbi.nlm.nih.gov/pmc/articles/PMC3042247/

+ Molecular function:
- Cobalamin binding
- Metal ion binding

+ Biological process:
- Cobalamin metabolic process
- Cobalamin transport
- Cobalt ion transport
- Small molecule metabolic process
- Vitamin metabolic process
- Water-soluble vitamin metabolic process

+ Subcellular location:
- Secreted

+ Cellular component:
- Endosome
- Extracellular exosome

- Extracellular region

http://www.uniprot.org/uniprot/P20062

TYMS

+ <u>**Overview for TYMS**</u> *Thymidylate synthetase.* TYMS, rs502396 (aka, C6633T), encodes thymidylate synthetase.

- TYMS catalyzes the conversion of deoxyuridine monophosphate (dUMP) to deoxythymidine monophosphate (dTMP).
- Contributes to the de novo mitochondrial thymidylate biosynthesis pathway.
- dTMP is one of the three nucleotides (dTMP, dTTP, and dTDP) that form thymine.

*Recall that 5,10-methyleneTHR results from the third step of MTHFD1 activity. That, plus dUMP (not shown in FIG. 4), are used by TYMS to generate DHF plus dTMP -> **thymine,** in a "feedback" pathway. Some of the 5,10-methyleneTHR is converted by MTHFR to form 5MTHF, in a "feedforward" pathway.

+ With inhibition of thymidylate synthetase, an imbalance of deoxynucleotides can result and cause DNA damage and impaired cell growth.

https://en.wikipedia.org/wiki/Thymidylate_synthase
https://www.ncbi.nlm.nih.gov/pubmed/12084461

+ For this reason, **thymidylate synthetase** has become an important target for chemotherapy cancer agents to address colorectal, pancreatic, ovarian, gastric, and breast cancers.

+ Catalytic activity:

- 5,10-methylenetetrahydrofolate + dUMP = dihydrofolate + dTMP

+ Molecular function:

- Cofactor binding
- Drug binding
- Folic acid binding
- mRNA binding
- Nucleotide binding
- Thymidylate synthase activity

+ Biological process:

- Aging
- Cartilage development
- Circadian rhythm
- Deoxyribonucleoside monophosphate biosynthetic process
- Development growth

- dTMP biosynthetic process
- dTTP biosynthetic process
- dUMP metabolic process
- G1/S transition of mitotic cell cycle
- Immortalization of host cell by virus
- Intestinal epithelial cell maturation
- Mitotic cell cycle
- Nucleobase-containing compound metabolic process
- Nucleobase-containing small molecule metabolic process
- Organ regeneration
- Pyrimidine nucleobase metabolic process
- Pyrimidine nucleoside metabolic process
- Regulation of transcription involved in G1/S transition of mitotic cell cycle
- Response to cytokine
- Response to drugs
- Response to ethanol
- Response to folic acid
- Response to glucocorticoid
- Response to organophosphorus
- Response to progesterone
- Response to toxic substance
- Response to vitamin A
- Small molecule metabolic process
- Tetrahydrofolate metabolic process
- Uracil metabolic process

+ Subcellular location:

- Nucleus
- Cytoplasm
- Mitochondrial inner membrane
- Mitochondria matrix
- Mitochondrian

+ Cellular component:

- Cytoplasm

- Cytosol
- Mitochondrial inner membrane
- Mitochondria matrix
- Mitochondrian
- Nucleolus
- Nucleoplasm
- Nucleus

http://www.uniprot.org/uniprot/P04818

VDR Bsm

+ Overview for VDR Bsm *Vitamin D-3 receptor (1,25-dihydroxyvitamin D-3 receptor, nuclear receptor subfamily 1 group I member 1)*

- VDR Bsm, rs1544410 (aka, VDR:BsmI), provides instructions for making nuclear vitamin D receptors.
- VDR is a member of the nuclear receptor family of transcription factors, sometimes called a sequence-specific DNA-binding factor. Recall that a transcription factor is a protein that binds to specific DNA sequences, thereby controlling the rate of transcription of genetic information from DNA to messenger RNA.

https://www.ncbi.nlm.nih.gov/pubmed/17132852

- Nuclear hormone receptor (in nucleus). Recruited to promoters via its interaction with BAZ1B/WSTF that mediates the interaction with acetylated histones, an essential step for VDR-promoter association. Plays a central role in calcium homeostasis.

http://www.uniprot.org/uniprot/P11473

- This gene encodes the nuclear hormone receptor for vitamin D-3. This receptor also functions as a receptor for the secondary bile acid, lithocholic acid. The receptor belongs to the family of trans-acting, transcriptional regulatory factors and shows similarity of sequence to the steroid and thyroid hormone receptors.
- According to Dr Yasko, VDR/Taq mutations oppose COMT mutations in the regulation of dopamine and epinephrine levels. In other words, having a VDR mutation in concert with a COMT mutation, "balances out" higher dopamine and epinephrine tendencies in those with COMT mutations. Additionally, VDR mutation confers less sensitivity to methyl group supplement levels (e.g., "mood swings"). Therefore, a person who has COMT SNPs and no VDR SNPs is most at risk for higher dopamine and epinephrine levels and higher sensitivity to methyl group supplementation.

> **Our Two Cents:** Consideration of DDC (enzyme responsible for tyrosin to dopamine conversion), DBH (enzymes responsible for dopamine to norepinephrine), and PNMT (norepinepherine to epinephrine conversion), and receptor sensitivity (e.g., DRD2 SNP status) factor into dopamine and epinephrine levels.

+ Molecular function:
    - Calcitriol binding
    - Calcitrol receptor activity
    - DNA binding
    - Lithocholic acid binding
    - Lithocholicacid acid receptor activity
    - Retinoid x receptor binding
    - Sequence specific DNA binding
    - Steroid hormone receptor activity
    - Zinc ion binding

+ VDR Bsm biological processes:
    - Bile acid signaling pathway
    - Calcium ion transport
    - Cell morphogenesis
    - Cellular calcium ion homeostasis
    - Decidualization
    - Gene expression
    - Intestinal absorption
    - Lactation
    - Mammary gland branching invovlved with pregnanacy
    - Negative regulation of cell proliferation
    - Negative regulation of keratinocyte proliferation
    - Negative regulation of transcription, DNA-templated
    - Negative regulation of transcription from RNA polymerase II promoter
    - Positive regulation of apoptitic process involved in mammary gland involution
    - Positive regulation of gene expression
    - Positive regulation of keratinocyte differentiation
    - Positive regulation of transcription from RNA polymerase II promoter
    - Positive regulation of vitamin D 24-hydroxylase activity
    - Regulation of calcidiol 1-monooxygenase activity
    - Signal transduction
    - Transcription initiation from RNA polymerase II promoter

- Vitamin D receptor signaling pathway

+ Subcellular location:
  - Nucleus

+ Cellular component:
  - Nucleoplasm
  - Nucleus
  - Receptor complex
  - RNA polymerase II transcription factor complex

http://www.uniprot.org/uniprot/P11473

Section 2.3.6.3 – Other SNPs Related to Methylation

DAO

+ **<u>Overview for DAO</u>** *Diamine Oxidase* (aka, AOC1, hDAO, ABP1 [old days]) DAO, rs3741775 (aka, A14747C), rs3918347 (aka, A24464G), rs2070586 (aka, G8864A), rs2070587 (aka, T8887G), rs2111902 (aka, T9891G), DAO/ABP1, rs1049742 (aka, C995T)

- The DAO gene provides instructions for producing the enzyme diamine oxidase, involved in the metabolism, oxidation, and inactivation of histamine within the digestive tract.

http://www.ncbi.nlm.nih.gov/pubmed/19764817

- Regulates the level of the neuromodulator D-serine in the brain and has high activity towards D-DOPA and contributes to dopamine synthesis. D-amino-acid oxidase acts as a detoxifying agent that removes D-amino acids accumulated during aging. Acts on a variety of D-amino acids with a preference for those having small hydrophobic side chains followed by those bearing polar, aromatic, and basic groups.
- Supplements that augment DAO are available to assist with histamine breakdown in the GI tract.

+ DAO Deficiency is an alteration in the metabolism of food histamine that appears when diamine oxidase (DAO) enzyme activity is low (SNPs); in other words, when for some reason there is a significant deficiency in the functional activity of the main enzyme in the metabolism of histamine. The imbalance between ingested histamine and the histamine released from the histamine storage cells, and the capacity for histamine degradation, leads to histamine accumulation in plasma and the occurrence of adverse effects on health.

http://www.deficitdao.org/dao-deficiency/#.VUpolKaZ6kU [Good reference]

+ Non-steroidal anti-inflammatory drugs (NSAIDs) are the drugs most frequently involved in hypersensitivity drug reactions. Histamine is released in the allergic response to NSAIDs and is responsible for some of the clinical symptoms. Some DAO polymorphisms cause impaired metabolism of resulting released/circulating histamine and is associated with the clinical response in crossed-hypersensitivity to NSAIDs.

http://www.ncbi.nlm.nih.gov/pubmed/23152756

+ Homozygous leads to reduced DAO activity and rs10156191 is associated with histamine intolerance (HIT).

+ There was an association of moderate significance of drug intolerance with rs1049793.

+ rs10156191 showed strong and highly significant effects on DAO serum activity and were associated with HIT symptoms in patients with decreased DAO levels.

(NB The researchers state: A reliable biomarker for the diagnosis is missing, as plasma histamine is very unstable and DAO serum activity is decreased only in half of the patients with HIT)

http://onlinelibrary.wiley.com/doi/10.1111/j.1398-9995.2011.02548.x/full

+ SNPs in rs10156191, which is related to decreased DAO enzyme activity, is associated with the risk of developing migraine, particularly in women.

http://www.deficitdao.org/docs/Diamine_Oxidase_rs10156191.pdf

+ Humans have three functioning genes that code for copper-containing amine oxidases. The product of the AOC1 gene is a so-called diamine oxidase (hDAO), named for its substrate preference for diamines, particularly histamine. Two active sites, one in each subunit, are characterized by the presence of a copper ion (type II copper ion) and a topaquinone residue formed by the post-translational modification of a tyrosine. They catalyze the oxidative deamination of primary amines to the corresponding aldehydes with the concomitant production of hydrogen peroxide and ammonia.

http://www.ncbi.nlm.nih.gov/pmc/articles/PMC2791411/

*Recall that histamine is an in important neurotransmitter and immune messenger molecule. It is associated with processes involving hydrochloric acid secretion for digestion. Histamine only becomes a problem when we have metabolic disturbances that do not allow us to effectively metabolize histamine. When histamine is formed, it is broken down by histamine N-methyltransferase (HMT) in the central nervous system and by DAO in the digestive tract. The experts state that DAO is the major enzyme involved in histamine metabolism. The enzyme converts the (reactive) histamine into imidazole acetaldehyde (non-reactive). As a result, DAO is responsible for ensuring a steady histamine level required for the balance of numerous chemical reactions taking place in the body.

- A DAO SNP may confer a tendency for histamine intolerance to histamine foods (e.g., fermented foods, "left-overs"). Small intestinal bacterial overgrowth (SIBO) and leaky gut can further contribute to poor DAO function.
- Use of certain medications can also contribute to poor DAO function:
    - Non-steroidal anti-inflammatory drugs (ibuprofen, aspirin)
    - Antidepressants (Cymbalta, Effexor, Prozac, Zoloft)
    - Immune modulators (Humira, Enbrel, Plaquenil)
    - Antiarrhythmics (propanolol, metaprolol, Cardizem, Norvasc)
    - Antihistamines (Allegra, Zyrtec, Benadryl)
    - Histamine (H2) blockers (Tagamet, Pepcid, Zantac)
- Alcohol is a DAO inhibitor. Endogenous histamine release foods: alcohol, citrus fruits, strawberries, pineapple, kiwi, tomato sauce, seafood, chocolate, fish, mushrooms, pig, cereals, and egg white.
- Common symptoms of histamine intolerance are:
    - Headaches/migraines
    - Difficulty falling asleep/easy arousal
    - Hypertension
    - Vertigo or dizziness
    - Arrhythmia
    - Difficulty regulating body temperature
    - Anxiety
    - Abdominal cramps
    - Flushing
    - Nasal congestion
    - Difficulty breathing
    - Abnormal menstrual cycle
    - Hives
    - Fatigue
    - Tissue swelling
    - Inability to be in the sun
    - Frequent sneezing

http://www.naturalnews.com/047470_DAO_enzymes_histamine_intolerance_immune_system.html#ixzz3ZO2QVBwz

+ Diseases associated with DAO are:
- Schizophrenia
- Primary hyperoxaluria

http://www.genecards.org/cgi-bin/carddisp.pl?gene=DAO

+ The following diseases are related to DAO:

Primary Hyperoxaluria
http://diseases.jensenlab.org/Entity?textmining=12&type1=-26&type2=9606&id1=DOID:2977
Hyperoxaluria, Primary http://www.medical-language-international.com/index-umls.php?C0020501

Kidney Disease
http://www.medical-language-international.com/index-umls.php?C0022658
Hp1http://ghr.nlm.nih.gov/con

Kidney Diseases http://www.medical-language-international.com/index-umls.php?C0022658

Kidney Failure http://www.medical-language-international.com/index-umls.php?C0035078

Oxalosis http://www.medical-language-international.com/index-umls.php?C1298681

Peroxisomal Alanine:glyoxylate Aminotransferase Deficiency http://ghr.nlm.nih.gov/condition/primary-hyperoxaluria

D-Glycerate Dehydrogenase Deficiency http://ghr.nlm.nih.gov/condition/primary-hyperoxaluria

Hepatic Agt Deficiency http://ghr.nlm.nih.gov/condition/primary-hyperoxaluria

Glyceric Aciduria http://ghr.nlm.nih.gov/condition/primary-hyperoxaluria

Glycolic Aciduria http://ghr.nlm.nih.gov/condition/primary-hyperoxaluria

Oxaluria, Primary http://ghr.nlm.nih.gov/condition/primary-hyperoxaluria

dition/primary-hyperoxaluria

Hp2

Primary Hyperoxaluria

Abnormal Renal Function http://www.medical-language-international.com/index-umls.php?C0151746

Hyperoxaluria Primary

Kidney Dysfunction

Renal Anomaly

Renal Failure

Schizophrenia http://www.malacards.org/card/primary_hyperoxaluria

+ Ketamine enhances the expression of serine racemase and DAO.
https://www.wikigenes.org/e/ref/e/16716293.html

+ Research suggests that schizophrenia may result from a hypofunction of glutamatergic neurotransmission.
https://www.wikigenes.org/e/ref/e/12625025.html

+ The following DAO SNPs have been related to NSAID sensitivity:
- rs17740607
- rs2073440
- rs1801105
- rs2052129
- rs10156191
- rs1049742
- rs1049793

+ Catalytic activity:
- A D-amino acid + H2O + O2 = a 2-oxo acid + NH3 + H2O2

+ Cofactor:
- FAD (vitamin B-2 derivative).

+ Molecular function:
- Cofactor binding
- FAD binding
- Receptor binding
- D-amino-acid oxidase activity
- Protein dimerization activity

+ Biological process:
- Cellular nitrogen compound metabolic process
- D-alanine catabolic process
- Dopamine biosynthetic process
- D-serine metabolic process
- D-serine catabolic process
- Glyoxylate metabolic process
- Proline catabolic process
- Small molecule metabolic process

+ Subcellular location:
- Peroxisome

+ Cellular component:
- Cytosol
- Peroxisomal matrix
- Peroxisomal membrane
- Peroxisome

http://www.uniprot.org/uniprot/P14920

FUT2

+ **Overview for FUT2** *Galactoside 2-alpha-L-fucosyltransferase 2* (aka, secretor blood group Alpha-2-Fucosyltransferase). *FUT2*, **rs492602** (aka, A12190G), rs1047781 (aka, A12404T), rs281377 (aka, C12376T), **rs601338** (aka, G12447A), **rs602662** (G12758A)

- ***This is a big SNP for GI issues, especially if many IgA SNPs.***

http://en.wikipedia.org/wiki/FOLR2 - cite_note-entrez-3

- FUT2 expresses in the small intestine, mouth, colon, and lungs.

> **Our Two Cents**: FUT2 SNPs, plus a high number or severe IgA SNPs are associated with autoimmune conditions. At a minimum, homozygous FUT2 SNPs often result in poor GI mucosa health.

- FUT2 encodes the enzyme, galactoside 2-alpha-L-fucosyltransferase 2 inmans.
- This gene is part of the protein modification; protein glycosylation pathway.

+ FUT2 affects the Lewis blood group system, which is a classification of human blood based on the expression of glycoproteins called, Lewis (Le) antigens, on the surfaces of red blood cells or in body fluids, or both.

- The Lewis antigen system is intimately associated with the secretor system and ABO blood group system biochemically, though the genetic loci are not linked.

http://www.britannica.com/EBchecked/topic/338252/Lewis-blood-group-system

+ Synthesis of soluble A, B, H, and Lewis b blood group antigens in humans is determined by the secretor (Se) (FUT2) blood group locus.

http://www.uniprot.org/citations/7876235

+ The protein encoded by this gene is a golgi stack membrane protein that is involved in the creation of a precursor of the H antigen, which is required for the final step in the soluble A and B antigen synthesis pathway.

http://www.genecards.org/cgi-bin/carddisp.pl?gene=FUT2

Role of FUT2 in the gut

FUT2 is involved in the formation of an immune complex, H antigen. FUT2 forms a sugar-polymer known as oligosaccharide (a few monosaccharides covalently linked), which then becomes "food" for gut flora. FUT2 regulates the expression of certain "blood-group antigens", and as such, directly influence bowel flora concentrations. Approximately twenty percent of the population has FUT2 gene mutations.

Carriers of the FUT2 genetic mutations have been shown to have lower concentrations of the gut microbe, bifidobacterium; a key beneficial microbial colony that lines the gut. Carriers of FUT2 genetic mutations confer a greater predisposition towards Crohn's disease and elevated serum concentrations of vitamin B-12. These FUT2 "non-secretors" however appear to have a greater resistance towards certain pathogenic infections such as H Pylori, as well as protection against certain viruses, but there is conflicting data with the norovirus.

http://www.ncbi.nlm.nih.gov/pmc/articles/PMC3098274/

> **Our Two Cents**: Homozygous FUT2 SNPs -- Dietary adjustments may be key; grains, dairy, legumes, eggs, nuts, yeast, and soy are often "no-no's", but there are exceptions to eliminating one or more food categories.

- Check vitamin B-6, magnesium, and zinc levels as they are depleted, inter alia, by higher *oxalate* foods. Unfortunately, they are found in some healthy leafy greens, sweet potatoes, and more. **Great Plains** OATs test can shed some light on whether an oxalate issue exists and whether the oxalate issue is gut yeast driven (and too much vitamin C consumption), genetically driven, or simply dietary driven (e.g., juicing greens daily) and individual is depleted of nutrients for oxalate-breakdown enzymes to do their job.

http://www.lowoxalate.info

    - Recall that vitamin B-6 and zinc and magnesium are key nutrient cofactors for neurotransmitter production and breakdown enzymes.
- Besides oxalates, lectins are another source of "anti-nutrients" used by the plant kingdom to protect themselves from predators. They also pose a problem for many with FUT2 SNPs.
- Nightshades are another type of food that can cause issues, especially if autoimmune issues are present. RA is a classic example.
- Consider the Elimination Diet. A good starting point is the IFM Elimination Diet, plus eliminating legumes.

http://www.harpersvillefamilymedicine.com/attachments/File/Comprehensive_Elimination_Diet.pdf

- If autoimmune issues are in play and/or many IgA SNPs in addition to FUT2 SNPs, **Cyrex Labs** offers panels to determine which antibodies have been created (Array 5), what foods may be triggering (Array 3, 4 and 10), and what chemicals may be triggering (Array 11).

https://www.cyrexlabs.com

> **Our Two Cents**: For those that have difficulty giving up cow dairy, consider camel milk as a temporary transitional milk source (e.g., A2 beta-casein in camel milk, similar to breast milk, vs A1 beta casein in cow and goat milk). Desert Farms brand has milk and kefir. Amazon is now carrying Desert Farms.

+ Common polymorphisms in FUT2 define the vitamin B-12 plasma level quantitative trait locus 1 (B12QTL1). Vitamin B-12 is necessary for the formation of red blood cells, DNA synthesis during cell division, and maintenance of the myelin nerve sheath, among other functions.

+ Approximately fifteen percent of the population have homozygous FUT2 rs1047781 and/or rs602662 polymorphisms and are referred to as, "non-secretors of H antigen". Dr. Peter J. D'Adamo states the following:

- "The gene coding for your blood type lies on chromosome *9q34*. However, a separate gene (*FUT2*) actually interacts with your blood type gene, and determines your ability to *secrete* your blood type antigens into body fluids and tissues. A person can be either a *Secretor* or a *Non-secretor*. This is completely independent of whether you are a blood type A, B, AB, or O. This means that someone can be an A Secretor or an A Non-secretor, a B Secretor or a B Non-secretor etc. http://www.ncbi.nlm.nih.gov/pmc/articles/PMC2916706/
- A Secretor is defined as a person who secretes their blood type antigens into body fluids and secretions like the saliva in your mouth, the mucus in your digestive tract and respiratory cavities, etc. Basically what this means is that a secretor puts their blood type into these body fluids. A Non-secretor on the other hand puts little to none of their blood type into these same fluids. As a general rule, in the U.S. about 20% of the population are Non-secretors (with the remaining 80% being Secretors).
- As a generality, being a Non-secretor appears to be a potential health disadvantage. At a very basic level, being a Secretor and able to secrete blood type into your saliva, mucus, etc. allows for an added degree of protection against the environment, particularly with respect to microorganisms and **lectins**. An additional advantage of being a Secretor might be a generalized tendency to promote a stabilized, blood-type friendly intestinal bacterial ecosystem. Many of the friendly (probiotic) bacteria in your digestive system actually use your blood type as one of their preferential foods. Since Secretors have a steady supply of blood type in the mucus that lines the digestive tract; their bacteria have a much more constant food supply.
- Non-secretors also tend to have more digestive problems. Several studies have indicated that Non-secretors have a significantly higher rate of duodenal and peptic ulcers. Non-secretors are also less resistant to infection by Helicobacter pylori (a microbe associated with ulcers). It appears that this organism can colonize more readily and generate more inflammation in individual's incapable of secreting their blood type into the digestive tract."

http://www.dadamo.com/txt/index.pl?2000

- FUT2 non-secretors have a higher susceptibility to the following:
    - Norovirus
    - HIV infection
    - Colorectal carcinomas
    - Staphylococcus aureus

- Early tooth decay

https://www.wikigenes.org/e/gene/e/2524.html

http://chriskresser.com/is-a-low-carb-diet-ruining-your-health/

+Catalytic activity:

- GDP-beta-L-fucose + beta-D-galactosyl-(1->3)-N-acetyl-beta-D-glucosaminyl-(1->3)-beta-D-galactosyl-(1->4)-beta-D-glucosyl-(1<->1)-ceramide

+ Molecular function:
- Fucosyltransferase activity
- Galactoside 2-alpha-L-fucosyltransferase activity

+ Biological process:
- Carbohydrate metabolic process
- L-fucose catabolic process
- Fucosylation
- Protein glycosylation

+ Cellular component:
- Extracellular exosome
- Golgi apparatus
- Golgi cisterna membrane
- Integral component of membrane

http://www.uniprot.org/uniprot/Q10981

❖ **NOTE: The following four SNPs are related to the metabolism of histamine.**

HDC

+ <u>**Overview for HDC**</u> *Histidine decarboxylase* HDC, rs2073440 (aka, A1932C), rs17740607 (aka, C92T), rs854158 (aka, T10086C), rs16963486 (aka, T1657C)

- HDC catalyzes the biosynthesis of histamine from histidine.
- <u>**Our Two Cents**</u>: Look at histamine SNPs (this and next three listed) when dealing with skin issues and/or leaky gut (histamine inducing foods). Histamine SNPs may also be in play if allergies are present. DAO SNPs are also part of the "histamine picture", as are IgE SNPs.
- <u>**Our Two Cents:**</u> There is interplay between histamine SNPs (e.g., DAO, HDC, HNMT, HRH1, HRH4) and COMT, via catechol<u>amine</u> breakdown.

- Histamine regulates several physiologic processes, including neurotransmission, gastric acid secretion, inflammation, and smooth muscle tone.

+ Diseases associated with HDC are:
- Gilles de la Tourette syndrome
- Intestinal obstruction

http://www.genecards.org/cgi-bin/carddisp.pl?gene=HDC

+ Catalytic activity:
- L-histidine = histamine + CO_2

+ Cofactor:
- Pyridoxal 5' phosphate

+ Pathway biosynthesis:
- Histidine decarboxylase is part of the subpathway that synthesizes histamine from L-histadine, which is part of amine and polyamine biosynthesis.

+ Molecular function:
- Histadine decarboxylase activity
- Pyridoxal phosphate binding

+ Biological process:
- Catecholamine biosynthetic process
- Cellular nitrogen compound metabolic process
- Histamine biosynthetic process
- Histadine catabolic/metabolic process
- Small molecule metabolic process

+ Cellular component:
- Cytosol

http://www.uniprot.org/uniprot/P19113

HNMT

+ **Overview for HNMT** *Histamine N-methyltransferase HNMT*, rs1378321 (aka, A47507G), rs17583889 (aka, C29232A), rs6430764 (aka, C3616T), rs1050891 (aka, T939C). This gene encodes one of the two enzymes involved in the metabolism of histamine, and requires SAM to donate its methyl group. The other enzyme is diamine oxidase or DAO **(See above).**
- The HNMT enzyme is present in most body tissues, but not serum.
- HNMT inactivates histamine by N-methylation. This gene plays an important role in degrading histamine and in regulating the airway response to histamine.

+ Neurotransmitter activity of histamine in brain is controlled by N(tau)-methylation via histamine N-methyltransferase.

+ Histamine is metabolized by two major pathways: N(tau)-methylation via histamine N-methyltransferase and oxidative deamination via diamine oxidase.

+ HNMT encodes the first enzyme that is found in the cytosol and uses S-adenosyl-L-methionine (SAMe) as the methyl donor. The neurotransmitter activity of histamine is controlled by N(tau)-methylation as diamine oxidase and is not found in the central nervous system. A common genetic polymorphism affects the activity levels of this gene product in red blood cells. Multiple alternatively spliced transcript variants that encode different proteins have been found for this the HNMT gene.

http://www.genecards.org/cgi-bin/carddisp.pl?gene=HNMT

+ HNMT is decreased in the brain of people with Down syndrome and increased in individuals with Pick's disease.

https://www.wikigenes.org/e/gene/e/3176.html

+ HNMT plays the dominant role in histamine biotransformation in bronchial epithelium.

http://www.omim.org/entry/605238

- ❖ NOTE: Histamine is derived from the amino acid histidine that acts as a neurotransmitter mediating arousal and attention, as well as a pro-inflammatory signal released from mast cells in response to allergic reactions or tissue damage. Histamine is also an important stimulant of HCl secretion by the stomach through histamine H_2 receptors (HRH2).

+ Potent HNMT inhibitor:
- Diphenhydramine
- Amodiaquine
- Antifolate drug metropine
- Tacrine

+ Catalytic activity:
- S-adenosyl-L-methionine + histamine = S-adenosyl-L-homocysteine + N(tau)-methylhistamine.

+ Molecular function:
- Histamine N-methyltransferase activity

+ Biological process:
- Brain development
- Hyperosmotic response
- Methylation

- Positive regulation of protein targeting to mitochondrian
- Repiratory gaseous exchange
- Response to amine
- Response to cocaine
- Response to glucocorticoid
- Response to immobilization stress
- Response to interleukin-1
- Response to tumor cell

+ Subcellular location:
- Cytoplasm

+ Cellular component:
- Cytoplasm
- Extracellular exosome
- Neuron projection
- Nucleoplasm

http://www.uniprot.org/uniprot/P50135

+Diseases related to HNMT are:
- Nasal polyps
- Gastric ulcer
- Ulcerative colitis
- Septic shock
- Other intestinal diseases

HRH1

+ **Overview for HRH1** *Histamine receptor H1*, *HRH1*, rs347591 (aka, G11290122T), rs2067466 (aka, G57C), rs346070 (aka, T*1687C), rs901865 (aka, T-17C).

- The **H$_1$ receptor** is a histamine receptor belonging to the family of rhodopsin-like G-protein-coupled receptors. The receptor is activated by the biogenic amine, histamine (a nitrogenous compound).

+ HRH1 has been associated with multiple processes, including memory and learning, circadian rhythm, and thermoregulation. It is also known to contribute to the pathophysiology of allergic diseases, such as, atopic dermatitis, asthma, anaphylaxis, and allergic rhinitis. Multiple alternatively spliced variants, encoding the same protein, have been identified.

+ Histamine H1 receptors are Galphaq/11-protein-coupled receptors that mediate allergic responses. These receptors are expressed in a wide variety of tissues including the gastrointestinal tract, central nervous system, airway, and vascular smooth muscle cells, endothelial cells, chondrocytes, monocytes, neutrophils, dendritic cells, T and B lymphocytes, adrenal medulla, and the cardiovascular and genitourinary systems. H1 receptor activation induces a wide range of biological responses due to their widespread distribution.

+ In smooth muscle, H1 activation increases tension and the contractile response and in vascular endothelial cells receptor activation increases cell permeability.

+ In the adrenal medulla, histamine acting at H1 receptors stimulates both adrenalin and noradrenalin release. Furthermore, H1 activation induces prostacyclin and platelet-activating factor synthesis, promotes von Willebrand factor and nitric oxide release, liberates arachidonic acid from phospholipids, and causes vasodilation of capillaries and arterioles.

+ At a physiological level, H1 receptors are involved in a wide array of processes including thermal regulation, memory and learning, and control of the sleep-wake cycle, food intake, and emotional and aggressive behaviors. Histamine acting through the H1 receptor has proinflammatory effects and is involved in the development of various aspects of the antigen-specific immune response.

+ Activation of these receptors triggers maturation of dendritic cells and modulates the balance of Th1 and Th2 cells. H1 receptors are involved in the pathological process of allergy, including allergic rhinitis, atopic dermatitis, anaphylaxis and asthma, and also have a role in autoimmune diseases and malignancy.

http://www.genecards.org/cgi-bin/carddisp.pl?gene=HRH1

+ Drugs that are used to treat HRH1 dysfunction are:

Aceprometazine.	Alcaftadine
Alimemazine	Amitriptyline
Amoxapine	Antazoline
Aripiprazole	Asenapine
Astemizole	Azatadine
Azelastine	Benzatropine
Bepotastine	Betahistine
Bromodiphenhydramine	Brompheniramine
Buclizine	Butriptyline
Carbinoxamine	Cetirizine
Chlorcyclizine	Chloropyramine
Chlorphenamine	Chlorpromazine
Chlorprothixene	Cinnarizine
Citalopram	Clemastine
Clofedanol	Clozapine

Cyclizine	Cyproheptadine
Desipramine	Desloratadine
Dexbrompheniramine	Dimenhydrinate
Dimetindene	Diphenhydramine
Diphenylpyraline	Doxepin
Doxylamine	Emedastine
Epinastine	Escitalopram
Fexofenadine	Flunarizine
Histamine Phosphate	Hydroxyzine
Iloperidone	Imipramine
Isothipendyl	Ketotifen
Levocabastine	Loratadine
Loxapine	Maprotiline
Meclizine	Mepyramine
Mequitazine	Methdilazine
Methotrimeprazine	Mianserin
Mirtazapine	Nortriptyline
Olanzapine	Olopatadine
Orphenadrine	Paliperidone
Phenindamine	Pheniramine
Promazine	Promethazine
Propiomazine	Quetiapine
Risperidone	Tolazoline
Trazodone	Trimipramine
Tripelennamine	Triprolidine
Ziprasidone	Zuclopenthixol

http://www.uniprot.org/uniprot/P35367

+ Diseases related to HRH1 are:
- Mast cell
- Urticaria
- Pruritus
- Pronchospasm
- Edema
- Inflammation
- Anaphylaxis
- Asthma
- Autoimmune diseases
- Cancer
- Tachycardia
- Astrocytoma

https://www.wikigenes.org/e/gene/e/3269.html

+ Molecular function:
- G protein-coupled receptor activity
- Histamin binding
- Histamine receptor activity

+ Biological process:

Cellular response to histamine
- Eosinophil chemotaxis
- G protein-coupled receptor signaling pathway
- Inflammatory response
- Inositol phosphate-mediated signaling
- Memory
- Phospholipase C-activating G protein-coupled receptor signaling pathway
- Positive regulation of vasoconstriction
- Positive regulation of inositol triphosphate biosynthetic process
- Regulation of synaptic plasticity
- Regulation of synaptic transmission
- Regulation of vascular permeability
- Regulation of vasoconstriction
- Sensory perception of chemical stimulus
- Visual learning

+ Cellular component:
- Cytoplasm
- Integral component of plasma membrane
- Nucleoplasm
- Plasma membrane

http://www.uniprot.org/uniprot/P35367

HRH4

+ **Overview for HRH4** *Histamine receptor H4*, *HRH4*, rs11662595 (aka, A617G), rs4800573 (aka, G*2144A), rs16940765 (aka, T3537649C), rs901865 (aka, T-17C).

- The **H₄ receptor** is a histamine receptor that is predominantly expressed in haematopoietic cells.

+ Histamine is a ubiquitous messenger molecule released from mast cells, enterochromaffin-like cells, and neurons.

+ Its various actions are mediated by a family of histamine receptors that are a subset of the G protein-coupled receptor superfamily.

+ The protein is thought to play a role in inflammation and allergy responses.

+ H4 receptors are expressed at high levels in the gastrointestinal tract, spleen, thymus, medullary cells, bone marrow, and peripheral haematopoietic cells, including eosinophils, basophils, mast cells, T lymphocytes, leukocytes, and dendritic cells. Moderate expression levels are detected in the brain, heart, liver, and lung.

+ H4 receptors have an important role in inflammation, haematopoiesis, and immunity and their expression is regulated by stimuli such as IFN, TNF-alpha, and IL-6.

+ Activation of this receptor mediates chemotaxis of mast cells and eosinophils and also controls cytokine release from dendritic and T-cells. Furthermore, H4 receptors have a role in the differentiation of myeloblasts and promyelocytes.

http://www.genecards.org/cgi-bin/carddisp.pl?gene=HRH4

+ Molecular function:
- Histamine binding
- Histamine receptor activity

+ Biological process:
- Inflammatory response
- Negative regulation of adenylate cyclase activity
- Positive regulation of cytosolic calcium ion concentration
- Regulation of MAPK cascade
- Sensory perception of chemical stimulus

+ Cellular component:
- Cytosol
- Integral component of plasma membrane
- Plasma membrane

http://www.uniprot.org/uniprot/Q9H3N8

+ Drugs that are used to address HRH4 dysfunction are:
- Amitriptyline
- Amoxapine
- Chlorpromazin
- Clozapine
- Doxepin
- Histamine Phosphate
- Loxapine

- Mianserin
- Olanzapine

http://www.uniprot.org/uniprot/Q9H3N8

Section 2.3.7 – Related to Liver Detox
Section 2.3.7.1 – Figures Related to Liver Deto

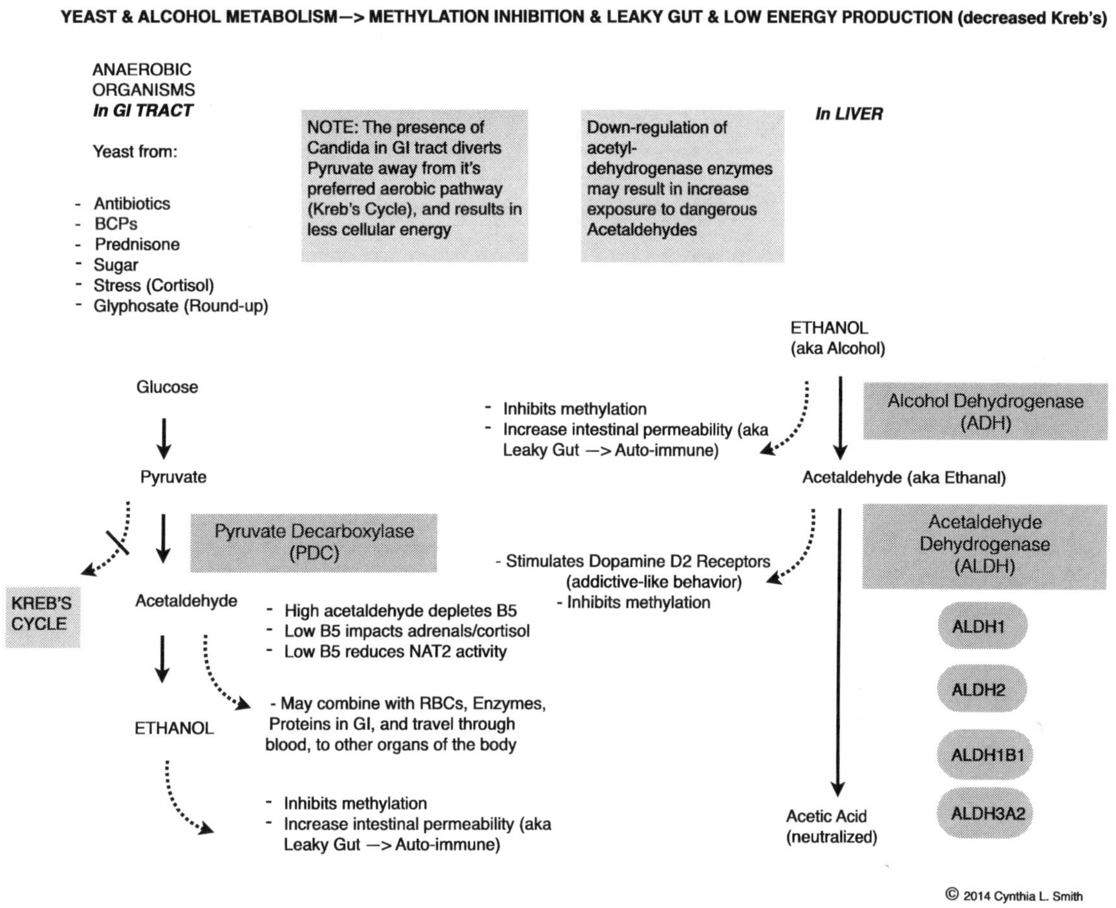

YEAST & ALCOHOL METABOLISM—> METHYLATION INHIBITION & LEAKY GUT & LOW ENERGY PRODUCTION (decreased Kreb's)

ANAEROBIC ORGANISMS *In GI TRACT*

Yeast from:
- Antibiotics
- BCPs
- Prednisone
- Sugar
- Stress (Cortisol)
- Glyphosate (Round-up)

NOTE: The presence of Candida in GI tract diverts Pyruvate away from it's preferred aerobic pathway (Kreb's Cycle), and results in less cellular energy

Down-regulation of acetyl-dehydrogenase enzymes may result in increase exposure to dangerous Acetaldehydes

In LIVER

Glucose → Pyruvate

Pyruvate Decarboxylase (PDC)

KREB'S CYCLE

Acetaldehyde
- High acetaldehyde depletes B5
- Low B5 impacts adrenals/cortisol
- Low B5 reduces NAT2 activity

ETHANOL
- May combine with RBCs, Enzymes, Proteins in GI, and travel through blood, to other organs of the body

- Inhibits methylation
- Increase intestinal permeability (aka Leaky Gut —> Auto-immune)

- Stimulates Dopamine D2 Receptors (addictive-like behavior)
- Inhibits methylation

- Inhibits methylation
- Increase intestinal permeability (aka Leaky Gut —> Auto-immune)

ETHANOL (aka Alcohol) → Alcohol Dehydrogenase (ADH) → Acetaldehyde (aka Ethanal) → Acetaldehyde Dehydrogenase (ALDH)

ALDH1
ALDH2
ALDH1B1
ALDH3A2

Acetic Acid (neutralized)

© 2014 Cynthia L. Smith

FIGURE 10 – Yeast/Alcohol Pathway

Alcohol Metabolism - 3 options to breakdown

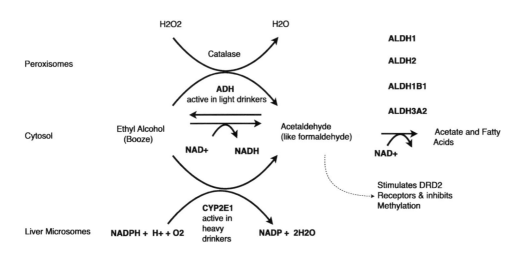

FIGURE 11 – Alcohol Breakdown Pathway

Section 2.3.7.2 – SNPs Related to Liver Detox

ADH1B

+ <u>**Overview for ADH1B**</u> *Alcohol dehydrogenase 1B*, ADH1B, rs17028834 (aka, A14973G), rs6413413 (aka, A178T), rs1042026 (aka, A19107G), rs2066702 (aka, A396C), rs1353621 (aka, A5998G), rs1229983 (aka, A7571G), rs2075633 (aka, A8575G), rs1789883 (aka, C11198T), rs1235416 (aka, C6652A), rs1041969 (aka, C8282A).

- The enzyme encoded by ADH1B is a member of the alcohol dehydrogenase family. Members of this enzyme family metabolize a wide variety of substrates, including ethanol, retinol, other aliphatic alcohols, hydroxysteroids, and lipid peroxidation products.

http://www.ncbi.nlm.nih.gov/gene/125

- Converts alcohol to acetaldehyde (ALDH then converts acetaldehyde to H_2O and CO_2).
- Previously, *ADH1B* was called *ADH2*. There are more genes in the family of alcohol and aldehyde dehydrogenase genes. These genes are now referred to as, ADH1A, ADH1C, ADH4, ADH5, ADH6 and ADH7.

http://www.ncbi.nlm.nih.gov/pubmed/3006456

+ ADH1B is related to alcohol sensitivity, which may be due to increased formation of acetaldehyde by persons with the atypical ADH1B.

+ ADH1B isoform was much higher in Japanese compared to Caucasians.

http://www.omim.org/entry/103720

+ Acetaldehyde is a colorless volatile liquid aldehyde obtained by oxidizing ethanol.

+ ADH1B may be related to alcohol allergies.

http://pubs.niaaa.nih.gov/publications/arh301/5-13.htm

+ Genetic differences in these enzymes may help to explain why some ethnic groups have higher or lower rates of alcohol-related problems. For example, one version of the ADH enzyme, called *ADH1B*2*, is common in people of Chinese, Japanese, and Korean descent but rare in people of European and African descent. Another version of the ADH enzyme, called *ADH1B*3*, occurs in fifteen to twenty-five percent of African Americans. These enzymes protect against alcoholism (14) by metabolizing alcohol to acetaldehyde very efficiently, leading to elevated acetaldehyde levels that make drinking alcohol unpleasant.

http://pubs.niaaa.nih.gov/publications/AA72/AA72.htm

+ *ADH1B* SNP rs1229984, causes a change from arginine to histidine. The 'typical' variant of this has been referred to as, ADH2(1) or ADH2*1, while the 'atypical' has been referred to as, e.g., ADH2(2), ADH2*2, ADH1B*47his, or ADH1B arg47-to-his. This SNP may be related to alcohol consumption with the atypical genotype having **reduced** risk of alcoholism.

http://www.ncbi.nlm.nih.gov/pubmed/7635462

+ rs2066702 – Risk allele A confers an increased risk for alcohol dependence in African Americans.

http://www.ncbi.nlm.nih.gov/pubmed/26036284

+ rs6413413 – Risk allele A confers decreased alcohol metabolic rate.

http://www.ncbi.nlm.nih.gov/pubmed/?term=rs6413413

+ rs17028834 – Risk allele C confers a higher risk of alcohol use and sub-site tumor from squamous cell carcinoma of the head and neck.

http://www.ncbi.nlm.nih.gov/pubmed/?term=rs17028834

+ rs1042026 – Risk allele C confers an association between higher alcohol intake and esophageal cancer.

http://www.ncbi.nlm.nih.gov/pubmed/?term=rs1042026+esopogeal+cancer

+ Catalytic activity:

- An alcohol + NAD+ = an aldehyde or ketone + NADH

+ Cofactor:
- Zinc

+ Molecular function:
- Alcohol dehydrogenase activity, zinc-dependant
- Zinc ion binding

+ Biological process:
- Ethanol oxidation
- Small molecule metabolic process
- Xenobiotic metabolic process

+ Cellular component:
- Cytoplasm
- Cytosol

http://www.uniprot.org/uniprot/P00325

ALDH2

+ **Overview for ALDH2** Alcohol dehydrogenase 2 family (mitochondrial), ALDH2, rs4767939 (aka, A7550G), rs4648328 (aka, A23443T), rs7311852 (aka, C25959G), rs4646778 (aka, C36438A), rs16941667 (aka, C45068T), rs671 (aka, G1369A), rs2238152 (aka, G15114T), rs2238151 (aka, T12488C), rs441 (aka, T29504C), rs968529 (aka, T35023C).

- The enzyme encoded by ALDH2 belongs to the aldehyde dehydrogenase family of enzymes that catalyze the chemical transformation of acetaldehyde to acetic acid (the last step in alcohol breakdown). Aldehyde dehydrogenase is the second enzyme of the major oxidative pathway of alcohol metabolism. Additionally, ALDH2 functions as a protector against oxidative stress.

https://www.ncbi.nlm.nih.gov/pubmed/15126281

+ Most Europeans have two major isozymes, while approximately fifty percent of Northeast Asians have one normal copy of the ALDH2 gene and one variant copy that encodes an inactive mitochondrial isoenzyme. In native Japanese, this variant ALDH2 gene encodes lysine instead of glutaminc acid at AA location 487 and therefore, encodes a product protein that is completely inactive in metabolizing acetaldehyde to acetic acid. Accordingly, Japanese individuals heterozygous or homozygous for the abnormal gene metabolize ethanol to acetaldehyde normally but metabolize acetaldehyde poorly and are thereby susceptible to certain adverse effects of alcoholic (i.e., ethanol-containing) beverages; these effects include the transient accumulation of acetaldehyde in blood and tissues; facial flushing, urticarial, systemic dermatitis, and alcohol-induced respiratory reactions such as rhinitis and asthma.

https://www.ncbi.nlm.nih.gov/pubmed/15126281

http://www.ncbi.nlm.nih.gov/gene?Db=gene&Cmd=ShowDetailView&TermToSearch=217

+ rs16941667 – Risk allele T confers a higher risk of gastric cancer in the case of higher alcohol consumption.

http://www.ncbi.nlm.nih.gov/pubmed/24633362

+ rs671 – Risk allele A confers a higher risk of colorectal cancer, coronary artery disease, pharyngeal cancer, benign prostate hyperplasia in the case of higher alcohol consumption.

http://www.ncbi.nlm.nih.gov/pubmed/26284938

+ rs2238151 – Risk allele T confers a higher risk of squamous cell carcinoma of the head and neck in the case of higher alcohol consumption.

http://www.ncbi.nlm.nih.gov/pubmed/?term=rs2238151

+ rs441 – Risk allele G confers a higher risk of Parkinson's disease with pesticide exposure.

http://www.ncbi.nlm.nih.gov/pubmed/26130061

+ Catalytic activity:
    - An aldehyde + NAD+ + H2O = a carboxylate + NADH

+ Pathway: ethanol degradation
  - This protein is involved in step two of the subpathway that synthesizes acetate from ethanol.
  - Aldehyde dehydrogenase, mitochondrial (ALDH2), Aldehyde dehydrogenase X, mitochondrial (ALDH1B1), Aldehyde

dehydrogenase family 3 member B1 (ALDH3B1), Aldehyde dehydrogenase family 3 member B2 (ALDH3B2).

This subpathway is part of ethanol degradation, which is part of alcohol metabolism.

+ Molecular function:
- Aldehyde dehydrogenase (NAD) activity
- Aldehyde dehydrogenase [NAD(P)+] activity
- Electron carrier activity

+ Biological process:
- Alcohol metabolic process
- Carbohydrate metabolic process
- Ethanol catabolic process
- Ethanol oxidation
- Neurotransmitter biosynthetic process
- Small molecule metabolic process
- Synaptic transmission
- Xenobiotic metabolic process

+ Cellular component:
- Mitochondrial matrix
- Extracellular exosome

http://www.uniprot.org/uniprot/P05091

ALDH3A2

+ **Overview for ALDH3A2** Aldehyde Dehydrogenase 3 Family, Member A2 (aka, Fatty Aldehyde Dehydrogenase, Microsomal Aldehyde Dehydrogenase, Long-chain-aldehyde dehydrogenase), *ALDH3A2*, rs72547575 (aka, A1157G), rs8069576 (aka, A23257G), rs72547566 (aka, C13996T), rs1800869 (aka, C17571G), rs72547564 (aka, G641A) encodes for the enzyme, fatty aldehyde dehydrogenase.

- Fatty aldehyde dehydrogenase isozymes play a major role in the detoxification of aldehydes generated by alcohol metabolism and lipid peroxidation. In other words, they function to remove toxic aldehydes.
- Fatty aldehyde dehydrogenase does this via catalyzing the oxidation of long-chain aliphatic aldehydes into fatty acids and acts on a variety of both saturated and unsaturated aliphatic aldehydes between six to twenty-four carbons in length, as well as dihydrophytal, a 20-carbon branched chain aldehyde.

https://www.ncbi.nlm.nih.gov/pubmed/9133646

> **Our Two Cents**: In addition to its role in alcohol detoxification, fatty aldehyde dehydrogenase plays an important role in the metabolism of catecholamines, specifically dopamine and epinephrine (to **vanillylmandelic acid**). Therefore, in addition to COMT, MAOA, and MAOB and associated DRD receptor SNPs, ALDH3A2 SNPs and their impact on catecholamine aldehydes should be considered when addresssing catecholamine breakdown issues. Similarly, additional aldehyde dehydrogenases are part of other neurotransmitter breakdown pathways. **(See FIGS. 8 and 9)** The following is a link to a good paper on the subject.

http://pharmrev.aspetjournals.org/content/59/2/125.long

+ Absence or insufficiency of ALDH3A2 protein products in mutant cells are known to cause abnormal metabolism of sphingosine 1-phosphate to ether-linked glycerolipids and the abnormal accumulation of lipid precursors.

+ Mutations in the gene cause Sjogren-Larsson syndrome (combination of severe mental retardation, spastic di- or tetraplegia, and congenital ichthyosis).

https://www.ncbi.nlm.nih.gov/pubmed/22633490

http://www.ncbi.nlm.nih.gov/pubmed/9829906

+ Other perturbations in aldehyde metabolism may manifest as type II hyperprolinemia, γ-hydroxybutyric aciduria, pyridoxine-dependent seizures, and hyperammonemia and hypoprolinemia.

http://pharmrev.aspetjournals.org/content/59/2/125.full

http://omim.org/entry/271980

http://www.omim.org/entry/266100

http://omim.org/entry/138250

+ Catalytic activity:

- An aldehyde + NAD+ + H2O = a carboxylate + NADH

+ Molecular function:
- 3-chloroallyl aldehyde dehydrogenase activity
- Aldehyde dehydrogenase (NAD) activity
- Aldehyde dehydrogenase [NAD(P)+] activity
- Long chain alcohol oxidase activity
- Long chain aldehyde dehydrogenase activity
- Medium chain aldehyde dehydrogenase activity

+ Biological process:
- Cellular aldehyde dehydrogenase process
- Central nervous system development

- Epidermis development
- Oxidation-reduction process
- Peripheral nervous system development
- Phytol metabolic process
- Sesquiterpenoid metabolic process

+ Cellular component:
- Endoplasmic reticulum membrane
- Extracellular exosome
- Integral component of membrane
- Intracellular membrane-bound organelle
- Mithochondrial inner membrane
- Peroxisome

http://www.uniprot.org/uniprot/P05091

ADP1

+ **<u>Overview for ADP1</u>** *Amiloride-sensitive amine oxidase* [copper-containing] (aka, AOC1 and DAO1), *ADP1/DAO*, rs1049793 (aka, C1933G), rs10156191 (aka, C47T)
- This gene encodes a metal-binding membrane glycoprotein that catalyzes the degradation of compounds such as putrescine, histamine, spermine, and spermidine, substances involved in allergic and immune responses, cell proliferation, tissue differentiation, tumor formation, and possibly apoptosis. Placental DAO is thought to play a role in the regulation of the female reproductive function.
- The encoded protein is inhibited by amiloride, a diuretic that acts by closing epithelial sodium ion channels.

http://www.genecards.org/cgi-bin/carddisp.pl?gene=AOC1

+Diseases associated with AOC1 include diabetic autonomic neuropathy, radiation proctitis, mast cell, mastocytosis, urticaria, allergic reaction, food allergy, bowel disease, short bowel syndrome, bladder carcinoma, multiple organ failure, nasal polyps, intestinal ischemia, and schizophrenia.

http://www.wikigenes.org/e/gene/e/26.html

+This gene is involved in:
    Tryptophan metabolism
    Tyrosine metabolism p.1 dopamine
    Histadine metabolism
    Histamine metabolism

Beta alanine metabolism

http://www.genecards.org/cgi-bin/carddisp.pl?gene=AOC1

+ Catalytic activity:

- Histamine + H2O + O2 = (imidazol-4-yl) acetaldehyde + NH3 + H2O2

+ Cofactor:

- Copper cation
- Calcium
- L-topaquinone

+ Molecular function:

- Calcium ion binding
- Cation channel activity
- Copper ion binding
- Diamine oxidase activity
- Drug binding
- Heparin binding
- Histamine oxidase activity
- Methylputrescine oxidase activity
- Primary amine oxidase activity
- Propane-1,3-diamine oxidase activity
- Protein complex binding
- Protein homodimerization activity
- Quinone binding
- Receptor activity
- Sodium ion channel
- Zinc ion binding

+ Biological process:

- Amine metabolic process
- Cellular response to azide
- Cellular response to copper ion
- Cellular response to copper ion starvation
- Cellular response to heparin
- Cellular response to histamine
- Oxidation-reduction process
- Response to antibiotic
- Response to drug

- Sodium ion transmembrane transport

+ Subcellular location
- Secreteted> extracellular space

+ Cellular component:
- Bicellular tight junction
- Extracellular exosome
- Extracellular space
- Peroxisome
- Plasma membrane

http://www.uniprot.org/uniprot/P19801

ACAT1

+ <u>**Overview for ACAT1**</u> *Acetyl-CoA acetyltransferase 1* (aka, Sterol O-acyltransferase 1), *ACAT1*, rs3741049 (aka, G22670A)

- The ACAT1 gene provides instructions for making an enzyme that is found in the energy-producing centers within cells (mitochondria). This enzyme plays an essential role in breaking down proteins and fats from the diet.

http://ghr.nlm.nih.gov/gene/ACAT1

+ ACAT1 catalyzes the formation of fatty acid-cholesterol esters, which are less soluble in membranes than cholesterol. Plays a role in lipoprotein assembly and dietary cholesterol absorption. In addition to its acyltransferase activity, it may act as a ligase.

www.uniprot.org

+ A deficiency in macrophage ACAT1 disrupts the efflux of cellular cholesterol.

http://atvb.ahajournals.org/content/25/1/128.full.pdf

+ Leptin accelerates cholesteryl ester accumulation in human monocyte-derived macrophages by increasing ACAT-1.

http://www.ncbi.nlm.nih.gov/pubmed/19625677

+ Defects in this gene are associated with the alpha-methylacetoaceticaciduria disorder, an inborn error of isoleucine catabolism characterized by urinary excretion of 2-methyl-3-hydroxybutyric acid, 2-methylacetoacetic acid, tiglylglycine, and butanone.

http://www.mybiosource.com/prods/Antibody/Monoclonal/ACAT1/datasheet.php?products_id=246376&att=5

+ It is suspected (Dr. Yasko) that those with ACAT1 SNPs may be prone to hosting increased clostridia species in the GI tract. Some individuals may need adenosyl B12 support.

+ Recall that Clostridium difficile toxin (CDT) is a binary actin-ADP-ribosylating toxin that causes depolymerization of the actin cytoskeleton and formation of microtubule-based membrane protrusions, which are suggested to be involved in enhanced bacterial adhesion and colonization of hypervirulent C. difficile strains.

http://www.jbc.org/lens/jbc/286/33/29356

+ Purified 2-methyleneglutarate mutase from Clostridium barkeri contains adenosylcobalamin (coenzyme B12) and varying amounts of oxygen-stable cob(II)alamin.

http://www.ncbi.nlm.nih.gov/pubmed/8382495

+ Catalytic activity:
    - Acyl-CoA + cholesterol = CoA + cholesterol ester

+ Molecular function:
    - Cholesterol binding
    - Cholesterol O-acyltransferase activity
    - Fatty-acyl-CoA binding
    - Sterol O-acyltransferase activity

+ Biological process:
    - Lipid metabolic process
    - Steroid metabolic process
    - Cholesterol metabolic process
    - Macrophage derived foam cell differentiation
    - Cholesterol storage
    - Cholesterol efflux
    - Very-low-density lipoprotein particle assembly
    - Cholesterol esterification
    - Cholesterol homeostasis
    - Positive regulation of amyloid precursor
    - Protein biosynthetic process

http://www.ebi.ac.uk/QuickGO/GProtein?ac=P35610

+ Cellular component:
    - Endoplasmic reticulum
    - Endoplasmic reticulum membrane
    - Cholesterol metabolic Integral component of membrane
    - Membrane

http://www.uniprot.org/uniprot/P35610

APOC3

+ **Overview for APOC3** *Apolipoprotein C3* (aka, Apolipoprotein C-III), *APOC3* rs5128 (aka, 3u386), rs4520 (aka, G34G)

- Apolipoprotein C3 is a protein that in humans is encoded by the APOC3 gene. Apolipoprotein C3 is a component of triglyceride-rich very-low-density lipoprotein (VLDL). Apolipoprotein C3 is also a component of high-density lipoproteins (HDL) in plasma. Apolipoprotein C3 plays a multifaceted role in triglyceride homeostasis. Intracellularly, it promotes hepatic very low-density lipoprotein 1 (VLDL1) assembly and secretion; extracellularly, attenuates hydrolysis and clearance of triglyceride-rich lipoproteins (TRLs). Impairs the lipolysis of TRLs by inhibiting lipoprotein lipase and the hepatic uptake of TRLs by remnant receptors.

http://www.uniprot.org/uniprot/P02656

+ Apolipoprotein C3 modulates triglyceride metabolism through inhibition of lipoprotein lipase, but is itself regulated by insulin, so that APOC3 represents a potential mechanism by which glucose metabolism may affect lipid metabolism. Unfavorable lipoprotein profiles and impaired glucose metabolism are linked to cognitive decline, and all three conditions may decrease lifespan. Associations between apolipoprotein C3 gene polymorphisms and impaired lipid and glucose metabolism are well established.

http://www.ncbi.nlm.nih.gov/pmc/articles/PMC2674932/

+ APOC3 inhibits lipoprotein lipase and hepatic lipase; it is thought to inhibit hepatic uptake of triglyceride - rich particles. Mendivil CO, Zheng C, Furtado J, Lel J, Sacks FM (Feb 2010).

http://atvb.ahajournals.org/content/30/2/239

+ An increase in Apolipoprotein C3 levels induces the development of hypertriglyceridemia. Recent evidences suggest an intracellular role for Apolipoprotein C3 in promoting the assembly and secretion of triglyceride-rich VLDL particles from hepatic cells under lipid-rich conditions.

http://www.ncbi.nlm.nih.gov/pubmed/20097930

http://www.snpedia.com/index.php/Rs5128

+ Molecular function:
- Cholesterol binding
- Enzyme regulator activity
- High-density lipoprotein particle receptor binding
- Lipase inhibitor activity
- Phospholipid binding

+ Biological process:
- Cholesterol efflux

- Cholesterol homeostasis
- Chylomicron remnant clearance
- G protein-coupled receptor signaling pathway
- High-density lipoprotein particle remodeling
- Lipoprotein metabolic process
- Negative regulation of cholesterol inport
- Negative regulation of high-density lipoprotein particle clearance
- Negative regulation of lipid catabolic process
- Negative regulation of lipid metabolic process
- Negative regulation of lipoprotein lipase activity
- Negative regulation of low-density lipoprotein particle clearance
- Negative regulation of receptor-mediated endocytosis
- Negative regulation of triglyceride catabolic process
- Negative regulation of of very-low-density lipoprotein particle clearance
- Negative regulation of of very-low-density lipoprotein particle remodeling
- Phospholipid efflux
- Phototransduction, visible light
- Regulation of Cdc42 protein signal transduction
- Retiniod metabolic process
- Reverse cholesterol transport
- Small molecule metabolic process
- Triglyceride catabolic process
- Triglyceride homeostatis
- Triglyceride metabolic process
- Very-low-density lipoprotein particle assembly

http://www.uniprot.org/uniprot/P02656

+ Subcellular location:
    - Secreted

+ Cellular component:
    - Chylomicron
    - Early endosome
    - Extracellular exosome
    - Extracellular region
    - Extracellular space
    - Intermediate-density lipoprotein particle
    - Spherical high-density

- Very low-density lipoprotein particle

http://www.uniprot.org/uniprot/P02656

+ Related diseases:

- Hyperalphalipoproteinemia 2 - A condition characterized by high levels of high-density lipoprotein (HDL) and increased HDL cholesterol levels.

http://www.ncbi.nlm.nih.gov/pubmed/2022742

CAT

+ **Overview for CAT** *Catalase*, *CAT* rs480575 (aka, A12175G), rs7943316 (aka, A5001T), rs11604331 (aka, A5298G), rs11032703 (aka, C14185T), rs17880442 (aka, C1476T), rs2300181 (aka, C21068T, rs10836235, (aka, C5233T), rs2420388 (aka, G35066A), rs7947841 (aka, 36209A), rs12272630 (aka, G6194C), rs2284365 (aka, T29502C), rs499406, (aka, T36470C), rs1049982 (aka, T5070C).

- The CAT gene provides instructions for making pieces (subunits) of an enzyme called, catalase. Four identical subunits, each attached (bound) to an iron-containing molecule, called a heme group, form the functional enzyme.
- Catalase is active in cells and tissues throughout the body, where it breaks down hydrogen peroxide (H_2O_2) molecules into oxygen (O_2) and water (H_2O). Hydrogen peroxide is produced through chemical reactions within cells. At low levels, it is involved in several chemical-signaling pathways, but at high levels it is toxic to cells. If hydrogen peroxide is not broken down by catalase, additional reactions convert it into compounds called reactive oxygen species that can damage DNA, proteins, and cell membranes.

http://ghr.nlm.nih.gov/gene/CAT

- Catalase is also utilized as part of the breakdown of alcohol to acetaldehyde.
+ At least 13 mutations in the CAT gene have been found to cause acatalasemia, a condition characterized by very low catalase activity. Many people with acatalasemia never have any related health problems, although the condition has occasionally been associated with open sores (ulcers) inside the mouth leading to the death of soft tissue (gangrene). Acatalasemia also appears to increase the risk of developing type II diabetes mellitus (the most common form of diabetes).
+ The mutations that cause acatalasemia occur in both copies of the CAT gene in each cell, and they reduce the activity of catalase to less than 10 percent of normal. A shortage of this enzyme can allow hydrogen peroxide to build up to toxic levels in certain cells. For example, hydrogen peroxide produced by bacteria in the mouth may accumulate in and damage soft tissues, leading to mouth ulcers and gangrene. A

buildup of hydrogen peroxide may also damage beta cells of the pancreas, which release a hormone called insulin that helps control blood sugar. Malfunctioning beta cells are thought to underlie the increased risk of type II diabetes mellitus in people with acatalasemia. It is unclear why some people have no health problems associated with a shortage of catalase activity.

+ CAT gene polymorphisms may also be associated with high blood pressure (hypertension), a skin condition called vitiligo, thinning of the bones (osteoporosis), and elevated levels of cholesterol and other fats (lipids) in the blood, which increase the risk of heart attack and stroke. However, it is unclear how polymorphisms in the CAT gene impact catalase activity and how changes in the activity of this enzyme might influence a person's risk of developing these diseases. A large number of genetic and lifestyle factors, many of which remain unknown, likely determine the risk of developing most common complex conditions.

http://www.ncbi.nlm.nih.gov/pubmed/25576221
http://www.ncbi.nlm.nih.gov/pubmed/24825136
http://www.ncbi.nlm.nih.gov/pubmed/24915010

+ Catalytic activity:
  - $2 H_2O_2 = O_2 + 2 H_2O$

+ Cofactor:
  - Heme
  - NADP(+)

+ Molecular function:
  - Aminoacylase activity
  - Anitoxidant activity
  - Catalase activity
  - Enzyme binding
  - Heme binding
  - Metal ion binding
  - NADP binding
  - Oxireductase activity, acting on peroxide acceptor
  - Protein homodimerization activity
  - Receptor binding

+ Biological process:
  - Aerobic respiration
  - Aging

- Cellular response to growth factor stimulus
- Cholesterol metabolic process
- Hemoglobin metabolic process
- Hydrogen peroxide catabolic process
- Negative regulation of apoptotic process
- Negative regulation of NF-kappaB transcription factor activity
- Nucleobase-containing small molecule metabolic process
- Osteoblast differentiation
- Positive regulation of cell division
- Positive regulation of NF-kappaB transcription factor activity
- Positive regulation of phosphatidylinositol 3-kinase signaling
- Protein homotetramerization
- Purine nuceobase metabolic process
- Purine nucleotice catabolic process
- Response to activity
- Response to cadmium ion
- Response to drug
- Response to Estradiol
- Response to ethanol
- Response to fatty acid
- Response to hypoxia
- Response to inactivity
- Response to insulin
- Response to L-ascorbic acid
- Response to lead ion
- Response to light intensity
- Response to ozone
- Response to phenylpropanoid
- Response to reactive oxygen species (ROS)
- Response to toxic substance
- Response to vitamin A
- Response to vitamin E
- Small molecule metabolic process
- Triglyceride metabolic process
- Ureteric bud development
- UV protection

+ Subcellular location:
- Peroxisome

+ Cellular component:
- Cytosol
- Endoplasmic reticulum
- Extracellular exosome
- Extracellular space
- Intermediate-density
- Focal adhesion
- Golgi apparatus
- Intracellular membrane-bounded organelle
- Lysosome
- Membrane Mitochondrial intermembrane space
- Peroxisomal matrix
- Peroxisomal membrane
- Peroxisome
- Plasma membrane

http://www.uniprot.org/uniprot/P04040

G6PD

+ **Overview for G6PD** *Glucose-6-phosphate 1-dehydrogenase G6PD*, rs1050757 (aka, A*357G), rs2230037 (aka, C1311T), rs72554664 (aka, G1478A), rs1050829 (aka, G6PD-A[+]), G6PD/IKBKG rs1050828 (aka, G6PD-A[-], rs5030868 (aka, G6PD-Mediterranean).

+ Glucose-6-phosphate dehydrogenase deficiency (G6PD deficiency), also known as, favism (after the fava bean), is an X-linked recessive genetic condition that predisposes to hemolysis (spontaneous destruction of red blood cells (RBC)) and resultant jaundice in response to a number of triggers, such as certain foods, illness, or medication. It is particularly common in people of Mediterranean and African origin. The condition is characterized by abnormally low levels of glucose-6-phosphate dehydrogenase, an enzyme involved in the pentose phosphate pathway that is especially important in the RBC. G6PD deficiency is the most common human enzyme defect. http://g6pddeficiency.org/wp/#.VhlkuMvY69Y

http://www.ncbi.nlm.nih.gov/pubmed/16225031

+ Carriers of the G6PD allele appear to be protected to some extent against malaria and in some cases dominant males have shown complete immunity to the disease.

+ Glucose-6-phosphate dehydrogenase (G6PD) deficiency is the most common human enzyme defect, being present in more than 400 million people worldwide. The global distribution of this disorder is remarkably similar to that of malaria, lending support to the so-called malaria protection hypothesis. G6PD deficiency is an X-linked, hereditary genetic defect due to mutations in the G6PD gene, which cause functional variants with many biochemical and clinical phenotypes. About 140 mutations have been described: most are single base changes, leading to aminoacid substitutions. The most frequent clinical manifestations of G6PD deficiency are neonatal jaundice, and acute haemolytic anaemia, which is usually triggered by an exogenous agent. Some G6PD variants cause chronic haemolysis, leading to congenital non-spherocytic haemolytic anaemia. The most effective management of G6PD deficiency is to prevent haemolysis by avoiding oxidative stress.

(See GSR below)

http://www.ncbi.nlm.nih.gov/pubmed/18177777

G6PD Deficiency:

+ A G6PD deficiency is the most common human enzyme defect, affecting more than 400 million people worldwide. G6PD is negatively regulated by acetylation on lysine. G6PD is a key enzyme in the pentose phosphate pathway and plays an essential role in the oxidative stress response by producing NADPH.

http://emboj.embopress.org/content/33/12/1304

+ Human glucose-6-phosphate dehydrogenase (G6PD) is $NADP^+$-dependent and catalyzes the first and rate-limiting step of the pentose phosphate shunt.

http://scripts.iucr.org/cgi-bin/paper?S0907444905002350

+G6PD deficiency was discovered during an investigation of hemolytic anemia occurring in some individuals treated for malaria with 6-methoxy-8-aminoquinoline drugs in 1926.

+ Ingesting fava beans has been known to induce hemolytic anemia in some individuals. Of note, Pythagoras warned his disciples not to eat beans. All patients with favism are G6PD deficient, but many individuals can eat fava beans without falling ill.

http://www.bloodjournal.org/content/111/1/16?sso-checked=true

+ G6PD deficiency may destroy red blood cells (RBC) and oxidatively-damage reduced glutathione. This is due to RBCs bursting because there is not enough reduced glutathione to protect them.

http://g6pddeficiency.org/wp/

+ In addition, iron overload may occur. In one study, the iron status of fifty Sicilian patients with G6PD deficiency under steady-state conditions was studied and compared to results with those for fifty control patients. Haemolysis and iron indices were considered to evaluate the iron balance. These patients could be considered to be at risk of iron overload as a result of increased bone marrow activity.

http://www.ncbi.nlm.nih.gov/pubmed/823727

+ Exposure to large amounts of naphthalene may damage or destroy red blood cells. Humans, particularly children, have developed hemolytic anemia after ingesting mothballs or deodorant blocks containing naphthalene. Those with glucose-6-phosphate dehydrogenase (G6PD) deficiency are especially susceptible. Trace amounts of naphthalene are produced by magnolias and specific types of deer, as well as the Formosan subterranean termite (likely as a repellant against ants), poisonous fungi, and nematode worms. Some strains of the endophytic fungus muscodor albus produce naphthalene among a range of volatile organic compounds, while muscodor vitigenus produces naphthalene almost exclusively.

http://www.medical-library.net/content/view/1698/41/

+ G6PD is a key enzyme in the pentose phosphate pathway and carbohydrate metabolism.

+ Some drugs to avoid if you have G6PD SNPs:

- Chloroquine
- Chlorpropamide (antidiabetic)
- Dabrafenib (regulates cell growth)
- Dapsone (antibiotic)
- Glibenclamide (antidiabetic)
- Glimepiride
- Glipizide (antidiabetic)
- Mafenide (sulfonamide-type antibiotic)
- **Methylene blue**
- Nalidixic acid (quinolone antibiotic)
- Nitrofurantoin (UTI antibiotic)
- Norfloxacin
- Pegloticase (gout treatment)
- Primaquine (malaria treatment)
- Probenecid (gout treatment)
- Quinine (analgesic, **tonic water**)
- Rasburicase (uric acid metabolizer)
- Nitrite
- Succimer (DMSA, chelator)
- **Sulfadiazine** (sulfonamide antibiotic)
- Sulfasalazine
- Sulfisoxazole
- **Vit C** (ascorbic acid)
- Sulfamethoxazole
- **Trimethoprim** (UTI antibiotic)

http://g6pddeficiency.org/wp/living-with-g6pd-deficiency/drugs-to-avoid-list/
https://www.pharmgkb.org/gene/PA28469#tabview=tab0&subtab=32

+ Aspirin has also been known to compromise red blood cells in G6PD deficient individuals.

http://www.g6pd.org/en/g6pddeficiency/researchpapers/Meloni_02.aspx

+ G6PD A*357G, rs1050757:

In a 2013 study, a total of 48 individuals (46.6%) were G6PD deficient, 83.3% of these carried G6PD 1311T/93C with enzyme activity ranging from 1.8 to 4.8 U gHb(-1). Three novel single-nucleotide polymorphisms (SNPs), rs112950723, rs111485003 and rs1050757, were found in the G6PD 3'-untranslated region (UTR). Strong association was observed between haplotype 1311T/93C and rs1050757G, which is located inside the 35 bp AG-rich region.

http://www.ncbi.nlm.nih.gov/pubmed/23389243?dopt=Abstract

+ 25% of the American population, 12% of the European population, 94% of the African population and 15% of the Asian population has a C allele for G6PD rs1050757. In an anecdotal study comprised of those who have shared their findings with Sterling Erdei, approximately 80% of people injured by a class of antibiotics called fluoroquinolones have the C allele as revealed via "Sterling's app" at www.mthfrsupport.com.

+ Fluoroquinolones have been labeled as a risk for folks with G6PD deficiency.

http://g6pddeficiency.org/wp/drug-detail/?g6pdid=3

G6PD G1478A rs72554644

+ The prevalence of G6PD variants in the Thai and Burmese populations:
    - Name of Variant: Kaiping
    - Thai population: 1 (0.3, 4.8%) [1:0]
    - Burmese population: 1 (0.5, 3.8%) [1:0]

http://www.biomedcentral.com/content/pdf/1475-2875-10-368.pdf

+ G6PD G6PD-A(+) rs1050829

Both males and females with this SNP are vulnerable to anemia.

+ G6PD G6PD-A(+) rs1050829

Both female and males are more vulnerable to hemolytic anemia.

http://www.ncbi.nlm.nih.gov/pmc/articles/PMC3382019/

http://www.ncbi.nlm.nih.gov/pmc/articles/PMC4077225/

+ Other genes that may impact G6PD deficient individuals are:
    - HFE; may confer a difficult time in metabolizing iron (hereditary hemochromatosis).
    - SOD2 A16V; SOD2 is iron binding, and therefore, when down-regulated, may contribute to an iron overload condition.
    - RAB6B; has been associated with elevated serum transferrin saturation.

+ Glucose-6-phosphate 1-dehydrogenase pathways affected:
    - Carbohydrate degradation
    - Pentose Phosphate pathway
    - D-ribulose 5-phosphate from D-glucose 6-phosphate (oxidative stage): step 1/3

http://www.uniprot.org/uniprot/P11413

+ Catalytic activity:
    - D-glucose 6-phosphate + NADP+ = 6-phospho-D-glucono-1,5-lactone + NADPH

+ Molecular function:
    - Glucose-6-phosphate dehydrogenase activity
    - Glucose binding
    - Identical protein binding
    - NADP binding

- Protein homodimerization

+ Biological process:
- Carbohydrate metabolic process
- Cellular response to oxidative stress
- Cholesterol biosynthetic process
- Cytokine production
- Erythrocyte maturation
- Gene expression
- Glucose 6-phosphate metabolic process
- Glucose metabolic process
- Glutathione metabolic process
- Lipid metabolic process
- NADPH regeneration
- NADP metabolic process
- Negative regulation of protein glutathionylation
- Oxidation-reduction process
- Pentose biosynthetic process
- Pentose-phosphate shunt
- Pentose-phosphate shunt, oxidative branch
- Regulation of neuron apoptotic process
- Response to ethanol
- Response to food
- Response to organic cyclic compound
- Ribose phosphate biosynthetic process
- Substantia nigra development
- Transcription initiation from RNA polymerase II promoter

+ Cellular component:
- Centrosome
- Cytoplasm
- Cytoplasmic side of plasma membrane
- Cytosol
- Extracellular exosome
- Intracellular membrane-bounded organelle
- Membrane

- Microtubule organizing center
- Nucleus

http://www.uniprot.org/uniprot/P11413

+ Associated disease:

> Anemia, non-spherocytic hemolytic, due to G6PD deficiency - deficiency of G6PD is associated with hemolytic anemia in two different situations. First, in areas in which malaria has been endemic, G6PD-deficiency alleles have reached high frequencies (1% to 50%) and deficient individuals, though essentially asymptomatic in the steady state, have a high risk of acute hemolytic attacks. Second, sporadic cases of G6PD deficiency occur at very low frequencies and usually present a more severe phenotype. Several types of NSHA are recognized. Class-I variants are associated with severe NSHA; class-II variants have an activity <10% of normal; class-III variants have an activity of 10% to 60% of normal; class-IV variants have near normal activity.

- The disease characterized by G6PD deficiency, presents with acute hemolytic anemia, fatigue, back pain, and jaundice. In most patients, an exogenous agent, such as, a drug, a food, or an infection, triggers the disease. Increased unconjugated bilirubin, lactate dehydrogenase, and reticulocytosis are markers of the disorder. Although G6PD deficiency can be life threatening, most patients are asymptomatic throughout their life.

http://www.ncbi.nlm.nih.gov/pubmed/1611091

MPO

+ **Overview for MPO** *Myeloperoxidase* MPO, rs2071409 (aka, A15067C), rs2759 (aka, A15191G), rs28730837 (aka, MMC7900T), rs7208693 (aka, G5479T).

- MPO is a heme protein synthesized during myeloid differentiation that constitutes the major component of neutrophil azurophilic granules.
- This enzyme produces hypohalous acids central to the microbicidal activity of neutrophils.

http://www.ncbi.nlm.nih.gov/gene/4353

- Myeloperoxidase is part of the host defense system of polymorphonuclear leukocytes (PMN). It is responsible for microbicidal activity against a wide range of organisms. PMN is

a category of white blood cells characterized by the presence of granules in their cytoplasm.
- In the stimulated PMN, MPO catalyzes the production of hypohalous acids, primarily hypochlorous acid in physiologic situations, and other toxic intermediates that greatly enhance PMN microbicidal activity.

+ MPOD Myeloperoxidase deficiency is a disorder characterized by decreased myeloperoxidase activity in neutrophils and monocytes that results in disseminated candidiasis.

http://www.uniprot.org/uniprot/P05164

+ Idiopathic edema, Alzheimer's disease, psoriasis, and vascular disease are related to the MPO gene.

http://www.genecards.org/cgi-bin/carddisp.pl?gene=MPO
http://ghr.nlm.nih.gov/gene/MPO
https://www.wikigenes.org/e/gene/e/4353.html

+ MPO could serve as a sensitive predictor for myocardial infarction in patients presenting with chest pain. Measuring both MPO and CRP provided added benefit for risk prediction than just measuring CRP alone.

+ Myeloperoxidase staining is still important in the diagnosis of myeloid sarcoma, contrasting with the negative staining of lymphomas.

+ Myeloperoxidase is the first, and so far the only, human enzyme known to break down carbon nanotubes. The concern here is that using nanotubes for targeted delivery of medicines would lead to an unhealthy buildup of nanotubes in tissues.

https://en.wikipedia.org/wiki/Myeloperoxidase

+ Inhibitors of MPO are:
- Azide and
- 4-aminobenzoic acid hydrazide

+ Cofactors:
- Calcium
- Heme b

+ Molecular function:
- Chromatin binding
- Heme binding
- Heparin binding
- Metal ion binding and
- Peroxidase activity

+ Biological process:

- Aging
- Defense response
- Defense response to fungus
- Hydrogen peroxide catabolic process
- Hypochlorous acid biosynthetic process
- Low-density lipoprotein particle remodeling
- Negative regulation of apoptotic process
- Negative regulation of growth of symbiont in host
- Oxidation-reduction process
- Removal of superoxide radicals
- Respiratory burst involved in defense response
- Response to food
- Response to gold nanoparticle
- Response to lipopolysaccharide
- Response to mechanical stimulus
- Response to oxidative stress and
- Response to yeast

http://www.uniprot.org/uniprot/P05164

NQO1

+ **Overview for NQO1** *NAD(P)H dehydrogenase [quinone] 1* NQO1, rs10517 (aka, C494+), rs1800566 (aka, C609T), rs689452 (aka, G13070C), rs689453 (aka, G13161A), rs34755915 (aka, G13528A), rs2917669 (aka, T6314C), rs1437135 (aka, T7706C)

- NQO1 is a member of the NAD(P)H dehydrogenase (quinone family) and encodes a 2-electron reductase (enzyme).
- This FAD binding protein forms homodimers and performs two-electron reduction of quinones to hydroquinones.

https://www.ncbi.nlm.nih.gov/pubmed/1657151

+ NQO1 enzyme expression can be induced by dioxin and inhibited by dicoumarol.

+ This protein's enzymatic activity prevents the one electron reduction of quinones that results in the production of radical species. The ubiquitin-independent p53 degradation pathway is regulated by NQO1. NQO1 stabilizes p53, protecting it from degradation. Individuals with decreased NQO1 expression/activity have reduced p53 stability, which may lead to resistance to drugs such as chemotherapeutics.

  ❖ **NOTE**: Tumor protein p53, also known as p53, cellular tumor antigen p53, phosphoprotein p53, the tumor suppressor p53. This homolog (originally thought to be, and often spoken of as, a single protein) is crucial in multicellular organisms where it prevents cancer formation, thus, functions as a tumor suppressor. As such, p53 has been described as "the guardian of the genome" because of its role in conserving stability by preventing genome mutation.

https://www.ncbi.nlm.nih.gov/pubmed/24379683

+ The enzyme is also involved in biosynthetic processes such as the vitamin K-dependent gamma-carboxylation of glutamate residues in prothrombin synthesis.

+ Catalytic activity:

- NAD(P)H + a quinone = NAD(P)+ + a hydroquinone

+ Cofactor:

- FAD

+ Molecular function:
- Cytochrome-b5 reductase activity, acting on NAD(P)H
- Identical protein binding
- NAD(P)H dehydrogenase (quinone) activity
- Poly(A) RNA binding
- Superoxide dismutase activity

+ Biological process:
- Aging
- Cellular nitrogen compound metabolic process
- Negative regulation of catalytic activity
- NO biosynthetic process
- Positive regulation of neuron apoptotic process
- Regulation of cellular AA metabolic process
- Response to ethanol
- Response to estradiol
- Response to nutrients
- Small molecule metabolic process
- Synaptic transmission, cholinergic
- Xenobiotic metabloc process

+ Cellular component:
- Cytoploasm
- Cytosol
- Extracellular exosome
- Neuronal cell body

http://www.uniprot.org/uniprot/P15559#section_comments

Neurotransmitters
Chapter 3

Section 3.1 – Neurotransmitter Pathway Figures

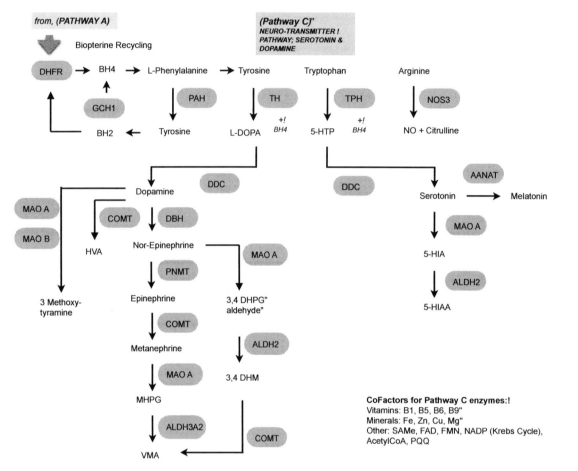

FIGURE 6 – Neurotransmitter Pathway

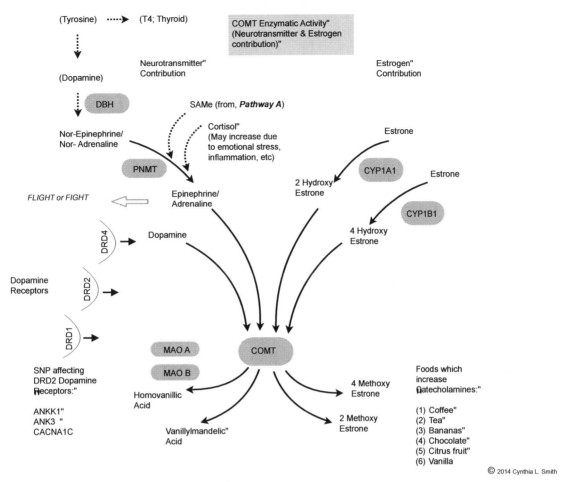

FIGURE 9 – COMT Pathway

Section 3.2 – Neurotransmitter SNPs

AANAT

+ Overview for AANAT *Serotonin N-acetyltransferase* (aka, aralkylamine N-acetyltransferase, AA-NAT) *AANAT*, rs11077820 (aka, C10236T), rs28697191 (aka, C735T), rs3760138 (aka, G18677AT)

- AANAT encodes an enzyme serotonin N-acetyltransferase and is the key regulator of day-night cycle (circadian rhythm).
- Catalyzes the N-acetylation of serotonin into N-acetylserotonin, a step in the synthesis of melatonin.
- Serotonin N-acetyltransferase controls the night/day rhythm in melatonin production in the pineal gland. (Recall that melatonin is essential for the function of the circadian clock that influences activity and sleep.)

http://www.ncbi.nlm.nih.gov/gene/15

+ In a study, there appeared to be a link between genetic variability in the AANAT gene with susceptibility to major depression (MD). The study's results support the hypothesis that the melatonin-signaling pathway and circadian clock mechanisms may contribute to the pathophysiology of MD.

http://www.ncbi.nlm.nih.gov/pubmed/20459461

+ Catalytic activity:

- Acetyl-CoA + a 2-arylethylamine = CoA + an N-acetyl-2-arylethylamine

+ Molecular function:

- Aralkylamine N-acetyltransferase activity
- Arylamine N-acetyltransferase activity

+ Biological process:

- Cellular nitrogen compound metabolic process
- Cellular response to cAMP
- Circadian rhythm
- Indolalkylamine biosynthetic process
- Melatonin biosynthetic process
- N-terminal protein amino acid acetylation
- Response to calcium ion
- Response to copper ion
- Response to corticosterone

- Response to cytokine
- Response to insulin
- Response to light stimulus
- Response to prostaglandin E
- Response to zine
- Small molecule metabolic process

+ Subcellular component:
- Cytoploasm

+ Cellular component:
- Cytosol
- Perinuclear region of cytoplasm

http://www.uniprot.org/uniprot/Q16613

+ Associated disease:
- Delayed sleep phase syndrome - A circadian rhythm sleep disorder characterized by sleep-onset insomnia and difficulty in awakening at the desired time. Patients with DSPS have chronic difficulty in adjusting their sleep-onset and wake-up times to occupational, school, and social activities.

http://www.ncbi.nlm.nih.gov/pubmed/12736803

ADH1B

+ **Overview for ADH1B** *Alcohol dehydrogenase 1B*, ADH1B, rs17028834 (aka, A14973G), rs6413413 (aka, A178T), rs1042026 (aka, A19107G), rs2066702 (aka, A396C), rs1353621 (aka, A5998G), rs1229983 (aka, A7571G), rs2075633 (aka, A8575G), rs1789883 (aka, C11198T), rs1235416 (aka, C6652A), rs1041969 (aka, C8282A).

- The enzyme encoded by ADH1B is a member of the alcohol dehydrogenase family. Members of this enzyme family metabolize a wide variety of substrates, including ethanol, retinol, other aliphatic alcohols, hydroxysteroids, and lipid peroxidation products.

http://www.ncbi.nlm.nih.gov/gene/125

- Converts alcohol to acetaldehyde (ALDH then converts acetaldehyde to H_2O and CO_2).
- Previously *ADH1B* was called *ADH2*. There are more genes in the family of alcohol and aldehyde dehydrogenase genes. These

genes are now referred to as ADH1A, ADH1C, ADH4, ADH5, ADH6 and ADH7.

http://www.ncbi.nlm.nih.gov/pubmed/3006456

+ See page 219 for full write-up

ALDH2

+ Overview for ALDH2 *Alcohol dehydrogenase 2 family (mitochondrial)*, ALDH2, rs4767939 (aka, A7550G), rs4648328 (aka, A23443T), rs7311852 (aka, C25959G), rs4646778 (aka, C36438A), rs16941667 (aka, C45068T), rs671 (aka, G1369A), rs2238152 (aka, G15114T), rs2238151 (aka, T12488C), rs441 (aka, T29504C), rs968529 (aka, T35023C).

- The enzyme encoded by ALDH2 belongs to the aldehyde dehydrogenase family of enzymes that catalyze the chemical transformation of acetaldehyde to acetic acid (the last step in alcohol breakdown). Aldehyde dehydrogenase is the second enzyme of the major oxidative pathway of alcohol metabolism. Additionally, ALDH2 functions as a protector against oxidative stress.

https://www.ncbi.nlm.nih.gov/pubmed/15126281

+ See page 220 for full write-up

ALDH3A2

+ Overview for ALDH3A2 *Aldehyde dehydrogenase 3 family, member A2* (aka, fatty aldehyde dehydrogenase, microsomal aldehyde dehydrogenase, long-chain-aldehyde dehydrogenase), ALDH3A2, rs72547575 (aka, A1157G), rs8069576 (aka, A23257G), rs72547566 (aka, C13996T), rs1800869 (aka, C17571G), rs72547564 (aka, G641A) encodes for the enzyme, fatty aldehyde dehydrogenase.

- Fatty aldehyde dehydrogenase isozymes play a major role in the detoxification of aldehydes generated by alcohol metabolism and lipid peroxidation. In other words, they function to remove toxic aldehydes.
- Fatty aldehyde dehydrogenase does this via catalyzing the oxidation of long-chain aliphatic aldehydes into fatty acids and acts on a variety of both saturated and unsaturated aliphatic aldehydes between six to twenty-four carbons in length, as well as dihydrophytal, a 20-carbon branched chain aldehyde.

https://www.ncbi.nlm.nih.gov/pubmed/9133646

> **Our Two Cents**: In addition to its role in alcohol detoxification, fatty aldehyde dehydrogenase plays an important role in the metabolism of catecholamines, specifically dopamine and epinephrine (to vanillylmandelic acid). Therefore, in addition to COMT, MAOA and MAOB, and associated DRD receptor SNPs, ALDH3A2 SNPs and their impact on catecholamine aldehydes should be considered when addresssing catecholamine breakdown issues. Similarly, additional aldehyde dehydrogenases are part of other neurotransmitter breakdown pathways. **(See FIGS. 8 and 9)** The following is a link to a good paper on the subject.

http://pharmrev.aspetjournals.org/content/59/2/125.long

+ See page 222 for full write-up

ANK3

+ Overview for ANK3 *Ankyrin 3, nodes of Ranvier (Ankyrin G)*, ANK3, rs11599164 (aka, C666301A), rs10994397 (aka, G219161A), rs10994336 (aka, G318473A), rs9804190 (aka, G658454A), rs1938526 (aka, T197902C), rs10761482 (aka, T62085337C)

- Ankyrins are a family of proteins that are believed to link the integral membrane proteins to the underlying spectrin-actin cytoskeleton.
- Ankyrins play key roles in activities such as cell motility, activation, proliferation, contact, and the maintenance of specialized membrane domains. Multiple isoforms of ankyrin with different affinities for various target proteins are expressed in a tissue-specific, developmentally regulated manner. Most ankyrins are typically composed of three structural domains: an amino-terminal domain containing multiple ankyrin repeats; a central region with a highly conserved spectrin binding domain; and a carboxy-terminal regulatory domain which is the least conserved and subject to variation. Ankyrin 3 is an immunologically distinct gene product from ankyrins 1 and 2, and was originally found at the axonal initial segment and nodes of Ranvier of neurons in the central and peripheral nervous systems.

http://www.genecards.org/cgi-bin/carddisp.pl?gene=ANK3

+ In skeletal muscle, ankyrin 3 is required for costamere localization of DMD and betaDAG1 (by similarity). May participate in the maintenance/targeting of ion channels and cell adhesion molecules at the nodes of Ranvier and axonal initial segments. Ankyrin 3 regulates KCNA1 channel activity in function of dietary Mg^{2+} levels and thereby contributes to the regulation of renal Mg^{2+} reabsorption.

+ Genetic variations in ANK3 may be associated with autism spectrum disorders susceptibility. https://www.ncbi.nlm.nih.gov/pubmed/?term=23390136

+ Molecular function:
- Cadherin binding
- Cytoskelton
- Ion channel binding
- Protein binding, bridging
- Spectrin binding
- Structural constituent of cytoskeleton

+ Biological process:
- Axon guidance
- Axonogenesis
- Cellular response to magnesium ion
- Cytoskeletal anchoring at plasma membrane
- Establishment of protein localization
- Golgi to plasma membrane transport
- Magnesium ion homeostasis
- Maintenance of protein location in plasma membrane
- Membrane assembly
- Mitiotic cytokinesis
- Negative regulation of delayed rectifier potassium channel activity
- Neuronal action potential
- Plasma membrane organization
- Positive regulation of gene expression
- Positive regulation of membrane depolarization during cardiac muscle cell action potential
- Positive regulation of membrane potential
- Positive regulation of sodium ion transmembrane transporter activity
- Positive regulation of sodium ion transport

- Protein localization to plasma membrane
- Protein targeting to plasma membrane
- Regulation of potassium ion transport
- Signal transduction
- Synapse organization

+ Subcellular location:
- Cytoploasm > cytoskeleton
- Cell projection > axon
- Cell membrane > sarcolemma
- Cell junction > synapse > postsynaptic cell membrane
- Lysosome

+ Cellular component:
- Axon initial segment
- Basolateral plasma membrane
- Cell surface
- Costamere
- Endoplasmic reticulum
- Golgi apparatus
- Intercalated disc
- Lateral plasm membrane
- Lysosome
- Node of Ranvier
- Paranode region of axon
- Plasma membrane
- Postsynaptic membrane
- Sarcolemma
- Spectrin-associated cytoskeleton
- T-tubule

http://www.uniprot.org/uniprot/Q12955

+ Associated disease:
- Mental retardation - A homozygous deletion in ANK3 predicted to result in frameshift and premature truncation, has been shown to be the cause of moderate intellectual disability, an ADHD-like phenotype, and behavioral problems in a consanguineous family. A disorder characterized by significantly below-average general

intellectual functioning associated with impairments in adaptive behavior and manifested during the developmental period. MRT37 patients manifest delayed global development with speech delay, hypotonia, spasticity, and a sleep disorder. Severe behavioral abnormalities include aggression, hyperactivity, and teeth grinding.

http://www.omim.org/entry/615493

ANKK1

+ **Overview for ANKK1** *Ankyrin repeat and kinase domain containing 1* (aka, protein kinase PKK2 or sugen kinase 288 (SgK288))**,** ANKK1, rs1800497 (aka, E713K), rs11604671 (aka, G318R)

- Ankyrins are a family of proteins that are believed to link the integral membrane proteins to the underlying spectrin-actin cytoskeleton.
- ANKK1 rs1800497 is a SNP that causes an amino acid substitution within the 11th of 12 ankyrin repeats of ANKK1 (Glu713Lys of 765 residues). This polymorphism, which is commonly referred to as Taq1A, is located in the coding region of the ANKK1 gene that controls the synthesis of dopamine in the brain.

❖ **NOTE**: DRD2/ANKK1-TaqIA is also refered to the "A1-allele".

The A1 allele is associated with increased activity of striatal L-amino acid decarboxylase. Changes in ANKK1 activity may provide an alternative explanation for previously described associations between the DRD2 Taq1A RFLP (i.e., A1-allele) and neuropsychiatric disorders such as addiction.

https://www.ncbi.nlm.nih.gov/pubmed/15146457

- The A1 allele of the human dopamine D2 receptor gene (DRD2) is associated with a low density of D2 dopamine receptors in the striatum.

https://www.ncbi.nlm.nih.gov/pubmed/15900211

+ The A1-allele of the DRD2/ANKK1-TaqIA gene has been associated with addictive disorders, obesity, and with the performance in executive functions.

http://www.ncbi.nlm.nih.gov/pubmed/22848508

+Other disorders associated with the A1-allele include: anti-social personality disorder, borderline personality disorder, dissocial personality disorder, schizoid/avoidant behavior, and Hep C risk increase due to persistant drug use.

https://www.ncbi.nlm.nih.gov/pubmed/21070510

https://www.ncbi.nlm.nih.gov/pubmed/18669994

https://www.ncbi.nlm.nih.gov/pubmed/20575771

+ Catalytic activity:
- ATP + a protein = ADP + a phosphoprotein

+ Molecular function:
- ATP binding
- Protein serine/threonine kinase activity

http://www.uniprot.org/uniprot/Q8NFD2

CACNA1C

+ **Overview for CACNA1C** *Voltage-dependent L-type calcium channel subunit alpha-1C,* CACNA1C, rs216013 (aka, A2729632G), rs2159100 (aka, C271442T), rs1006737 (aka, G115699A), rs2302729 (aka, T709021C)

- Voltage-sensitive calcium channels (VSCC) mediate the entry of calcium ions into excitable cells and are also involved in a variety of calcium-dependent processes, including muscle contraction, hormone or neurotransmitter release, gene expression, cell motility, cell division, and cell death. The isoform alpha-1C gives rise to L-type calcium currents. Long-lasting (L-type) calcium channels belong to the 'high-voltage activated' (HVA) group—excitatory. Calcium channels containing the alpha-1C subunit play an important role in excitation-contraction coupling in the heart. The various isoforms display marked differences in the sensitivity to DHP compounds. Binding of calmodulin or CABP1 at the same regulatory sites results in an opposit effects on the channel function.
- **NOTE**: L-type calcium channels are blocked by dihydropyridines (DHP), phenylalkylamines, benzothiazepines, and by omega-agatoxin-IIIA (omega-Aga-IIIA). They are however, insensitive to omega-conotoxin-GVIA (omega-CTx-GVIA) and omega-agatoxin-IVA (omega-Aga-IVA).

http://www.ncbi.nlm.nih.gov/pubmed/9607315

+ Molecular function:
- Alpha actinin binding
- Calmodulin binding

- High voltage-gated calcium channel activity
- Metal ion binding
- Voltage-gated calcium channel activity

+ Biological process:
- Adult walking behavior
- Axon guidance
- Calcium ion-dependant exocytosis
- Calcium ion import
- Calcium ion transport into cytosol
- Calcium-mediated signaling using extracellular calcium source
- Energy reserve metabolic process
- Glucose homeostasis
- Growth hormone secretion
- Insulin secretion
- Ion transmembrane transport
- Membrane depolarization during action potential
- Positive regulation of cytosolic calcium ion concentration
- Regulation of blood pressure
- Regulation of cardiac muscle contraction
- Regulation of organ growth
- Regulation of vasoconstriction
- Smooth muscle contraction involved in micturition
- Synaptic transmission
- Visual learning

+ Subcellular location:
- Membrane; Multipass membrane protein
- Cell membrane

http://www.uniprot.org/uniprot/Q12955

+ Cellular component:
- Caveolar macromolecular signaling complex
- Cytoplasm
- Cytosol
- Dendritic shaft
- Integral component of membrane

- Neuronal cell body
- Plasma membrane
- Postsynaptic density
- T-tubule
- Voltage gated calcium channel complex
- Z disc

http://www.uniprot.org/uniprot/Q13936

+ Associated disease:

- Timothy syndrome – A disorder characterized by multiorgan dysfunction including, lethal arrhythmias, webbing of fingers and toes, congenital heart disease, immune deficiency, intermittent hypoglycemia, cognitive abnormalities, and autism.

http://www.ncbi.nlm.nih.gov/pubmed/15454078

- Brugada syndrome 3 - A heart disease characterized by the association of Brugada syndrome with shortened QT intervals. Brugada syndrome is a tachyarrhythmia characterized by right bundle branch block and ST segment elevation on an electrocardiogram (ECG). It can cause the ventricles to beat so fast that the blood is prevented from circulating efficiently in the body. When this situation occurs, the individual will faint and may die in a few minutes if the heart is not reset.

http://www.ncbi.nlm.nih.gov/pubmed/17224476

COMT

+ **Overview for COMT/TXNRD2** *Catechol-O-methyltransferase, COMT* **rs769224 (aka, -61 P199P)**, rs2239393 (aka, A 26166G), **rs6269 (aka, A-1324G)**, rs933271 (aka, A2953G), rs174675 (aka, A309G), rs1544325 (aka, A7406G), rs4646316 (aka, C27870T), rs174696 (aka, C28914T), rs174699, (aka, C30196T), rs9332377 (aka, C31430T). rs8192488 (aka, C438T), rs165599 (aka, G*522A), rs739368 (aka, G14834A), rs165656 (aka, G24601C), rs165774 (aka, G28299A0, **rs4633 (aka, H62H)**, rs5993883 (aka, T13376G), rs4646312 (aka, T24075C), rs740601 (aka, T26501G), **rs4680 (aka, V158M)**. COMT/TXNRD2 rs737866 (aka, A4251G), rs2020917 (aka, C4622T), rs737865 (aka, T4239C).

- Catechol-*O*-methyltransferase is encoded by COMT and is one of several enzymes that degrade catecholamines such as dopamine, epinephrine, and norepinephrine.

http://www.ncbi.nlm.nih.gov/pubmed/1572656

- Catechol-O-methyltransferase also plays a role in estrogen breakdown.
- ❖ **NOTE**: Recall that GABA may be called into action to keep high dopamine levels in-check. As a result, GABA levels may be low in those with COMT V158M/H62H homozygous SNPs. (GABA is our calming neurotransmitter). The sympathetic nervous system may dominate over parasympathetic nervous system in those with COMT V158M/H62H homozygous SNPs, so stress management techniques (e.g., life style and dietary changes to remove extraneous inflammatory influences, jettisoning toxic relationships, Heart Math techniques, yoga, etc.) are helpful. Adrenal support (e.g., glandulars, vitamin B-5 and vitamin B-6, adpatogens, etc.) may also be key to reversing affects of stress/sympathetic nervous system tendency conferred by long-term, poor catecholamine breakdown due to COMT V158M/H62H homozygous SNPs.

+ See page 128 for full write-up

CSAD

+ <u>Overview for CSAD</u> *Cysteine Sulfinic Acid Decarboxylase* (aka, Cysteine-Sulfinate Decarboxylase), CSAD rs1006959 (aka, C13258T), rs11170453 (aka, C15829T), rs2272306 (aka, C25411T), rs12161793 (aka, T7219C), rs2293429 (aka, T5791G), encodes the enzyme, Cysteine-Sulfinate Decarboxylase.

- CSAD encodes a member of the group 2-decarboxylase family. A similar protein in rodents plays a role in multiple biological processes as the rate-limiting enzyme in taurine biosynthesis, catalyzing the decarboxylation of cysteinesulfinate to hypotaurine.

http://www.genecards.org/cgi-bin/carddisp.pl?gene=CSAD&search=CSAD

- ❖ **NOTE**: Taurine is a sulfur containing amino acid; it also functions with glycine and GABA as an inhibitory neurotransmitter. Taurine is found in many areas of our body, including our central nervous system, skeletal muscle, and in even greater concentration, in our heart, and brain. As a powerful inhibitory neurotransmitter, one of taurine's uses has been that of an anticonvulsant. These anticonvulsant effects come from its ability to stabilize nerve cell membranes, which prevents the erratic firing of nerve cells. Therefore, it is also used to calm excitable tissues such as, the heart, skeletal muscles, and central nervous system.

+ See page 125 for full write-up

DBH

+ <u>Overview for DBH</u> *Dopamine-β-hydroxylase,* DBH, rs1611115, rs77905 (aka, A1410G), rs1108580 (aka, A486G), rs1108581 (aka, A8757G), rs1611123 (aka, C12599T), rs1611125 (aka, C12828T), rs2283123 (aka, C18813T), rs129882 (aka, C27185T), rs1611114 (aka, C3719T), rs5324 (aka, G12174A), rs1541332, (aka, G15032A), rs3025382 (aka, G5837A), rs5320 (aka, G631A), rs5321 (aka, G717C), rs4531 (aka, G952T), rs2519152 (aka, T13150C), rs2519154 (aka, T15791C), rs2797853 (aka, T16031C), rs2097628 (aka, T2145C), rs2007153 (aka, T7335C), rs2519155 (aka, T8114C), rs2873804 (aka, T9160C)

- Encodes the neurotransmitter synthesizing enzyme *Dopamine-β-hydroxylase,* which catalyzes the formation of norepinephrine from dopamine, ultimately leading to the formation of epinephrine (aka, adrenaline) by the enzyme phenylethanolamine-N-methyl transferase (PNMT) in the mammalian tissues and serum.

http://www.ncbi.nlm.nih.gov/pmc/articles/PMC3614808/

- ❖ **NOTE**: Norepinephrine plays an important role in the autonomic nervous system, which controls involuntary body processes such as, the regulation of blood pressure and body temperature.

+ At least six mutations in the DBH gene have been found to cause dopamine β-hydroxylase deficiency. The most common mutation (usually written as IVS1+2T>C) interferes with the normal processing of dopamine β-hydroxylase. As a result of this mutation, an abnormally short, nonfunctional version of the enzyme is produced. A lack of functional dopamine β-hydroxylase leads to a shortage of norepinephrine, which causes difficulty with regulating blood pressure and other autonomic nervous system problems seen in dopamine β-hydroxylase deficiency.

+ Studies have also shown certain variations (polymorphisms) in the *DBH* gene to be associated with increased risk of attention deficit hyperactivity disorder (ADHD). *DBH* gene polymorphisms are also thought to increase the risk of psychotic symptoms in people with schizophrenia or unipolar major depression. Other studies, however, have not supported these findings. Many genetic and environmental factors are believed to contribute to these complex conditions.

http://ghr.nlm.nih.gov/gene/DBH

+ Catalytic activity:

- 3,4-dihydroxyphenethylamine + ascorbate + O_2 = noradrenaline + dehydroascorbate + H_2O

+ Cofactor:

- Pyrroloquinoline quinone   Binds one PQQ per subunit

- Copper   Binds two copper ions per subunit

+ Pathway: (R)-noradrenaline biosynthesis from dopamine
  - This protein is involved in step one of the subpathway that synthesizes (R)-noradrenaline from dopamine.
  - This subpathway is part of the pathway (R)-noradrenaline biosynthesis, which is part of catecholamine biosynthesis.

+ Molecular function:
  - Catalytic activity
  - Copper ion binding
  - Dopamine beta-monooxygenase activity
  - L-ascorbic acid binding

+ Biological process:
  - Behavioral response to ethanol
  - Blood vessel remodeling
  - Catecholamine biosynthetic process
  - Cellular nitrogen compound metabolic process
  - Cytokine production
  - Dopamine catabolic process
  - Fear response
  - Glucoase homeostasis
  - Homoiothermy
  - Leukocyte mediated immunity
  - Leukocyte migration
  - Locomotory behavior
  - Maternal behavior
  - Memory
  - Norepinepherine biosynthetic process
  - Positve regulation of vasoconstriction
  - Regulation of cell proliferation
  - Regulation of extrinsic apoptotic signaling pathway
  - Response to amphetamine
  - Response to pain
  - Small molecule metabolic process
  - Synaptic transmission
  - Visual learning

+ Subcellular location:

- Cytoplasmic vesicle > secretory vesicle lumen
- Cytoplasmic vesicle > secretory vesicle > chromaffin granule lumen
- Cytoplasmic vesicle > secretory vesicle membrane; single-pass type II membrane protein
- Cytoplasmic vesicle > secretory vesicle > chromaffin granule membrane; single-pass type II membrane protein

http://www.uniprot.org/uniprot/P09172

+ Cellular component:

- Chromaffin granule lumen
- Chromaffin granule membrane
- Cytoplasm
- Extracellular region
- Integral component of membrane
- Secretory granule lumen
- Transport vesicle membrane
- Dendritic shaft
- Integral component of membrane

http://www.uniprot.org/uniprot/P09172

+ Associated disease:

- Dopamine beta-hydroxylase deficiency – characterized by profound deficits in autonomic and cardiovascular function, but apparently only subtle signs, if any, of central nervous system dysfunction.

http://www.ncbi.nlm.nih.gov/pubmed/11857564

DDC

+ **Overview for DDC** *Dopa Decarboxylase (Aromatic L-Amino Acid Decarboxylase)* (aka, AADC), DDC, **rs921451 (aka, A14870G)**, rs3779084 (aka, A158104G), rs880028 (aka, A159505G), rs10499695 (aka, A19551G), rs6263 (A415G), rs1451371 (aka, A85104G), rs11575543 (aka, C107286T), rs11575537 (aka, C121254T), rs11575522 (aka, C124764T), rs1470750 (aka, C166017G), rs3735273 (aka, C186233T), rs12669770 (aka, C209826T), rs11575340 (aka, C41684A0, rs2242041 (aka, G108706C), rs11575542 (aka, G1385A), rs1451375 (aka, G15443T), rs998850 (aka, G196757C), rs3829897 (aka, G219133T), rs11575551 (aka, T111892C), rs11575552 (aka, T111909C), rs2167364 (aka, T155196C), rs6264 (aka, T201104C/G49G), rs10235796 (aka, T52006C), rs12718541 (aka, T88011C), rs732215 (aka, T94092G), Encodes the neurotransmitter synthesizing enzyme Dopa Decarboxylase (Aromatic L-Amino Acid Decarboxylase), which catalyzes the decarboxylation of L-3,4-dihydroxyphenylalanine (DOPA) to dopamine, L-5-hydroxytryptophan to serotonin and L-tryptophan to tryptamine.

http://www.genecards.org/cgi-bin/carddisp.pl?gene=DDC

- ❖ **NOTE**: Dopamine is a neurotransmitter of the catecholamine and phenethylamine families, and plays a number of important roles in the human brain and body. Its name derives from its chemical structure; it is an amine that is formed by removing a carboxyl group from a molecule of L-DOPA. In the brain, dopamine functions as a neurotransmitter, a chemical released by nerve cells to send signals to other nerve cells. The brain includes several distinct dopamine systems, one of which plays a major role in reward-motivated behavior. Most types of reward increase the level of dopamine in the brain, and a variety of addictive drugs increase dopamine neuronal activity. Other brain dopamine systems are involved in motor control and in controlling the release of several other important hormones.

https://en.wikipedia.org/wiki/Dopamine

- ❖ **NOTE:** Serotonin is primarily found in the GI tract, blood platelets, and the central nervous system (CNS). It is popularly thought to be a contributor to feelings of well-being and happiness. Approximately ninety percent of the human body's serotonin is located in the enterochromaffin cells in the GI tract, where it is used to regulate intestinal movements. The remainder is synthesized in serotonergic neurons of the CNS, where it has various functions, including the regulation of mood, appetite, and sleep. Serotonin also has some cognitive functions, including memory and learning.

https://en.wikipedia.org/wiki/Serotonin

+ Parkinson's and DDC - Dopa-decarboxylase gene polymorphisms affect the motor response to l-dopa in Parkinson's disease. The rs921451 and rs3837091 polymorphisms of the DDC gene promoter influence the motor response to l-dopa but do not significantly change peripheral pharmacokinetic parameters for l-dopa and dopamine. Results from this study suggest that DDC may be a genetic modifier of the l-dopa response in Parkinson's disease.
http://www.prd-journal.com/article/S1353-8020(13)00380-5/abstract

+ Catalytic activity:

- L-dopa = dopamine + CO_2
- 5-hydroxy-L-tryptophan = 5-hydroxytryptamine + CO_2

+ Cofactor:
- Pyridoxal 5'-phosphate (derived from vitamin B-6)

+ Pathway: Dopamine biosynthesis
- This protein is involved in step two of the subpathway that synthesizes dopamine from L-tyrosine.
- Proteins known to be involved in the two steps of the subpathway in this organism are:
  - Tyrosine 3-monooxygenase (TH)
  - Aromatic-L-amino-acid decarboxylase (DDC)

+ Molecular function:
- Amino acid binding
- Aromatic-Lamino-acid decarboxylase activity
- Enzyme binding
- L-dopa decarboxylase activity
- Pyridoxal phosphate binding

+ Biological process:
- Catecholamine biosynthetic process
- Cellular amino acid metabolic process
- Cellular nitrogen compound metabolic process
- Cellular response to alkaloid
- Cellular response to drug
- Cellular response to growth factor stimulus
- Circadian rhythm
- Dopamine biosynthetic process
- Indolalkylamine biosynthetic process
- Isoquinoline alkaloid metabolic process
- Multicellular aging
- Phytoalexin metabolic process
- Response to pyrethroid
- Serotonin biosynthetic process
- Small molecule process
- Synaptic vesicle amine transport

+ Cellular component:
- Axon
- Cytosol

- Extracellular exosome
- Neuronal cell body
- Synaptic vesicle

http://www.uniprot.org/uniprot/P20711

+ Associated disease:

- Aromatic L-amino-acid decarboxylase deficiency – An inborn error in neurotransmitter metabolism that leads to combined serotonin and catecholamine deficiency. It causes developmental and psychomotor delay, poor feeding, lethargy, ptosis, intermittent hypothermia, and gastrointestinal disturbances. The onset is early in infancy and inheritance is autosomal recessive.

http://www.ncbi.nlm.nih.gov/pubmed/14991824
http://www.ncbi.nlm.nih.gov/pubmed/15079002

DHFR

+ **Overview for DHFR** *Dihydrofolate Reductase*, DHFR, rs7387 (aka, A*115T), rs10072026 (aka, A10661G), rs1643649 (aka, A16352G), rs1643659 (aka, A20965G), rs1677693 (aka, C19483A), DHFR/MSH, rs1650697 (aka, T-473A)

- The DHFR gene provides instructions for producing the enzyme dihydrofolate reductase that converts dihydrofolate into tetrahydrofolate using NADPH (electron donor) as a cofactor. While the functional dihydrofolate reductase gene has been mapped to chromosome 5, multiple intronless processed pseudogenes or dihydrofolate reductase-like genes have been identified on separate chromosomes.
- Recall that tetrahydrofolate is a methyl group shuttle required for the de novo synthesis of purines, thymidylic acid, and certain amino acids.

http://www.genecards.org/cgi-bin/carddisp.pl?gene=DHFR
http://www.ncbi.nlm.nih.gov/gene/1719

+ **See page 134 for full write-up**

DISC1

+ **Overview for DISC1** *Disrupted in schizophrenia 1*, DISC1, rs823162 (aka, C14853T), rs373401 (aka, R264Q)

- Disrupted in schizophrenia 1 is a protein that is encoded by the DISC1 gene in humans.

http://www.ncbi.nlm.nih.gov/pubmed/10814723

- In coordination with a wide array of interacting partners, DISC1 has been shown to participate in the regulation of cell proliferation, differentiation, migration, neuronal axon, and dendrite outgrowth, mitochondrial transport, fission and/or fusion, and cell-to-cell adhesion.

+ Several studies have shown that unregulated expression or altered protein structure of DISC1 may predispose individuals to the development of schizophrenia, clinical depression, bipolar disorder, and other psychiatric conditions.

+ The protein encoded by DISC1 locates to the nucleus, centrosome, cytoplasm, mitochondria, axons, and synapses. Mitochondria are the predominant site of endogenous DISC1 expression, with at least two isoforms occupying internal mitochondrial locations. The DISC1 protein function appears to be highly diverse and its functional role in cellular processes is dependent upon the cellular domain it is located in. The presence or absence of certain protein interaction domains or targeting motifs may confer specific functions and influence subcellular targeting; therefore, it is probable that alternative splicing co-determines both the function and the intracellular location of DISC1.

http://www.ncbi.nlm.nih.gov/pubmed/15121183

+ Involved in the regulation of multiple aspects of embryonic and adult neurogenesis. Required for neural progenitor proliferation in the ventrical/subventrical zone during embryonic brain development and in the adult dentate gyrus of the hippocampus. Participates in the Wnt-mediated neural progenitor proliferation as a positive regulator by modulating GSK3B activity and CTNNB1 abundance. Plays a role as a modulator of the AKT-mTOR signaling pathway controlling the tempo of the process of newborn neurons integration during adult neurogenesis, including neuron positioning, dendritic development, and synapse formation. Inhibits the activation of AKT-mTOR signaling upon interaction with CCDC88A. Regulates the migration of early-born granule cell precursors toward the dentate gyrus during the hippocampal development. Plays a role, together with PCNT, in the microtubule network formation.

http://www.genecards.org/cgi-bin/carddisp.pl?gene=DISC1

+ Protein Interactions: The DISC1 protein has no known enzymatic activity; rather it exerts its effect on multiple proteins through interactions to modulate their functional states and biological activities in time and space.

http://www.ncbi.nlm.nih.gov/pubmed/21195721

These include:
- DISC1 has been shown to self-associate, to form dimers, multimers, and oligomers. The ability of DISC1 to form complexes with itself may be important in regulating its

affinity for interacting partners such as NDEL1. In postmortem brain samples of schizophrenia patients, there is an increase in insoluble DISC1 oligomer aggregates, indicative of a common link with other neurological disorders characterised by protein aggregation, namely Alzheimer's disease, Parkinson's disease, and Huntington's disease.

http://www.ncbi.nlm.nih.gov/pubmed/18400883

- Two DISC1 SNPs have been related to schizophrenia:
    - rs751229 and rs3738401

http://www.omim.org/entry/605210

- ATF4 and ATF5 are members of the leucine zipper activating transcription factor/CREB family. They are known to bind to and regulate the function of **GABA$_B$ receptors** in synapses and are involved in signal transduction from the cell membrane to the nucleus. Both proteins interact with DISC1 and GABA$_B$ receptors via their second C-terminal leucine zipper domain; therefore, DISC1 is able to regulate GABA$_B$ receptor function through its interaction with ATF4/ATF5.
- FEZ1 -- DISC1 participates in neurite outgrowth through its interaction with the fasciculation and elongation protein ζ-1 (FEZ1). FEZ1 is a mammalian homolog of the C. elegans UNC-76 protein involved in axonal outgrowth and fasciculation. DISC1-FEZ1 interaction is enhanced during neuro-differentiation and expression of the FEZ1-binding domain of DISC1 has a dominant negative effect on neurite outgrowth, which implies cooperation of DISC1 and FEZ1 in this process.

http://www.ncbi.nlm.nih.gov/pubmed/21195721

- Kalirin-7 -- DISC1 protein plays a role in the process of regulating spine form-and-function through its interactions with kalirin-7 (kal-7). Kal-7 is a regulator of spine morphology and synaptic plasticity in association with neuronal activity. Activation of **NMDA receptors** causes dissociation of DISC1 and kal-7, leaving kal-7 available to activate rac1.

http://www.ncbi.nlm.nih.gov/pubmed/19828788

- NDEL1/NUDEL -- DISC1 is localized to the centrosome, the primary microtubule organizing center of the cell, via interaction with nuclear distribution gene homologue-like 1 (NDEL1, aka, NUDEL), where it is part of a protein complex involved in cytoskeletal processes of neuronal migration, including nucleokinesis and neurite outgrowth. NUDEL is also known to play a role in axon regeneration and has an additional DISC1-modulated function as a cysteine endopeptidase.

http://www.ncbi.nlm.nih.gov/pubmed/19828788

- PCM1 -- The protein, pericentriolar material 1 (PCM1) that is associated with cilia development in the CNS interacts directly with the disrupted-in-schizophrenia 1 (DISC1) and calmodulin 1 (CALM1) proteins. Kamiya, et al., have shown that PCM1, DISC1 and BBS4 can all disrupt neuronal organisation in the mouse when their expression is down-regulated. Markers at the pericentriolar material 1 gene (PCM1) have shown genetic association with schizophrenia in several schizophrenia case control studies. The findings in relation to PCM1 support the role of DISC1 also being a susceptibility locus for schizophrenia.

http://www.ncbi.nlm.nih.gov/pubmed/18762586
http://www.ncbi.nlm.nih.gov/pubmed/20468070
http://www.ncbi.nlm.nih.gov/pubmed/16894060
http://www.ncbi.nlm.nih.gov/pubmed/19048012

+ Biological process:
    - Canonical Wnt signaling pathway
    - Cellular protein localization
    - Microtubule cytoskeleton organization
    - Neuron migration
    - Positive regulation of protein ubiquitination involved in ubiquitin-dependent protein catabolic process
    - Positive regulation of Wnt signaling pathway
    - Regulation of synapse maturation
    - Cell proliferation in forebrain
    - Cerebral cortex radially oriented cell migration
    - Mitochondrial calcium ion homeostasis
    - Positive regulation of neuroblast proliferation
    - Regulation of neuron projection development
    - TOR signaling

http://www.ebi.ac.uk/QuickGO/GTerm?id=GO:0051560

+ Cellular component:
    - Axon
    - Cell body
    - Cell junction
    - Centrosome
    - Ciliary basal body
    - Ciliary base
    - Dynein complex

- Endoplasmic reticulum
- Microtubule
- Mitochondrion
- Nucleus
- Perinuclear region of cytoplasm
- Postsynaptic density
- Postsynaptic membrane

http://www.uniprot.org/uniprot/Q9NRI5

+ Associated diseases:
- Schizophrenia 9 - A complex, multifactorial psychotic disorder or group of disorders characterized by disturbances in the form and content of thought (e.g., delusions, hallucinations), in mood (e.g., inappropriate affect), in sense of self and relationship to the external world (e.g., loss of ego boundaries, withdrawal), and in behavior (e.g., bizarre or apparently purposeless behavior). Although it affects emotions, it is distinguished from mood disorders in which such disturbances are primary. Similarly, there may be mild impairment of cognitive function and it is distinguished from the dementias in which disturbed cognitive function is considered primary. Some patients manifest schizophrenic as well as bipolar disorder symptoms and are often given the diagnosis of schizoaffective disorder.

http://www.ncbi.nlm.nih.gov/pubmed/11468279
http://www.ncbi.nlm.nih.gov/pubmed/14532331
http://www.ncbi.nlm.nih.gov/pubmed/15939883

DRD1

+ **Overview for DRD1** *Dopamine receptor D1* (aka, Dopamine D1 Receptor, D(1A) dopamine receptor, DADR), DRD1, rs4867798 (aka, A8265G), rs251937 (aka, A9244G), rs686 (aka, C7464T), rs5326 (G5968A), rs4532 (aka, G6014A), rs265981 (aka, T5262C), encodes the D1 subtype of the dopamine receptor.

- The D1 subtype is the most abundant dopamine receptor in the central nervous system. This G protein-coupled receptor stimulates adenylyl cyclase and activates cyclic AMP-dependent protein kinases. D1 receptors regulate neuronal growth and development, mediate some behavioral responses, and modulate dopamine receptor D2-mediated events.

http://www.genecards.org/cgi-bin/carddisp.pl?gene=DRD1

❖ **NOTE**: Dopamine is a neurotransmitter of the catecholamine and phenethylamine families and plays a number of important roles in the human brain and body. Its name derives from its chemical structure: it is an amine that is formed by removing a carboxyl group from a molecule of L-DOPA. In the brain, dopamine functions as a neurotransmitter, a chemical released by nerve cells to send signals to other nerve cells. The brain includes several distinct dopamine systems, one of which plays a major role in reward-motivated behavior. Most types of reward increase the level of dopamine in the brain and a variety of addictive drugs increase dopamine neuronal activity. Other brain dopamine systems are involved in motor control and in controlling the release of several other important hormones.

https://en.wikipedia.org/wiki/Dopamine

+ D1 and D5 receptors (also known as D1-like receptors) are a subset of the dopamine receptor G protein-coupled receptor family that also includes D2, D3, and D4. The two receptor subtypes are highly homologous and very few ligands have been identified that are selective between the D1 and D5 subtypes. D1 receptors are widely expressed throughout the brain, whereas D5 receptors show a restricted distribution (mainly limbic areas).

http://www.genecards.org/cgi-bin/carddisp.pl?gene=DRD1

+ SNPs rs4532 & rs5326 may contribute to schizophrenia by interacting with other genes.
http://www.ncbi.nlm.nih.gov/pubmed/?term=24790447

+ SNPs rs686 and 265981 significantly associated with less maternal orienting away from infant.
http://www.ncbi.nlm.nih.gov/pubmed/?term=22574669

+ Cofactor:
- Dopamine binding
- Dopamine neurotransmitter receptor activity
- Dopamine neurotransmitter activity, coupled via Gs
- Drug binding
- G protein-coupled amine receptor activity

+ Molecular function:
- Amino acid binding
- Aromatic-L-amino-acid decarboxylase activity
- Enzyme binding
- L-dopa decarboxylase activity
- Pyridoxal phosphate binding

+ Biological process:
- Activation of adenylate cyclase activity
- Adenylate cyclase-activating dopamine receptor signaling pathway
- Adenylate cyclase-activating G protein-coupled receptor signaling pathway
- Adult walking behavior
- Astrocyte development
- Behavioral fear response
- Behavioral response to cocaine
- Calcium-mediated signaling
- Cellular response to catecholamine stimulus
- Cellular response to hypoxia
- Cellular response to insulin stimulus
- Cerebral cortex GABAergic interneuron migration
- Conditioned tast aversion
- Dentate gyrus development
- Dopamine metabolic process
- Dopamine transport
- Glucose import
- G protein-coupled receptor signaling pathway, coupled to cyclic nucleotide second messanger
- Habituation
- Learning
- Long-term synaptic depression
- Long-term synaptic potentiation
- Maternal behavior
- Mating behavior
- Memory
- Negative regulation of cell migration
- Negative regulation of circadian cycle
- Negative regulation of protein kinase activity
- Neuronal action potential
- Operant conditioning

- Orbitofrontal cortex development
- Peristalsis
- Phospholipase C-activating dopamine receptor signaling pathway
- Positive regulation of adenylate cyclase activity involved in G protein-coupled receptor signaling pathway
- Positive regulation of of cAMP biosynthetic process
- Positive regulation of cell migration
- Positive regulation of cytosolic calcium ion concentration involved in phospholipase C-activating G protein-coupled signaling pathway
- Positive regulation of feeding behavior
- Positive regulation of long-term synaptic potentiation
- Positive regulation of membrane potential
- Positive regulation of potassium ion transport
- Positive regulation of release of sequestered calcium ion into cytosol
- Positive regulation of synaptic transmission, glutamatergic
- Prepulse inhibition
- Protein import into nucleus
- Regulation of dopamine metabolic process
- Regulation of dopamine uptake involved in synaptic plasticity
- Regulation of vasoconstriction
- Response to activity
- Response to amino acid
- Response to amphetamine
- Response to antidepressant
- Response to drug
- Response to estradiol
- Response to ethanol
- Response to food
- Response to morphine
- Response to nicotine
- Response to retinoic acid
- Sensitization

- Sensory perception of chemical stimulus
- Social behavior
- Striatum development
- Synapse assembly
- Synaptic transmission, dopaminergic
- Temperature homeostasis
- Transmission of nerve impulse
- Vasodilation
- Visual learning

+ Subcellular location:
- Cell membrane; Multi-pass membrane protein
- Endoplasmic reticulum membrane; Multi-pass membrane protein

❖ **NOTE:** Transport from the endoplasmic reticulum to the cell surface is regulated by interaction with DNAJC14.

http://www.uniprot.org/uniprot/P21728

+ Subcellular location:
- Axon terminus
- Caveola
- Ciliary membrane
- Cytosol
- Dendritic shaft
- Dendritic spine head
- Dendritic spine neck
- Endoplasmic reticulum membrane
- Integral component of plasma membrane
- Neuronal cell body
- Nonmotile primary cilium
- Nucleus
- Plasma membrane

http://www.uniprot.org/uniprot/P21728

DRD2

+ **Overview for DRD2** *Dopamine receptor D2 (aka, Dopamine D2 Receptor, D2R), DRD2, rs4936270 (aka, A32594G), rs4245146 (aka, A33029G), rs4648318 (aka, A37613G), rs1799978 (aka, A4651G), rs1125394 (aka, A53817G), rs1079727 (aka, A61820G),* rs2440390 (aka, A64124G), rs10891549 (aka, A72555G), rs4938019 (aka, A9611G), rs4648317 (aka, C19470T), rs4274224 (aka, C31550T), rs17529477 (aka, C33935T), rs4648319 (aka, C36639T), rs4620755 (aka, C41383T), rs2242592 (aka, C71572T), rs2234689 (aka, C72519G), rs6277 (aka, C957T), rs7125415 (aka, G40321A0, rs11214606 (aka, G41133A), rs4436578 (aka, G44237A), rs2471857 (aka, G52663A), rs1079596 (aka, G54383A), rs1079597 (aka, G54716A), rs2283265 (aka, G65466T), rs1076560 (aka, G67314T), rs7131056 (aka, T21228G), rs12364283 (aka, T4047C), rs1076563 (aka, T55093G), rs2734838 (aka, T64501C), rs6275 (aka, T852C), encodes the D(2) dopamine receptor

- The activity of the D(2) dopamine receptor is mediated by G proteins which inhibit adenylyl cyclase.

http://www.ncbi.nlm.nih.gov/pubmed/21645528

+ Schizophrenia may be treated by blocking the dopamine receptors type 2.

http://www.ncbi.nlm.nih.gov/pubmed/26290802

+ Dopamine and opioid neurotransmitter systems share many functions such as regulation of reward and pleasure.

http://www.ncbi.nlm.nih.gov/pubmed/26260431

> **Our Two Cents**: If you desire additional info on dopamine receptors, Dr. Deth is your guy. He assisted Dr. Yasko in her learning curve. Dr Yasko did much to bring SNPs and how they relate to health, to the fore. Dr Deth has a great book as well, but it is not for the faint-hearted. It is very technical, but his book includes much info on DRD2 and DRD. Warning…he is a trail-blazer and as such, many do not agree with his thimerosol/autism link. I have met with him, listened to him lecture, and he is a kind man. He knows his stuff and is very passionate (and correct, based on my clinical experience/observations).

> **Our Other Two Cents:** In my clinical experience, where I use a very comprehensive intake form (from IFM) and testing, my observation is that many children who present with autism spectrum traits are also on the autoimmune spectrum. They often have compromised GI health, they often have SNPs in neurotransmitter pathways that once conferred high IQ in past generations (e.g., COMT), and experience some sort of trigger. The trigger could be a vaccination, introduction of a GMO food, soy-milk, a virus, a bacteria, bovine growth hormone from cow milk, or others. There are now autism spectrum disorders that are "officially" linked to bacteria like strep. That same strep was a non-starter 20 years ago. What is the difference?

Wrt vaccines, followed up with baby acetaminophine drops, it's a double whammy if glutathione SNPs are an issue. Acetaminophine can impair glutathione production. Glutathione is a pathway to clear heavy metals, along with methylation. **(See phase II above)** I'm going out on a limb and saying that autism spectrum expression is grounded in autoimmune and epigenetic changes and poor phenotypic expression due to our foods, chemicals and EMF exposure and other environmental exposures (e.g., glyphosates) that alter our DNA **expression** and our gut bacteria. Mom, dad, and grandparent habits and exposures count too.

Our DNA has not changed in these last two generations; our environment has, like never before. It is the same with elder dementia and associated blood-brain barrier breaches, similar to leaky gut, and same triggers. I am stepping off my soapbox now…

+ rs4936270 - Its genotype frequency, allele frequency, and genotype distribution are associated with development of schizophrenia. A linkage disequilibrium block consisted of rs4648317, rs7131056, and rs4936270 weakly associated with schizophrenia.
http://www.ncbi.nlm.nih.gov/pubmed/?term=23429213

+ rs4245146 – is associated with generalized anxiety disorder. The association becomes stronger when anxiety with comorbid alcohol use, were considered.
http://www.ncbi.nlm.nih.gov/pubmed/?term=20122683

+ rs4648318 - There is interaction between the SNP and sex on pain scores: females with two minor alleles have increased pain intensity; while males with two minor alleles have less pain.
http://www.ncbi.nlm.nih.gov/pubmed/?term=25370144

+ rs1799978 - Association between sleep problems and overweight is stronger in children who were more impulsive and in G allele carriers.
http://www.ncbi.nlm.nih.gov/pubmed/?term=23828101 As predictor of schizophrenia treatment response to risperidone.
http://www.ncbi.nlm.nih.gov/pubmed/?term=18855532

+ rs4648317 - Its T allele is associated with higher rates of smoking and scored higher on nicotine dependence.
http://www.ncbi.nlm.nih.gov/pubmed/?term=18434921

+ rs17529477 - Association with increase in systolic blood pressure.
http://www.ncbi.nlm.nih.gov/pubmed/?term=24058526

+ rs2242592 - Associated with prediction of clinical improvement in psychotic treatment.
http://www.ncbi.nlm.nih.gov/pubmed/?term=22893251

+ rs4436578 - Association with significant four-way interaction of rs174675 (COMT), rs174697 (COMT), rs1076560 (DRD2), and rs4436578 (DRD2) on verbal fluency of creative potential.
http://www.ncbi.nlm.nih.gov/pubmed/?term=24782743

+ rs12364283 - Associated with transcription and D2 receptor density and strongly and selectively predictive of avoidance-based decision.
http://www.ncbi.nlm.nih.gov/pubmed/?term=19393722

+ Molecular function:
- Dopamine binding
- Dopamine neurotransmitter receptor activity, coupled via Gi/Go
- Drug binding
- Identical protein binding
- Potassium channel regulator activity

+ Biological process:
- Activation of adenylate cyclase activity
- Adenohypophysis development
- Adenylate cyclase-inhibiting dopamine receptor signaling pathway
- Adult walking behavior
- Arachidonic acid secretion
- Associative learning
- Auditory behavior
- Behavioral response to cocaine
- Behavioral response to ethanol
- Branching morphogenesis of a nerve
- Cellular calcium ion homeostasis
- Cerebral cortex GABAergic interneuron migration
- Circadian regulation of gene expression
- Dopamine metabolic process
- Feeding behavior
- G protein-coupled receptor internalization
- Grooming behavior
- Intracellular signal transduction
- Locomotory behavior
- Negative regulation of adenylate cyclase activity
- Negative regulation of blood pressure
- Negative regulation of cell migration
- Negative regulation of cell proliferation
- Negative regulation of circadian cycle
- Negative regulation of cytosolic calcium ion concentration
- Negative regulation of dopamine receptor signaling pathway

- Negative regulation of dopamine secretion
- Negative regulation of innate immune response
- Negative regulation of insulin secretion
- Negative regulation of protein kinase B signaling
- Negative regulation of protein sectretion
- Negative regulation of of synaptic transmission, glutamatergic
- Negative regulation of voltage-gated calcium channel activity
- Neurological sysem process involved in regulation of systemic arterial blood pressure
- Neuron-neuron synaptic transmission
- Orbitofrontal cortex development
- Peristalsis
- Phospholipase C-activating dopamine receptor signaling pathway
- Pigmentation
- Positive regulation of cytokinesis
- Positive regulation of cytosolic calcium ion concentration involved in phospholipase C-activating G protein-coupled signaling pathway
- Positive regulation of of cytokinesis
- Positive regulation of of cytosolic calcium ion concentration involved in phospholipase C-activating G protein-coupled signaling protein
- Positive regulation of dopamine uptake involved in synaptic transmission
- Positive regulation of glial cell line-derived neurotrophic factor secretion
- Positive regulation of G protein-coupled receptor protein signaling pathway
- Positive regulation of growth hormone secretion
- Positive regulation of long-term synaptic potentiation
- Positive regulation of multicellular organism growth
- Positive regulation of neuroblast proliferation
- Positive regulation of receptor internalization
- Positive regulation of renal sodium excretion

- Positive regulation of transcription from RNA polymerase II promoter
- Positive regulation of urine volume
- Prepulse inhibition
- Protein localization
- Regulation of cAMP metabolic process
- Regulation of dopamine secretion
- Regulation of dopamine uptake involved in synaptic transmission
- Regulation of heart rate
- Regulation of locomotion involved in locomotory behavior
- Regulation of long-term neuronal synaptic plasticity
- Regulation of phosphoprotein phosphate activity
- Regulation of potassium ion transport
- Regulation of sodium ion transport
- Regulation of synapse structural plasticity
- Regulation of synaptic transmission, GABAergic
- Release of sequestered calcium ion into cytosol
- Response to amphetamine
- Response to axon injury
- Response to cocaine
- Response to drug
- Response to histamine
- Response to hypoxia
- Response to inactivity
- Response to iron ion
- Response to light stimulus
- Response to morphine
- Response to nicotine
- Response to toxic substance
- Sensory perception of smell
- Striatum development
- Synapse assembly
- Synaptic transmission, dopaminergic
- Temperature homeostasis

- Visula learning
- Wnt signaling pathway (signal transduction)

+ Subcellular location:

- Acrosomal vesicle
- Axon
- Axon terminus
- Ciliary membrane
- Cytosol
- Dendrite
- Dendritic spine
- Endocytic spine
- Endocytic vesicle
- Integral component of plasma membrane
- Intracellular
- Lateral plasma membrane
- Nonmotile primary cilium
- Perikaryon
- Plasma membrane
- Postsynaptic density
- Sperm flagellum
- Synaptic vesicle membrane

http://www.uniprot.org/uniprot/P14416

+ Associated disease:

- Dystonia - A myoclonic dystonia. Dystonia is defined by the presence of sustained involuntary muscle contractions, often leading to abnormal postures. DYT11 is characterized by involuntary lightning jerks and dystonic movements and postures alleviated by alcohol. Inheritance is autosomal dominant. The age of onset, pattern of body involvement, presence of myoclonus, and response to alcohol are all variable.

http://www.ncbi.nlm.nih.gov/pubmed/10220438

DRD3

+ **Overview for DRD3** *Dopamine receptor D3* (DRD3 protein), DRD3, rs167771 (aka, C26625T), rs963468 (aka, C40013T), rs9828046 (aka, C44637T), rs10934256 (aka,

G17248T), rs1394016 (aka, G20405035A), rs6280 (aka, G25A), rs9824856 (aka, G50169T), rs1486009 (aka, T14368C), rs324029 (aka, T21277C), rs9825563 (aka, T2680C), rs2630351 (aka, T27841C), rs2630349 (aka, T29528C), rs3773678 (aka, T32822C), rs9288993 (aka, T43727C), encodes Dopamine Receptor D3.

- This gene encodes the D3 subtype of the five (D1-D5) dopamine receptors. The activity of the D3 subtype receptor is mediated by G proteins that inhibit adenylyl cyclase. This receptor is localized to the limbic areas of the brain, which are associated with cognitive, emotional, and endocrine functions. Genetic variation in this gene may be associated with susceptibility to hereditary essential tremor 1.

http://www.ncbi.nlm.nih.gov/gene/1814

+ rs167771 - Associated with striatum and stereotyped behaviour in autism spectrum disorders.
http://www.ncbi.nlm.nih.gov/pubmed/?term=25792691

+ rs963468 - Associated with schizophrenia risk.
http://www.ncbi.nlm.nih.gov/pubmed/?term=17125970

+ rs10934256 - Associated with other genes including COMT as risk factors for schizophrenia.
http://www.ncbi.nlm.nih.gov/pubmed/?term=18045777

+ rs6280 - Associated with a decreased risk of Parkinson's disease.
http://www.ncbi.nlm.nih.gov/pubmed/?term=21683922 May influence the binding affinity of D3 receptors as a result of serine to glycine substitution of the receptor protein.
http://www.ncbi.nlm.nih.gov/pubmed/?term=20860469

+ rs324029 - Associated with development of early-onset heroin dependence.
http://www.ncbi.nlm.nih.gov/pubmed/?term=24398431

+ rs2630351, rs3773678, rs2630349 - Associated with Fagerstrom test for nicotine dependence as individual SNP and haplotype.
http://www.ncbi.nlm.nih.gov/pubmed/?term=22309839

+ Molecular function:
- Dopamine neurotransmitter receptor activity

+ Biological process:
- Adenylate cyclase-inhibiting dopamine receptor signaling pathway

+ Subcellular location:
- Integral component of plasma membrane

+ Cellular component:

- Membrane

http://www.uniprot.org/uniprot/A1A4V4

DRD4

+ **Overview for DRD4** *Dopamine receptor D4* (D(4) dopamine receptor), DRD4, rs916457 (aka, C4710T), rs752306 (aka, C5318T), rs11246226 (aka, C8887A), rs3758653 (aka, T4095C), rs1800443 (aka, T581G), rs4331145 (aka, T643683C), encodes dopamine receptor D4.

- This dopamine receptor is responsible for neuronal signaling in the mesolimbic system of the brain, an area of the brain that regulates emotion and complex behavior. Its activity is mediated by G-proteins that inhibit adenylyl cyclase. It modulates the circadian rhythm of contrast sensitivity by regulating the rhythmic expression of NPAS2 in the retinal ganglion cells.

http://www.uniprot.org/uniprot/P21917

- Dopamine receptor D4 is linked to many neurological and psychiatric conditions including schizophrenia, bipolar disorder, addictive behaviors and eating disorders, such as, anorexia nervosa.

https://www.ncbi.nlm.nih.gov/pubmed/21873960

+ Dopamine receptor D4 is a target for drugs that treat schizophrenia and Parkinson's disease. The D_4 receptor is considered to be D_2-like, in which the activated receptor inhibits the enzyme adenylate cyclase, thereby reducing the intracellular concentration of the second messenger, cyclic AMP.

https://www.ncbi.nlm.nih.gov/pubmed/23469923

+ DRD4-7R, the 7-repeat (7R) variant of DRD4, has been linked to susceptibility for developing ADHA in several meta-analyses and other psychological traits and disorders.

https://www.ncbi.nlm.nih.gov/pubmed/11431226

+ The frequency of the alleles varies greatly between populations, e.g., the 7-repeat version has high incidence in America and low in Asia.

https://www.ncbi.nlm.nih.gov/pubmed/15077199

+ "Long" versions of polymorphisms are the alleles with six to ten repeats. 7R appears to react less strongly to dopamine molecules.

https://www.ncbi.nlm.nih.gov/pubmed/7643093

+ The 48-base pair VNTR has been the subject of much speculation about its evolution and role in human behaviors cross-culturally. The 7R allele appears to have been selected for about 40,000 years ago.

https://www.ncbi.nlm.nih.gov/pubmed/15077199

+ rs916457 - Associated with tardive dyskinesia in males in a Caucasian cohort as one of the four tag polymorphisms of DRD4 receptor gene.

http://www.ncbi.nlm.nih.gov/pubmed/?term=19238168

+ rs11246226 - A connection between the alleles of two SNPs (rs11246226, rs4331145) in the 3rd region of the DRD4 gene and schizophrenia.

http://www.ncbi.nlm.nih.gov/pubmed/?term=21874733

+ rs3758653 - Allele frequencies associated with more symptoms of bipolar I disorder.

http://www.ncbi.nlm.nih.gov/pubmed/?term=25233244

T allele associated with Alzheimer's disease.

http://www.ncbi.nlm.nih.gov/pubmed/?term=23034259

+ Molecular function:
- Dopamine binding
- Dopamine neurotransmitter receptor activity, coupled via Gi/Go
- Drug binding
- G protein-coupled amine receptor activity
- Identical protein binding
- Potassium channel regulator activity
- SH3 domaine binding

+ Biological process:
- Activation of MAPK activity
- Adenylate cyclase-inhibiting dopamine receptor signaling pathway
- Adult walking behavior
- Arachidonic acid secretion
- Behavioral fear response
- Behavioral response to cocaine
- Behavioral response to ethanol
- Cellular calcium ion homeostasis
- Circadian rhythm
- Dopamine metabolic process
- Dopamine receptor signaling

- Fear response
- Negative regulation of adenylate cyclase activity
- Negative regulation of cAMT biosynthetic process
- Negative regulation of protein secretion
- Negative regulation of voltage-gated calcium channel activity
- Olfactory learning
- Photoperiodism
- Positive regulation of dopamine uptake involved in synaptic transmission
- Positive regulation of excitatory postsynaptic membrane potential
- Positive regulation of kinase activity
- Positive regulation of penile erection
- Positive regulation of sodium: proton antiporter activity
- Regulation of calcium-mediated signaling
- Regulation of circadian rhythm
- Regulation of dopamine metabolic process
- Regulation of inhibitory postsynaptic membrane potential
- Regulation of neurotransmitter secretion
- Response to amphetamine
- Response to histamine
- Response steroid hormone
- Sensory perception of chemical stimulus
- Short-term memory
- Social behavior
- Synaptic transmission

+ Subcellular location:
- Cell membrane; Multipass membrane protein

http://www.uniprot.org/uniprot/P21917

+ Cellular component:
- Cell cortex
- Dedritic spine
- Integral component of plasma membrane
- Membrane
- Neuronal cell body

- Plasma membrane
- Terminal bouton
- Vesicle membrane

GAD1

+ <u>Overview for GAD1</u> *Glutamate decarboxylase 1 (brain, 67kDa) (GAD67)*, GAD, rs2241164 (aka, GAD1), rs769395 (aka, A48604A), rs2241165 (aka, C10180T), rs3828275 (aka, C14541T), rs12185692 (aka, C2627A), rs701492 (aka, C34281T), rs769407 (aka, G25509C), rs3791850 (aka, G39901A), rs3791878 (aka, G3992T), rs3749034 (aka, G5276A), rs2058725 (aka, T21922C), rs3791851 (aka, T30473C), GAD2, rs1805398 (aka, G264744809T)
Glutamate decarboxylase 2

- Catalyzes the production of GABA, our calming neurotransmitter.
- Deficiency of GAD1 enzyme has been shown to lead to pyridoxine dependency (vitamin B-6) seizures (a pyridoxine-dependent epilepsy that requires high levels of vitamin B-6 to mitigate, where standard anticonvulsant drugs are ineffective). Mutations in the ALDH7A1 gene may also cause pyridoxine-dependent epilepsy. ALDH7A1 is also another cause of pyridoxine-dependent epilepsy and is involved in the breakdown of lysine in the brain.

http://www.ncbi.nlm.nih.gov/pubmed/1339255

+ See page 141 for full write-up

GCH1

+ <u>Overview for GCH1</u> GTP cyclohydrolase 1 (Guanosine 5-Triphosphate Cyclohydrolase I), *GCH1*, rs2878169, rs3783642 (aka, A14340G), rs3783641 (aka, A14404T), rs12147422 (aka, A30528G), rs4411417 (aka, A53980G), rs8017210 (aka, C12707T), rs7147286 (aka, C15878T), rs8007267 (aka, C36378991T), rs7492600 (aka, C37668A), rs2878168 (aka, C53758T), rs841 (aka, C64051T), rs998259 (aka, G19512A), rs3783637 (aka, G26425A), rs9671371 (aka, G45908A), rs10483639 (aka, G55306457C), rs 752688 (aka, G62974A), rs8004018 (aka, T23847C), encodes GTP Cyclohydrolase 1, a member of the GTP cyclohydrolase family.

- GTP Cyclohydrolase 1 is the first and rate-limiting enzyme in tetrahydrobiopterin (BH4) biosynthesis, catalyzing the conversion of GTP into 7,8-dihydroneopterin triphosphate. BH4 is an essential cofactor required by aromatic amino acid hydroxylases (e.g., produce serotonin, dopamine, epi-, nor-epi), as well as, nitric oxide synthases.

Mutations in this gene are associated with malignant hyperphenylalaninemia and dopa-responsive dystonia.

http://www.genecards.org/cgi-bin/carddisp.pl?gene=GCH1

- GTP Cyclohydrolase 1 positively regulates nitric oxide synthesis in umbilical vein endothelial cells (HUVECs). It may be involved in dopamine synthesis and may modify pain sensitivity and persistence. Isoform GCH-1 is the functional enzyme. The potential function of the enzymatically inactive isoforms remains unknown.

http://www.ncbi.nlm.nih.gov/pubmed/8068008

+ Catalytic activity:
- GTP + H2O = formate + 2-amino-4-hydroxy-6-(erythro-1,2,3-trihydroxypropyl)-dihydropteridine triphosphate

+ Enzyme regulation:
- GTP shows a positive allosteric effect, and tetrahydrobiopterin inhibits the enzyme activity. Zinc is required for catalytic activity. Inhibited by Mg2+
- Optimum pH is 7.7 in phosphate buffer
- Relatively stable at high temperatures. Retains fifty percent of its activity after incubation at seventy degrees Celsius for fifteen minutes.

+ Pathway: 7,8-dihydroneopterin triphosphate biosynthesis
- This protein is involved in step one of the subpathway that synthesizes 7,8-dihydroneopterin triphosphate from GTP.
- Step one – GTP cyclohydrolase 1
- This subpathway is part of the pathway 7,8-dihydroneopterin triphosphate biosynthesis, which is part of cofactor biosynthesis.

+ Molecular function:
- Calcium ion binding
- Coenzyme binding
- GTP binding
- GTP cyclohydrolase I activity
- Protein homodimerization activity
- Zinc ion binding

+ Biological process:
- 7,8-dihydroneopterin 3'-triphosphate biosynthetic process
- Dopamine biosynthetic process

- Metabolic process
- Negative regulation of blood pressure
- Neuromuscular process controlling posture
- Nitric oxide metabolic process
- Positive regulation of nitric-oxide synthase activity
- Protein herooligomerization
- Protein homooligomerization
- Pteridine-containing compound biosynthetic process
- Regulation of blood pressure
- Regulation of lung blood pressure
- Regulation of nitric-oxide synthase activity
- Response to interferon-gamma
- Response to lipopolysaccharide
- Response to pain
- Response to tumor necrosis factor
- Small molecule metabolic process
- Tetrahydrobiopterin biosynthetic process
- Tetrahydrofolate biosynthetic process
- Vasodilation

+ Subcellular location:
- Cytoplasm
- Nucleus

+ Cellular component:
- Cytoplasm
- Cytoplasmic vesicle
- Cytosol
- Nuclear membrane
- Nucleoplas Nucleus
- Protein complex

http://www.uniprot.org/uniprot/P30793

+ Associated disease:
- Hyperphenylalaninemia, BH4 deficient - A disease characterized by malignant hyperphenylalaninemia due to tetrahydrobiopterin deficiency and defective neurotransmission due to depletion of the neurotransmitters dopamine and serotonin. The principal

symptoms include: psychomotor retardation, tonicity disorders, convulsions, drowsiness, irritability, abnormal movements, hyperthermia, hypersalivation, and difficulty swallowing. Some patients may present a phenotype of intermediate severity between severe hyperphenylalaninemia and mild dystonia. In this intermediate phenotype, there is marked motor delay, but no mental retardation and only minimal, if any, hyperphenylalaninemia.

http://www.ncbi.nlm.nih.gov/pubmed/9667588

HTR2A

+ **Overview for HTR2A** *5-Hydroxytryptamine (Serotonin) receptor 2A, G protein-coupled*, *HTR2A*, rs7997012 (aka, T64185C). Aka, 5-HT-2A, HTR2, 5-Hydroxytryptamine (Serotonin) Receptor 2A, 5-Hydroxytryptamine Receptor 2A, Serotonin 5-HT-2A Receptor, Serotonin Receptor 2A, 5-HT2 Receptor, 5-HT2A, 5-HT-2

- The mammalian **5-HT$_{2A}$ receptor** is a subtype that belongs to the serotonin receptor family and is a G protein-coupled receptor.
- Down-regulation of a post-synaptic 5-HT$_{2A}$ receptor is an adaptive process provoked by chronic administration of SSRIs and classical antipsychotics.

https://en.wikipedia.org/wiki/5-HT2A_receptor

+ Mutations in this gene are associated with susceptibility to schizophrenia and obsessive-compulsive disorder, and are also associated with response to the antidepressant citalopram in patients with major depressive disorder (MDD).
http://www.ncbi.nlm.nih.gov/pubmed/17691947
+ MDD patients who also have a mutation in intron 2 of this gene show a significantly reduced response to citalopram as this antidepressant down-regulates expression of this gene.
http://www.ncbi.nlm.nih.gov/gene/3356
+ 5-Hydroxytryptamine receptor 2A functions as a receptor for various drugs and psychoactive substances. These include, inter alia, mescaline, psilocybin, 1-(2,5-dimethoxy-4-iodophenyl)-2-aminopropane (DOI), and lysergic acid diethylamide (LSD).
+ HTR2A is involved in intestinal smooth muscle contraction and may play a role in arterial vasoconstriction.

+ This gene encodes for serotonin 2A receptor, one of the principle excitatory receptors in the serotonin system. Those with allele that causes a reduced response have an increased risk of side effects from SSRIs. G allele carries increased risk of adverse drug reactions with certain SSRIs.

+ Ligand binding causes a conformation change that triggers signaling via guanine nucleotide-binding proteins (G proteins) and modulates the activity of down-stream effectors.

+ Beta-arrestin family members inhibit signaling via G proteins and mediate activation of alternative signaling pathways.

+ Signaling activates phospholipase C and a phosphatidylinositol-calcium second messenger system that modulates the activity of phosphatidylinositol 3-kinase and promotes the release of $Ca(2+)$ ions from intracellular stores.

+ HTR2A affect neural activity, perception, cognition, and mood. Plays a role in the regulation of behavior, including responses to anxiogenic situations and psychoactive substances.

+ Serotonin 5-HT2A receptors are located primarily in the neocortex, caudate nucleus, nucleus accumbens, olfactory tubercle, hippocampus, and vascular and non-vascular smooth muscle cells.

+ HTR2A receptors play a role in appetite control, thermoregulation, and sleep.

+ The following diseases or traits (phenotypes of DNA expression), are known or believed to be associated with SNPs or SSRI effects in the HTR2A gene:

- Alcohol dependence
- Anorexia nervosa 1
- Major depressive disorder
- Obsessive-compulsive disorder
- Schizophrenia
- Cystic fibrosis
- Obstructive sleep apnea
- Cirrhosis
- Coronary artery spasm
- Prinzmental angina

https://www.wikigenes.org/e/gene/e/3356.htm
http://www.genecards.org/cgi-bin/carddisp.pl?gene=HTR2A
http://ghr.nlm.nih.gov/gene/HTR2A
https://www.pharmgkb.org/gene/PA193

❖ NOTE: **5-HTR2C** (serotonin receptor...OCD, Schizo). 5HT2C receptors [formerly termed 5HT1C], are widely expressed in the brain and spinal cord, are particularly enriched in the choroid plexus, and appear to mediate many important effects of 5HT.

http://www.ncbi.nlm.nih.gov/pmc/articles/PMC20038/#B8

http://www.ncbi.nlm.nih.gov/pmc/articles/PMC20038/#B9

+ Molecular function:
- 1-(4-iodo-2,5-dimethoxyphenyl)propan-2-amine binding
- Serotonin binding
- Drug binding
- Serotonin receptor activity

+ Biological process:
- Activation of phospholipase C activity
- Artery smooth muscle contraction
- Cell death
- Detection of mechanical stimulus involved in sensory perception of pain memory
- Negative regulation of synaptic transmission, glutamtergic
- Phospholipase C-activating serotonin receptor signaling pathway
- Positive regulation of ERK1 and ERK2 cascade
- Positive regulation of glycolytic process
- Positive regulation of peptidyl-tyrosine phosphorylation
- Positive regulation of vasoconstriction
- Positive regulation of behavior
- Regulation of hormone secretion
- Response to drugs
- Sleep
- Behavioral response to cocaine
- Aging
- Cellular calcium ion homeostasis
- Detection of temperature stimulus involved in sensory perception of pain
- Negative regulation of potassium ion transport
- Phosphatidylinositol 3-kinase signaling
- Positive regulation of fat cell proliferation
- Positive regulation of MAP kinase activity
- Positive regulation of phosphatidylinositol biosynthetic process
- Protein localization to cytoskeleton
- Regulation of dopamine secretion

- Release of sequestered calcium ion into cytosol
- Serotonin receptor signaling pathway
- Synaptic transmission
- Urinary bladder smooth muscle contraction

+ Medications/other used for the proper functioning of HTR2A:

- Acepromazine
- Amisulpride
- Amitriptyline
- Amoxapine
- Apomorphine
- Aripiprazole
- Asenapine
- Bromocriptine
- Butriptyline
- Cabergoline
- Chlorpromazine
- Chlorprothixene
- Cinitapride
- Cisapride
- Clomipramine
- Clozapine
- Cyclobenzaprine
- Cyproheptadine
- Desipramine
- Donepezil
- Doxepin
- Epinastine
- Ergoloid mesylate
- Ergotamine
- Flupentixol
- Fluspirilene
- Haloperidol
- Iloperidone
- Imipramine
- Ketamine
- Lisuride
- Loxapine
- Lurasidone
- Maprotiline
- Mesoridazine
- Methotrimeprazine
- Methysergide
- Mianserin
- Minaprine
- Mirtazapine
- Molindone
- Nefazodone
- Nortriptyline
- Olanzapine
- Paliperidone
- Paroxetine
- Pergolide
- Pipotiazine
- Pramipexole
- Promazine
- Promethazine
- Propiomazine
- Quetiapine
- Remoxipride
- Risperidone
- Ropinirole
- Sertindole
- Thioproperazine
- Thioridazine
- Thiothixene
- Trazodone
- Trimipramine
- Yohimbine
- Ziprasidone
- Zuclopenthixol

+ HTR2A interacts with the following genes:
- MPDZ
- INADL
- MPP3
- PRDX6
- DLG4
- DLG1
- CASK

- APBA1
- MAGI2
- GRM2
- DRD2

http://www.uniprot.org/uniprot/P28223

MAOA

+ **Overview for MAOA** *Monomine oxidase A* (aka, Amine oxidase [flavin-containing] A, MAOA), MAOA, rs5906883 (aka, A16535C), rs5906957 (aka, A36902G), rs909525 (aka, C42794T), rs5953210 (aka, C42794T), rs5953210 (aka, G3638A), rs6323 (aka, R297R/G492T/T941G), rs2072743 (aka, T89113C) encodes for the enzyme Monomine oxidase A.

- Monoamine oxidase A is an isozyme of monoamine oxidase. It preferentially deaminates (assists in the breakdown) of norepinephrine (noradrenaline), epinephrine (adrenaline), serotonin, and dopamine (which is equally deaminated by MAOA and MAOB).
- Catalyzes the oxidative deamination of biogenic and xenobiotic amines and functions in the metabolism of neuroactive and vasoactive amines in the central nervous system and peripheral tissues. MAOA preferentially oxidizes biogenic amines such as 5-hydroxytryptamine (5-HT), norepinephrine, and epinephrine.
- The protein localizes to the outer mitochondrial membrane. Its encoding gene is adjacent to MAOB on the opposite strand of the X chromosome.
- Monoamine oxidase A is inhibited by clorgyline and befloxatone. Inhibition of both MAOA and MAOB using a MAO inhibitor is used in the treatment of clinical depression, ED, and anxiety.
- ➤ **Our Two Cents**: In the case of inhibiting MAOA activity, clorgyline and befloxatone are used to treat depression, ED, and anxiety. This has an effect of slowing the breakdown of nor-epi, epi, serotonin, and dopamine. MAOB and COMT are also part of the picture. In the case of COMT, no SNPs (e.g., green on variant report) indicate maximum/fastest breakdown of epinepherine and dopamine. On the other hand, homozygous SNPs (e.g., red in the variant report) in COMT indicate the slowest breakdown of epinepherine and dopamine. Vitamin D is also in play, so look at VDR SNPs.

+ See page 154 for full write-up

MAOB

+ **Overview for MAOB** *Monomine oxidase B* (aka, Amine oxidase [flavin-containing] B, MAOB), MAOB, **rs1799836 (aka, A118723G)**, rs10521432 (aka, C112982T), rs6651806 (aka, T57758G), encodes for the enzyme Monomine oxidase B.

- Monoamine oxidase B is an isozyme of monoamine oxidase. It catalyzes the oxidative deamination of biogenic and xenobiotic amines and has important functions in the metabolism of neuroactive and vasoactive amines in the central nervous system and peripheral tissues. MAOB preferentially degrades benzylamine and phenylethylamin.
- In humans, MAOA preferentially oxidizes serotonin and noradrenaline, whereas MAOB oxidizes dopamine.
- More active polymorphisms of the MAOB gene have been linked to negative emotionality and suspected as an underlying factor in depression.
- Monoamine oxidase B inhibitors are typically used in the treatment of Parkinson's disease.

https://www.ncbi.nlm.nih.gov/pubmed/22110357

- Inhibition of MAOB in rats has been shown to prevent many age-related biological changes such as optic nerve degeneration and extend average lifespan by up to thirty-nine percent.

https://www.ncbi.nlm.nih.gov/pubmed/23082958

+ See page 156 for full write-up

NOS1

+ **Overview for NOS1** *Nitric oxide synthase 1 (neuronal)* (aka, nNOS, Nitric oxide synthase, brain), NOS1, rs7298903 (aka, A57373G), rs3782206 (aka, G59494A), rs2293054 (aka, T2202C), encodes for the enzyme, nitric oxide synthase 1.

- Nitric oxide (NO) is a messenger molecule with diverse functions throughout the body. In the brain and peripheral nervous system, NO displays many properties of a neurotransmitter.
- NO is implicated in neurotoxicity associated with stroke and neurodegenerative diseases, neural regulation of smooth muscle, including peristalsis, and penile erection. NO is also responsible for endothelium-derived relaxing factor activity regulating blood pressure.

https://www.ncbi.nlm.nih.gov/pubmed/1379716

- nNOS is one of three isoforms that synthesize nitric oxide, a small gaseous and lipophilic molecule that participates of several biological processes.

https://www.ncbi.nlm.nih.gov/pubmed/20388537

+ See page 179 for full write-up

NOS2

+ Overview for NOS2: *Nitric oxide synthase 2 (inducible)* (aka, Inducible NO synthase - iNOS), NOS2, rs2297518 (aka, C1823T), rs2248814 (aka, T32235C), rs2274894 (aka, T836165G), encodes for the enzyme, nitric oxide synthase 2 (NOS2).

- iNOS is a <u>reactive free radical</u> that acts as a biologic mediator in several processes, including neurotransmission and antimicrobial and antitumoral activities. It is inducible by a combination of lipopolysaccharides and particular cytokines. In other words, its expression is typically induced in inflammatory diseases.

http://www.uniprot.org/citations/7528267

- ❖ **NOTE**: Lipopolysaccharides are an endotoxin, found in the outer membrane of gram-negative bacteria and released into the surrounding environment (e.g., GI tract), which elicit a strong immune response. Detection of lipopolysaccharide antibodies as well as occluding and zonulin can be measured via **Cyrex Labs**, to determine if leaky gut has occured.

+ See page 182 for full write-up

NOS3

+ Overview for NOS3 *Nitric oxide synthase 3 (endothelial)* (aka, eNOS, Constitutive NOS), NOS3, rs1800783 (aka, A6251T), rs3918188 (aka, C19635T), rs7830 (aka, G10T), rs1800779 (G6797A), rs2070744 (aka, T786C) encodes for the enzyme, nitric oxide synthase 3 (NOS3).

- NOS3 produces nitric oxide (NO) that is implicated in <u>vascular smooth muscle relaxation</u> through a cGMP-mediated signal transduction pathway. NO mediates vascular endothelial growth factor (VEGF)-induced angiogenesis in coronary vessels and promotes blood clotting through the activation of platelets.

+ See page 185 for full write-up

PAH

+ Overview for PAH *Phenylalanine hydroxylase* (Phenylalanine-4-hydroxylase, PheOH, alternatively PheH or PAH), PAH, rs62507347 (aka, A27743C), rs10860936 (aka, A33429G), rs3817446 (aka, A55562G), rs1722387 (A75311G), rs5030858 (aka, C1222T), rs1522305 (aka, C35625G), rs2037639 (aka, C45031T), rs1718301 (aka, C45188T), rs1522296 (aka, C5594T), rs2245360 (aka, C81837T), rs1801153 (aka, G*187A), rs772897 (aka, G1155C), rs1722392 (aka, G37636A), rs1042503 (aka, G735A), rs5030849 (aka, G782A), rs1522307 (aka, T17864C), rs11111419 (aka, T31338A), rs10778209 (aka, T32409C), rs1718312 (aka, T75193C), encodes phenylalanine hydroxylase.

- Phenylalanine hydroxylase is an enzyme that catalyzes the hydroxylation of the aromatic side-chain of phenylalanine to generate tyrosine.
- Phenylalanine hydroxylase is one of three members of the biopterin-dependent aromatic amino acid hydroxylases, a class of nonooxygenase that uses tetrahydrobiopterin (BH4) and a non-heme iron for catalysis. During the reaction, molecular oxygen is heterolytically cleaved with sequential incorporation of one oxygen atom into BH_4 and a phenylalanine substrate.

https://www.ncbi.nlm.nih.gov/pubmed/10872454

+ Phenylalanine hydroxylase is the rate-limiting enzyme of the metabolic pathway that degrades excess phenylalanine. Research on phenylalanine hydroxylase, by Seymour Kaufman, led to the discovery of tetrahydrobiopterin as a biological cofactor.

https://www.ncbi.nlm.nih.gov/pubmed/13525410

+ Mutations in PAH, the encoding gene, can lead to phenylketonuria, a severe metabolic disorder. Deficiency in PheOH activity due to those mutations in the PAH gene can causes hyperphenylalaninemia (HPA), and when blood phenylalanine levels increase above twenty times the normal concentration, phenylketonuria (PKU) results.

https://www.ncbi.nlm.nih.gov/pubmed/10077654

+ Catalytic activity:

- L-phenylalanine + tetrahydrobiopterin + O2 = L-tyrosine + 4a-hydroxytetrahydrobiopterin

+ Cofactor:

- Iron (Fe 2+)

+ Enzyme regulation:

- N-terminal region of PAH is thought to contain allosteric binding regulation sites for phenylalanine and to constitute an "inhibitory" domain that regulates the activity of a catalytic domain in the C-terminal portion of the molecule.

+ Temperature dependence:

- Optimum temperature is fifty degrees Celsius.

+ Pathway: L-phenylalanine degradation

Step 1 – Phenylalanine-4-hydroxylase (PAH)

Step 2 – Tyrosine aminotransferase (TAT)

Step 3 – 4-hydroxyphenylpyruvate dioxygenase (HDP)

Step 4 – Homogentisate 1,2-dioxygenase (HGD)

Step 5 – Maleyacetoacetate isomerase (GSTZ1)

Step 6 – Fumaryacetoacetase (FAH)

+ Molecular function:

- Amino acid binding
- Cofactor binding
- Iron ion binding
- Phenylalanine 4-monooxygenase activity

+ Biological process:

- Catecholamine biosynthetic process
- Cellular amino acid metabolic process
- Cellular nitrogen compound metabolic process
- L-phenylalanine catabolic process
- Neurotransmitter biosynthetic process
- Protein hydroxylation
- Small molecule metabolic process
- Tetrahydrobiopterin metabolic process
- Tyrosine biosynthetic process

+ Cellular component:

- Cytosol
- Extracellular exosome

http://www.uniprot.org/uniprot/P00439

+ Associated disease:

- Phenylketonuria (PKU) – Autosomal recessive inborn error of phenylalanine metabolism, due to severe phenylalanine hydroxylase deficiency. It is characterized by blood concentrations of phenylalanine persistently above 1,200 mumol (normal concentration 100 mumol) that usually causes mental retardation (unless a low phenylalanine diet is introduced early in life). They tend to have light pigmentation, rashes similar to eczema, epilepsy, extreme hyperactivity, psychotic states, and an unpleasant 'mousy' odor.

http://www.ncbi.nlm.nih.gov/pubmed/2840952

http://www.ncbi.nlm.nih.gov/pubmed/1975559

PEMT

+ Overview for PEMT *Phosphatidylethanolamine N-methyltransferase,* PEMT, rs7946 (aka, G634A), rs4646406 (aka, T17020543A), rs4244593 (aka, T17023592G), encodes for the enzyme, phosphatidylethanolamine N-methyltransferase.

- PEMT is a transferase enzyme that converts phosphatidylethanolamine (PE) to phosphatidylethanolamine (PC) in the liver, via three sequential methylation steps by SAM (i.e., three molecules of SAM).
- PC made via PEMT plays a wide range of physiological roles, utilized in choline synthesis, hepatocyte membrane structure, bile secretion, and VLDL secretion.
- Although the CDP-choline pathway accounts for approximately seventy percent of PC biosynthesis in the liver, the PEMT pathway has been shown to play a critical (evolutionary) role in providing PC during times of starvation.

https://www.ncbi.nlm.nih.gov/pubmed/22877991

- ❖ **NOTE**: The CDP-choline pathway is one where choline is obtained either by dietary consumption (e.g., eggs) or by metabolism of choline-containing lipids is converted to PC.

+ See page 187 for full write-up

PNMT

+ Overview for PNMT *Phenylethanolamine N-methyltransferase,* PNMT, rs5638 (aka, A456G), rs876493 (aka, G-184A), encodes phenylethanolamine N-methyltransferase, an enzyme found in the adrenal medulla that converts norepinepherine (noradrenaline) to epinephrine (adrenaline).

https://en.wikipedia.org/wiki/Phenylethanolamine_N-methyltransferase

- SAMe is a required cofactor, as it is for all MT enzymes.
- PNMT catalyzes the transfer of a methyl group from SAM to norepinephrine, converting it into epinephrine (flight/fight neurotransmitter).
- It also shares many structural properties, like the shape of the folding lip with COMT, though it shares less sequence identity. Several features of the structure, like the folding lip, suggest that PNMT is a recent adaptation to the catecholamine synthesizing enzyme family, evolving later than COMT, but before other methyltransferases like GNMT.

https://www.ncbi.nlm.nih.gov/pubmed/11591352

+ The residue glutamine 185 is necessary in binding the catecholamine substrate. The replacement of this residue by another amino acid reduces the catalytic efficiency of PNMT by tenfold up to three-hundredfold. For example, if the critical Glu(185) catalytic residue is replaced by aspartic acid, a loss of a tenfold in catalytic efficiency results. This is because protein backbone movements place the Asp(185) carboxylate almost coincident with the carboxylate of Glu(185). Conversely, replacement of Glu(185) by glutamine reduces catalytic efficiency almost three-hundredfold, not only because of the loss of charge, but also because the variant residue does not adopt the same conformation as Glu(185).

https://www.ncbi.nlm.nih.gov/pubmed/19570037

+ In Caucasians, PNMT SNPs are associated with the development of acute kidney injury, disease severity, and in-hospital mortality.

https://www.ncbi.nlm.nih.gov/pubmed/?term=rs5638

+ Molecular function:

- Phenylethanolamine N-methylatransferase activity

+ Biological process:

- Catecholamine biosynthetic process
- Cellular nitrogen compound metabolic process
- Epinepherine biosynthetic process
- Small molecule process

+ Cellular component:

Cytosol

http://www.uniprot.org/uniprot/P11086

SLC6A2

+ **Overview for SLC6A2** *Solute carrier family 6 (Neurotransmitter Transporter), Member 2* (aka, Norepinephrine Transporter (NET), Solute Carrier Family 6 (Neurotransmitter Transporter, Noradrenalin), SLC6A2, rs4564560 (aka, A40223G), rs5568 (aka, A45583C), rs168924 (aka, A5003G), rs3785143 (aka, C10565T), rs36020 (aka, C28547T), rs10521329 (aka, C35917A), rs11568324 (aka, C41517T), rs3785157 (aka, C45295T), rs36009 (aka, C48079T), rs2242447 (aka, C51371T), rs2242446 (aka, C5884T), rs1532701 (aka, G13486A), rs40147 (aka, G32299A), rs1566652 (aka, G47034T), rs9998424 (aka, G47405A), rs3785152 (aka, T32009C), rs5558 (aka, T49018G), rs1800887 (aka, T49048C).

- SLC6A2 encodes a member of the sodium neurotransmitter symporter family, commonly referred to as, norepinephrine transporter (NET). This member is a multi-pass membrane protein that is responsible for the reuptake of norepinephrine into presynaptic nerve terminals and is a regulator of norepinephrine homeostasis.

+ NET is responsible for the sodium-chloride (Na^+/Cl^-)-dependent reuptake of extracellular norepinepherine (aka, noradrenaline).

+ NET is can also reuptake extracellular dopamine.

+ Mutations in SLC6A2, resulting in hypermethylation of CpG islands in the NET promoter region, may cause reduced expression of the noradrenaline (norepinephrine) transporter and consequently a phenotype of impaired neuronal reuptake of norepinephrine has been implicated in both postural orthostatic tachycardia syndrome and panic disorder.

> Postural orthostatic tachycardia syndrome (dysautonomia); a syndrome characterized by lightheadedness, fatigue, altered mentation, and syncope. Often, patients have high plasma norepinephrine concentrations (at least 600 pg/ml) in relation to sympathetic outflow upon standing, suggesting OI is a hyperandrenergic condition. The genetic defect in the NET protein results in decreased NET activity that could account for abnormally high NE plasma levels in OI. (Ala457Pro = an alanine residue replaces a proline residue).

https://www.ncbi.nlm.nih.gov/pubmed/16785272

> Mutations in SLC6A2 may cause general anxiety disorder and is one of many associated with ADHD.

http://www.genecards.org/cgi-bin/carddisp.pl?gene=SLC6A2

+ NETs constitute the primary mechanism for inactivation of synaptically released NE, are targets for multiple antidepressants and psychostimulants, and have been reported to be deficient in affective and autonomic disorders.

https://www.ncbi.nlm.nih.gov/pubmed/10753308

+ It has been suggested that the life-threatening cardiovascular effects of cocaine may involve the inhibition of NETs at sympathetic and CNS autonomic synapses. Similarly, amphetamines induce norepinephrine to build up in the synaptic cleft (due to inhibition of NETs).

http://www.acnp.org/g4/GN401000029/CH029.html

+ Many drugs exist in the treatment of ADHD. Dexedrine, Dextrostat, Ritalin, Metadate, Concerta, Daytrana, Vyvanse, etc., block reabsorption of the catecholamine neurotransmitters dopamine and norepinephrine via monoamine transporters, NET included, and thereby increase levels of these neurotransmitters in the brain. They basically block NETs activity. As a result, it is thought that one's ability to focus is increased, impulsiveness decreased, and hyperactivity lessened in those with ADHD.

https://www.ncbi.nlm.nih.gov/pubmed/14717619

❖ **NOTE**: See http://www.medscape.org/viewarticle/523887 for discussion of the functional roles of Dopamine and Epinepherine in ADHD.

+ Molecular function:
- Monoamine transmember transporter activity
- Norepinepherine: sodium symporter activity

+ Biological process:
- Monoamine transport
- Response to pain
- Synaptic transmission
- Transmembrane transport
- Transport

http://www.uniprot.org/uniprot/P23975

+ Subcellular location:
- Membrane; multi-pass membrane protein

+ Cellular component:
- Integral component of plasma membrane
- Membrane
- Plasma membrane

+ Associated disease:
- Orthostatic intolerance associated with norepinephrine transporter deficiency - syndrome characterized by lightheadedness, fatigue, altered mentation, and syncope. It is associated with postural tachycardia. Plasma norepinephrine concentration is abnormally high.

http://www.ncbi.nlm.nih.gov/pubmed/10684912

SLC6A3

+ **Overview for SLC6A3** *Solute carrier family 6 (Neurotransmitter Transporter), Member 3* (aka, Dopamine Transporter (DAT), Solute Carrier Family 6 (Neurotransmitter Transporter, Dopamine), SLC6A3, rs6347 (aka, A39132G), rs2617605 (aka, A8023G), rs460000 (aka, C17719T), rs11564771 (aka, C51747T), rs6350 (aka, C7345T), rs27048 (aka, G37899A), rs6869645 (aka, G45996T), rs11133767 (aka, G48964A), rs40184 (aka, G55467A), rs27072 (aka, G56022A), rs403636 (aka, T12190G), rs464049 (aka, T26639C), rs1042098 (aka, T55729C).

- SLC3A6 s a membrane-spanning protein that pumps the neurotransmitter dopamine out of the synapse back into cytosol,

- from which other transporters sequester dopamine and norepinephrine into vesicles for storage and later release.
- Dopamine reuptake via DAT provides the primary mechanism through which dopamine is cleared from synapses, although there may be an exception in the prefrontal cortex, where evidence points to a possibly larger role of the NET **(See SLC6A2 page 292)**

https://www.ncbi.nlm.nih.gov/pubmed/2117046

- DAT is implicated in a number of dopamine-related disorders, including ADHD, bipolar disorder, clinical depression, and alcoholism.

https://www.ncbi.nlm.nih.gov/pubmed/1478653

- Dopamine underlies several aspects of cognition, including reward, and DAT facilitates regulation of that signal.

https://www.ncbi.nlm.nih.gov/pubmed/9658025

- Sodium ions must bind to the extracellular domain of the transporter (DAT) before dopamine can bind. Once dopamine binds, the protein undergoes a conformational change, which allows both sodium and dopamine to unbind on the intracellular side of the membrane.

+ The rate at which DAT removes dopamine from the synapse can have a profound effect on the amount of dopamine in the cell. This is best evidenced by the severe cognitive deficits, motor abnormalities, and hyperactivity of mice with no dopamine transporters. These characteristics have striking similarities to the symptoms of ADHD.

https://en.wikipedia.org/wiki/Attention_deficit_hyperactivity_disorder

+ Cocaine blocks DAT by binding directly to the transporter and reducing the rate of transport resulting in less removal of dopamine from the synapse and increased signaling, which is thought to underlie the pleasurable feelings elicited by cocaine.

https://www.ncbi.nlm.nih.gov/pubmed/9658025

+ The SLC6A3 gene has been implicated in human disorders such as, Parkinsonism, Tourette syndrome, and substance abuse.

http://www.omim.org/entry/126455

+ Molecular function:
- Dopamine transmember transporter activity
- Dopamine: sodium symporter activity
- Monoamine transmember transporter activity

- Dopamine binding

+ Biological process:
- Adenohypophysis development
- Ammonium transmembrane transport
- Cation transmember transport
- Dopamine biosynthetic process
- Dopamine catabolic process
- Dopamine transport
- Lactation
- Locomotory behavior
- Monoamine transport
- Neurotransmitter biosynthetic process
- Positive regulation of multicellular organism growth
- Prepulse inhibition
- Regulation of dopamine metabolic process
- Response to cocaine
- Sensory perception of smell (loss often preceeds Parkinson's)
- Transmembrane transport

http://www.uniprot.org/uniprot/Q01959

+ Subcellular location:
- Cembrane; multi-pass membrane protein

+ Cellular component:
- Axon
- Cell surface
- Cytoplasm
- Flotillin
- Integral component of membrane
- Integral component of plasma membrane
- Neuronal cell body
- Plasma membrane

+ Associated disease:
- Parkinsonism-dystonia infantile - A neurodegenerative disorder characterized by infantile onset of Parkinsonism and dystonia. Other neurologic features include, global developmental delay, bradykinesia, and pyramidal tract signs.

http://www.ncbi.nlm.nih.gov/pubmed/19478460

SLC6A4

+ **Overview for SLC6A4** *Solute carrier family 6 (neurotransmitter transporter, serotonin), member 4* (aka, serotonin transporter, SERT **or** 5-HTT)

SLC6A4, rs25531 encodes aserotonin transporter protein

- SLC6A4 is a type of monoamine transporter protein that transports serotonin from the synaptic cleft to the presynaptic neuron.
- The serotonin transporter removes serotonin from the synaptic cleft back into the synaptic boutons. Thus, it terminates the effects of serotonin and simultaneously enables its reuse by the presynaptic neuron. (e.g., reuptake of serotonin)
- Variations of SLC6A4 are associated with decreased response to certain SSRIs; an SNP in the 5-HTTLPR rs25532 and another in the 5-HTTLPR.

https://www.ncbi.nlm.nih.gov/pubmed/1657151

+ The promotor region of the SLC6A4 gene contains a polymorphism with "short" and "long" repeats in a region: 5-HTT-linked polymorphic region (5-HTTLPR or *SERTPR*).

+ The short variation has fourteen repeats of a sequence, while the long variation has sixteen repeats. The short variation leads to less transcription for SLC6A4 and it has been found that it can partly account for anxiety-related personality-traits.

https://www.ncbi.nlm.nih.gov/pubmed/8632190

+ A repeat length polymorphism in the promoter of this gene has been shown to affect the rate of serotonin uptake and may play a role in sudden infant death syndrome, aggressive behavior in Alzheimer's disease patients, post-traumatic stress disorder, and depression-susceptibility in people experiencing emotional trauma.

+ Medical studies have shown that changes in serotonin transporter metabolism appear to be associated with many different phenomena, including alcoholism, clinical depression, obsessive-compulsive disorder (OCD), romantic love, hypertension, and generalized social phobia.

+ The serotonin transporter is also present in platelets; there, serotonin functions as a vasoconstrictive substance.

https://www.ncbi.nlm.nih.gov/pubmed/10405096
https://www.ncbi.nlm.nih.gov/pubmed/18413401

+ In addition to behavioral affects, phenotypic changes due to SLC6A4 may also promote increased gut dysfunction.

https://www.ncbi.nlm.nih.gov/pubmed/18209729

+ Some of the human genetic variations associated with the gene are:
  + Length variation in the serotonin-transporter-gene-linked polymorphic region (5-HTTLPR)
  * rs25531— an SNP in the 5-HTTLPR
  * rs25532— another SNP in the 5-HTTLPR
  * STin2 — a variable number of tandem repeats a (VNTR) in the functional intron 2
  * G56A on the second exon
  * I425V on the ninth exon
+ Molecular function:
  - Actin filament binding
  - Cocaine binding
  - Monoamine transmembrane transporter activity
  - Rab GTPase binding
  - Serotonin: sodium symporter activity
  - Serotonin transmembrane transporter activity
+ Biological process:
  - Brain morphogenesis
  - Cellular response to cGMP
  - Cellular response to retinoic acid
  - Circadian rhythm
  - Memory
  - Negative regulation of cerebellar granule cell precursor proliferation
  - Negative regulation of neuron differentiation
  - Negative regulation of organ growth
  - Negative regulation of gene expression
  - Protein homooligomerization
  - Response to drug
  - Response to estradiol
  - Response to hypoxia
  - Response to nutrient
  - Response to toxic substance
  - Serotonin uptake
  - Social behavior
  - Sperm ejaculation

- Thalamus
- Vasoconstriction

+ Cellular component:
- Cytosol
- Endomembrane system
- Endosome membrane
- Integral component of plasma membrane
- Membrane raft
- Neuron projection
- Plasma membrane

http://www.uniprot.org/uniprot/P31645

TH

+ **Overview for TH** *Tyrosine hydroxylase* (aka, tyrosine 3-monooxygenase), TH, rs28934581 (aka, A733C), rs28934580 (aka, G1010A/R337H), rs2070762 (aka, T1090C), rs7483056 (aka, T7517C), rs6356 (aka, V112M)

- Encodes tyrosine hydroxylase, which is important for functioning of the nervous system.

http://ghr.nlm.nih.gov/gene/TH

- Tyrosine hydroxylase takes part in the first step of the pathway that produces catecholamines– specifically conversion of tyrosine to L-dopa and then L-dopa to dopamine via the DDC enzyme.
- ❖ **NOTE**: Dopamine is a neurotransmitter of the catecholamine and phenethylamine families and plays a number of important roles in the human brain and body. Its name derives from its chemical structure: it is an amine that is formed by removing a carboxyl group from a molecule of L-DOPA. In the brain, dopamine functions as a neurotransmitter, a chemical released by nerve cells to send signals to other nerve cells. The brain includes several distinct dopamine systems, one of which plays a major role in reward-motivated behavior. Most types of reward increase the level of dopamine in the brain and a variety of addictive drugs increase dopamine neuronal activity. Other brain dopamine systems are involved in motor control and in controlling the release of several other important hormones.

https://en.wikipedia.org/wiki/Dopamine

- Tyrosine hydroxylase catalyzes the rate-limiting step in this synthesis of catecholamines.

- Tyrosine hydroxylase is present in the CNS, peripheral sympathetic neurons, and the adrenal medulla.

https://www.ncbi.nlm.nih.gov/pubmed/8822146

+ Because tyrosine hydroxylase catalyzes the rate-limiting step in the biosynthesis of catecholamines, alterations in the enzyme activity may be involved in disorders such as, Segawa's dystonia, Parkinson's, and schizophrenia.

https://www.ncbi.nlm.nih.gov/pubmed/9228951

+ Catalytic activity:
  - L-tyrosine + tetrahydrobiopterin + O_2 = L-dopa + 4a-hydroxytetrahydrobiopterin

+ Cofactor:
  - Iron (Fe^{2+})
  - BH4

+ Enzyme regulation:
  - Phosphorylation leads to an increase in the catalytic activity

+ Pathway: Dopamine biosynthesis
  - Step 1 – Tyrosine 3-monooxygenase (TH)
  - Step 2 – Aromatic-L-amino-acid decarboxylase (DDC)

+ Molecular function:
  - Amino acid binding
  - Dopamine binding
  - Enzyme binding
  - Ferric iron binding
  - Ferrous iron binding
  - Oxygen binding
  - Tetrahydrobiopterin binding
  - Tyrosine 3-monooxygenase activity

+ Biological process:
  - Anatomical structure morphogenesis
  - Catecholamine biosynthetic process
  - Cellular nitrogen compound metabolic process
  - Cellular reponse to drug
  - Cellular response to glucose stimulus
  - Cellular response to growth factor stimulus
  - Cellular response to manganese ion
  - Cellular response to nicotine

- Cerebral cortex development
- Circadian cycle
- Dopamine biosynthetic process
- Dopamine biosynthetic process from tyrosine
- Eating behavior
- Embryonic camera-type eye morphogenesis
- Epinepherine biosynthetic process
- Eye photoreceptor cell development
- Fatty acid metabolic process
- Glycoside metabolic process
- Heart development
- Heart morphogenesis
- Isoquinolin alkaloid metabolic process
- Learning
- Locomotory behavior
- Mating behavior
- Memory
- Multicellular organismal aging
- Neurotransmitter biosynthetic process
- Pigmentation
- Regulation of heart contraction
- Response to activity
- Response to amphetamine
- Response to corticosterone
- Response to electrical stimulation
- Response to estradiol
- Response to ethanol
- Response to ether
- Response to herbicide
- Response to hypoxia
- Response to immobilization stress
- Response to light stimulus
- Response to lipopolysaccharide
- Response to nutrient levels

- Response to peptide hormone
- Response to prethroid
- Response to salt stress
- Response to water deprivation
- Response to zinc
- Sensory perception of sound
- Small molecule metabolic process
- Social behavior
- Sphingolipid metabolic process
- Synaptic transmitssion, dopaminergic
- Synaptic vesicle amine transport
- Terpene metabolic process
- Visual perception

+ Cellular component:

- Cytoplasm
- Cytoplasmic side of plasma membrane
- Cytoplasmic vesicle
- Cytosol
- Dendrite
- Melanosome membrane
- Mitochondrian
- Neuron projection
- Nucleus
- Perikaryon
- Smooth endoplasmic reticulum
- Synaptic vesical
- Terminal bouton

http://www.uniprot.org/uniprot/P07101

+ Associated disease:

- Segawa syndrome autosomal recessive - A form of dystonia that presents in infancy or early childhood. Dystonia is defined by the presence of sustained involuntary muscle contractions, often leading to abnormal postures. Some cases present with Parkinsonian symptoms in infancy. Unlike all other forms of dystonia, it is a treatable condition, due to a favorable response to L-DOPA.

http://www.ncbi.nlm.nih.gov/pubmed/9613851

TPH1/TPH2

+ <u>Overview for TPH1</u> *Tryptophan 5-hydroxylase 1, Tryptophan 5-hydroxylase 2,* TPH1, encodes the neurotransmitter synthesizing enzyme tryptophan 5-hydroxylase 1 that synthesizes serotonin from L-tryptophan.

- ❖ **NOTE**: Serotonin is primarily found in the GI tract, blood platelets, and the central nervous system (CNS). It is popularly thought to be a contributor to feelings of well-being and happiness. Approximately ninety percent of the human body's serotonin is located in the enterochromaffin cells within the GI tract, where it is used to regulate intestinal movements. The remainder is synthesized in serotonergic neurons of the CNS, where it has various functions, including the regulation of mood, appetite, and sleep. Serotonin also has some cognitive functions, including memory and learning.

https://en.wikipedia.org/wiki/Serotonin

+ In nondiabetic controls, SNPs of TPH1 were associated with waist circumference and BMI. It was also found that a variant of TPH1 (rs623580) was associated with BMI in a genome-wide association study comprised of 8,842 subjects. Although genetic variants in HTR2B and TPH1 were not associated with risk of gestational diabetes mellitus, we found significant association of these variants with measures of obesity.

http://www.ncbi.nlm.nih.gov/pubmed/21836641

+ TPH1 was first discovered to synthesize serotonin in 1988. It was thought that there was only a single TPH gene until 2003, when a second form was found in the human brain (TPH2).

+ One human mutant of TPH1, A218C found in intron 7, is highly associated with schizophrenia. Introns are regions of DNA that do not code for the amino acid sequence of a protein and were long considered to be 'junk DNA', lacking purpose.

https://www.ncbi.nlm.nih.gov/pubmed/18583979

+ TPH1 is expressed in the body, but not the brain. Nevertheless the effect of variations in the TPH1 gene on brain-related variables, such as personality traits and neuropsychiatric disorders, has been studied. For example, one study (1998) found an association between a polymorphism in the gene with impulsive-aggression traits.

https://www.ncbi.nlm.nih.gov/pubmed/9514581

+ Catalytic activity:

- L-tryptophan + tetrahydrobiopterin + O2 = 5-hydroxy-L-tryptophan + 4a-hydroxytetrahydrobiopterin

+ Cofactor:

- Iron

+ Pathway: Serotonin biosynthesis
  - This protein is involved in the two steps of the subpathway that synthesizes serotonin from L-tryptophan.
  - Proteins known to be involved in the two steps of the subpathway in this organism are:
  –Tryptophan 5-hydroxylase 2 (TPH2), Tryptophan 5-hydroxylase 2 (TPH1)

+ Molecular function:
  - Amino acid binding
  - Iron ion binding
  - Tryptophan 5-monoxygenase activity

+ Biological process:
  - Aromatic amino acid family metabolic process
  - Bone remodeling
  - Cellular nitrogen coumpound metabolic process
  - Circadian rhythm
  - Indolalkylamine biosynthetic process
  - Mammary gland alveolus development
  - Negative regulation of ossification
  - Positive regulation of fat cell differentiation
  - Response to immobilization stress
  - Serotonin biosynthetic process
  - Small molecule process

+ Cellular component:
  - Cytosol
  - Neuron projection

http://www.uniprot.org/uniprot/P17752

Section 3.2.1 – Other SNPs Related to Neurotransmitters

DTNBP1

+ **Overview for DTNBP1** *Dystrobrevin binding protein* (aka, Alternative names for Dysbindin are Biogenesis of lysosome-related organelles complex 1 subunit 8, BLOC-1 subunit 8, Dysbindin-1, Dystrobrevin-binding protein 1, Hermansky-Pudlak syndrome 7 protein and HPS7 protein), DTNBP1, rs1018381 (aka, C11202T), rs2619522 (aka, T14623G)

- This gene encodes a protein that may play a role in organelle biogenesis associated with melanosomes, platelet dense granules, and lysosomes. A similar protein in mice is a component of a protein complex termed, biogenesis of lysosome-related organelles complex 1 (BLOC-1), and binds to alpha- and beta-dystrobrevins, which are components of the dystrophin-associated protein complex (DPC). Mutations in this gene are associated with Hermansky-Pudlak syndrome type 7.

http://www.genecards.org/cgi-bin/carddisp.pl?gene=DTNBP1

+ Dysbindin is a component of the BLOC-1 complex, a complex that is required for normal biogenesis of lysosome-related organelles (LRO), such as platelet dense granules and melanosomes. It plays a role in synaptic vesicle trafficking and in neurotransmitter release. DTPNBP1 also regulates cell surface exposure of DRD2. It may play a role in actin cytoskeleton reorganization and neurite outgrowth. And may modulate MAPK8 phosphorylation. This gene promotes neuronal transmission and viability through regulating the expression of SNAP25 and SYN1, modulating PI3-kinase-Akt signaling and influencing glutamatergic release. DTNPB1 regulates the expression of SYN1 through binding to its promoter. It modulates prefrontal cortical activity via the dopamine/D2 pathway.

http://www.uniprot.org/uniprot/Q96EV8

+ Hermansky-Pudlak syndrome, also known as, HPS, is a disorder characterized by oculocutaneous albinism, bleeding due to platelet storage pool deficiency, and lysosomal storage defects. Ceroid storage in the lungs is associated with pulmonary fibrosis and is common with HPS.

+ Defects in DTNBP1 are associated with susceptibility to schizophrenia.
    - Genetic mutations lead to alterations in the glutamatergic transmission in the brain and modified Akt signaling. Protein levels and expression are reduced in nerve terminals of the hippocampus and there is an increased release of glutamate in schizophrenic patients.

http://www.uniprot.org/uniprot/Q96EV8
    - Genetic variation dystrobrevin-binding protein 1 has recently been shown to be associated with schizophrenia.

http://www.ncbi.nlm.nih.gov/pubmed/15345706

+ DTNBP1 also plays a role in synaptic vesicle trafficking and in neurotransmitter release.
+ Plays a role in the regulation of cell surface exposure of DRD2.

http://www.genecards.org/cgi-bin/carddisp.pl?gene=DTNBP1

+ "Cognitive functions are highly heritable and the impact of complex genetic interactions.... In healthy volunteers (N=176) studied with functional magnetic resonance imaging during a working memory paradigm, individuals homozygous for the COMT rs4680 Met allele that reduces COMT enzyme activity showed a relatively more efficient prefrontal engagement. In contrast, we found that the same genotype was less efficient on the background of a dys haplotype associated with decreased DTNBP1 expression."

http://www.nature.com/mp/journal/v19/n3/full/mp2013133a.html

+ Biological process:
- Actin cytoskeleton reorganization
- Anterograde synaptic vesicle transport
- Melanosome organization
- Neuron projection development
- Platelet dense granule organization
- Positive regulation of neurotransmitter secretion
- Regulation of dopamine receptor signaling pathway
- Anterograde axon cargo transport
- Blood coagulation
- Membrane organization
- Neuron projection morphogenesis
- Positive regulation of gene expression
- Post-Golgi vesicle-mediated transport and
- Regulation of dopamine secretion

http://www.ebi.ac.uk/QuickGO/GTerm?id=GO:0014059

+ Subcellular location:
- Cytoplasm
- Cytoplasmic vesicle membrane; peripheral membrane protein; cytoplasmic side
- Endosome membrane; peripheral membrane protein; cytoplasmic side
- Melanosome membrane; peripheral membrane protein; cytoplasmic side
- Cell junction > synapse > postsynaptic cell membrane > postsynaptic density
- Endoplasmic reticulum
- Nucleus

❖ **NOTE**: There are three isoforms distributed between cytoplasm and nucleus.

+ Cellular component:
- Axon
- BLOC-1 complex
- Cell junction
- Cytoplasm
- Cytosol
- Dedritic spine

- Endoplasmic reticulum membrane
- Endosome membrane
- Growth cone
- Melanosome membrane
- Neuron projection
- Nucleus
- Postsynaptic density
- Postsynaptic membrane
- Sarcolemma
- Sarcoplasm
- Synaptic vesicle membrane

http://www.uniprot.org/uniprot/Q96EV8

+ Associated disease:

- Hermansky-Pudiak syndrome 7- A genetically heterogeneous autosomal recessive disorder characterized by oculocutaneous albinism, bleeding due to platelet storage pool deficiency, and lysosomal storage defects. This syndrome results from defects of diverse cytoplasmic organelles including melanosomes, platelet dense granules, and lysosomes. Ceroid storage in the lungs is associated with pulmonary fibrosis, a common cause of premature death in individuals with HPS.

http://www.ncbi.nlm.nih.gov/pubmed/12923531

- Defects in DTNBP1 are associated with susceptibility to schizophrenia, a mental disorder characterized by a breakdown of thought processes and by poor emotional responsiveness. Genetic mutations lead to alterations in the glutamatergic transmisssion in the brain and modified Akt signaling.

http://www.ncbi.nlm.nih.gov/pubmed/?term=15345706

- Protein levels and expression are reduced in nerve terminals of the hippocampus and there is an increased release of glutamate in schizophrenic patients.

http://www.ncbi.nlm.nih.gov/pubmed/?term=15124027

- Levels of isoform 1 are reduced in the pSTG, but not in HF, by about forty-eight percent in ninety-two percent of schizophrenic patients. In the HF, there is an average of thirty-three percent reduction in synaptic expression of isoform 2 in sixty-seven percent of cases, and of isoform 3, an average reduction of thirty-five percent, in eighty percent of cases. In the dorsolateral prefrontal cortex (DLPFC), significant reductions in levels of isoform 3 are observed; about seventy-one percent of schizophrenic patients showed an average reduction of about sixty percent of this isoform.

http://www.ncbi.nlm.nih.gov/pubmed/?term=19617633

IDO1

+ **Overview for IDO1** *Indoleamine 2,3-dioxygenase*, IDO1, rs7820268 (aka, 6202T), rs35099072 (aka, G344A). aka, Indoleamine 2,3-Dioxygenase 1, INDO, IDO, Indoleamine-Pyrrole 2,3-Dioxygenase, IDO-1, Indoleamine-Pyrrole 2,3 Dioxygenase, Indolamine 2,3 Dioxygenase, Indole 2,3-Dioxygenase (Note the connection to pyrroles)

- IDO1 is a heme enzyme that catalyzes the first and rate-limiting step in tryptophan catabolism to N-formyl-kynurenine, through the kynurenine pathway, thus causing depletion of tryptophan. It can also result in halted growth of microbes as well as T-cells, so has a protective role, but at the cost of lowering tryptophan.
- ➢ **Our Two Cents** – If you see a high kynurenic acid marker on a test such as, NutrEval from Genova Diagnostics, look for a source of inflammation/infection and address it. You may also see high quinolinic acid (produced by active microglia and macrophages) as well, which is an NMDA receptor stimulator (glutamate). I see this often in children on the spectrum, as it results in "stim" behavior. Calcium channels are involved as well. Again, look for source of inflammation; mostly GI. Dietary restriction of inflammatory foods that include gluten/gliadin and cow dairy is often helpful in reducing IDO activity that causes "high-jacking" of tryptophan away from serotonin and melatonin production.
- ❖ **NOTE**: Quinolinic acid has a potent neurotoxic effect. Studies have demonstrated that quinolinic acid may be involved in many psychiatric disorders, neurodegenerative processes in the brain, as well as other disorders.

+ The IDO enzyme is thought to play a role in a variety of pathophysiological processes such as antimicrobial and antitumor defense, neuropathology, immunoregulation, and antioxidant activity. Through its expression in dendritic cells, monocytes, and macrophages this enzyme modulates T-cell behavior by its peri-cellular catabolization of the essential amino acid tryptophan. Human tumors constitutively express IDO.
http://www.omim.org/entry/147435
+ IDO enzyme acts on multiple tryptophan substrates including D-tryptophan, L-tryptophan, 5-hydroxy-tryptophan, tryptamine, and serotonin.
http://www.ncbi.nlm.nih.gov/gene/3620
http://www.ncbi.nlm.nih.gov/pmc/articles/PMC3850167/
+ Gamma-interferon has an antiproliferative effect on many tumor cells and inhibits intracellular pathogens such as toxoplasma and chlamydia, at least partly because of the induction of

indoleamine 2,3-dioxygenase. This enzyme catalyzes the degradation of the essential amino acid, L-tryptophan to N-formyl-kynurenine.

+ When T-cells are deprived of tryptophan, they arrest at a mid-G1 phase of the cell cycle. Restoring tryptophan does not restore the activation process, which requires a second round of T-cell receptor signaling along with tryptophan. Together, this information has suggested that antigen-presenting cells can employ IDO1 to restrict T-cell activation by blocking T-cell proliferation, due to tryptophan catabolism.

http://atlasgeneticsoncology.org/Genes/IDO1ID40973ch8p11.html

+ A wide range of human cancers, such as, prostatic, colorectal, pancreatic, cervical, gastric, ovarian, head, lung, etc. overexpress human IDO1.

http://en.wikipedia.org/wiki/Indoleamine_2,3-dioxygenase

+ Catalytic activity:

D-tryptophan + O_2 = N-formyl-D-kynurenine

L-tryptophan + O_2 = N-formyl-L-kynurenine.

+ The catalytic efficiency for L-tryptophan is one-hundred fifty times higher than for D-tryptophan.

+ Cofactor
- Heme

+ Pathway:
- Amino-acid degradation
- L-tryptophan degradation via kynurenine pathway
- L-kynurenine from L-tryptophan

+ Molecular function:
- Electron carrier activity
- Indoleamine 2,3-dioxygenase activity
- Tryptophan 2,3-deoxygenase activity
- Heme binding
- Metal ion binding

+ Biological process:
- Cellular nitrogen compound metabolic process
- Female pregnancy
- Multicellular organismal response to stress
- Negative regulation of T-cell apoptotic
- Positive regulation of chronic inflammatory response

- Positive regulation of T-cell apoptotic process
- Positive regulation of type 2 immune response
- Small molecule metabolic process
- Tryptophen catabolic process
- Cytokine production involved in inflammatory response
- Kynurenic acid biosynthesis
- Negative regulation of interleukin-10 production
- Positive regulation of interleukin-12 production
- Positive regulation of T-cell tolerance induction
- Response to lipopolysaccharide
- Tryptophan catabolic process to kynurenine

http://www.uniprot.org/uniprot/P14902

+ The enzyme regulation activity for IDO1 is inhibited by and MTH-trp (methylthiohydantoin-DL-tryptophan), modestly inhibited by L-1MT (1-methyl-L-tryptophan).

http://www.omim.org/entry/147435

Chapter 4

Mitochodria – Electron Transport Chain (ETC)

Section 4.1 - Review of mitochondria basics

Mitochondria are the cell's power plants and convert energy from food (e.g., fatty acids, amino acids, and glucose) into adenosine triphosphate (ATP) a chemical energy usable by the cell. Located in the cytoplasm, they are the sites of cellular respiration, which ultimately generates fuel for the cell's activities and "housekeeping" for that particular cell.

Metabolic processes that use ATP as an energy source convert it back into its precursors. ATP is therefore, continuously recycled in organisms: the human body, which on average contains only 250 grams (8.8 oz) of ATP, turns over its own body weight equivalent in ATP each day. https://en.wikipedia.org/wiki/Adenosine_triphosphate

The number of mitochondria in a cell can vary widely by tissue and cell type. For example, red blood cells have no mitochondria, whereas liver cells can have more than two thousand.

Mitochondria are bounded by a double membrane, with each of these membranes composed of a phospholipid bilayer with embedded proteins. Mitochondrial proteins vary, depending on the tissue and the species. In humans, six hundred fifteen distinct types of protein have been identified from cardiac mitochondria.
https://www.ncbi.nlm.nih.gov/pubmed/12592411

The outermost membrane is smooth while the inner membrane has many folds. These folds are called cristae. The folds enhance the "productivity" of cellular respiration by increasing the available surface area.

The double membranes divide the mitochondrion into two distinct parts: the intermembrane space and the mitochondrial matrix. The intermembrane space is the narrow part between the two membranes while the mitochondrial matrix is the part enclosed by the innermost membrane. Several of the steps in cellular respiration occur in the matrix due to its high concentration of enzymes.

Mitochondria are semi-autonomous in that they are only partially dependent on the cell to replicate and grow. They have their own DNA and ribosomes; so can therefore make their own proteins. Further, its DNA shows substantial similarity to bacterial genomes.
https://www.ncbi.nlm.nih.gov/pubmed/12594925

In a nutshell, generation of ATP is a multistep process, but can be broken down into two primary steps; the Krebs cycle (aka, citric acid cycle) and the electron transport chain. The Krebs cycle has as its inputs, fatty acids, glucose, and amino acids and utilizes acetyl CoA to enable the molecules from fatty acids, glucose, and amino acids (digested food) to enter the cycle. Although many intermediary byproducts are generated, the primary output of the Krebs cycle is NADH and FADH2. NADH then enters complex 1 while FADH2 enter complex 2 of the electron transport chain. CoQ10 (ubiquinone) is a cofactor. The enzymes of each complex (e.g., NDUFS3) are used as NADH and FADH2 are passed and converted along the electron transport chain to eventually generate ATP. The electrical gradient provided by the inner and outer mitochondrial membrane is an important factor for electron transport chain function, so healthy cell membranes are key (SNPs associated with phospholipid transformation, and good bile production should be considered). In addition, antioxidants and SOD are utilized to quell oxidation that occurs during ATP production and to protect mitochondrial DNA from damage.

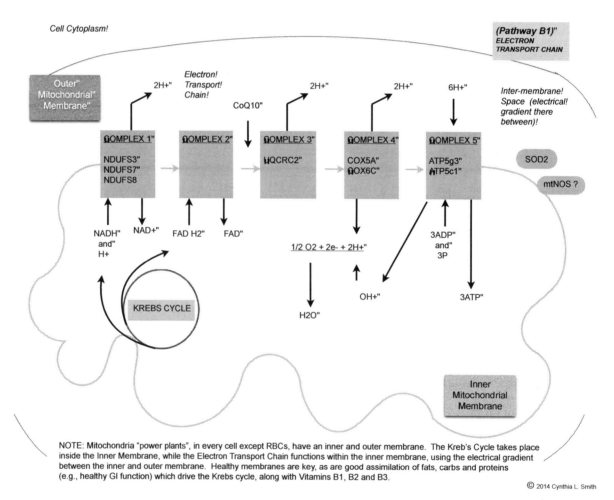

FIGURE 8 – Mitochondria- Electron Transport Chain

Section 4.2 – Mitochondria SNPs

Section 4.2.1 – Mitochondria SNPs Complex I – CoQ10 is required

NDUFS3

+ **Overview for NDUFS3** *NADH dehydrogenase [ubiquinone] iron-sulfur protein 3, mitochondrial,* NDUFS3, rs2233354, rs4147730, rs4147731, encode NADH dehydrogenase [ubiquinone] iron-sulfur protein 3, mitochondrial.

- NADH dehydrogenase [ubiquinone] iron-sulfur protein 3 is a core subunit of the mitochondrial membrane respiratory chain NADH dehydrogenase (complex I) that is believed to belong to the minimal assembly required for catalysis. Complex I functions in the transfer of electrons from NADH to the respiratory chain. The immediate electron acceptor for the enzyme is believed to be ubiquinone.

+ Mutations in the NDUFS3 gene are associated with mitochondrial complex I deficiency, which is autosomal recessive. This deficiency is the most common enzymatic defect of the oxidative phosphorylation disorders.

https://www.ncbi.nlm.nih.gov/pubmed/15372108

+ Mitochondrial complex I deficiency shows extreme genetic heterogeneity and can be caused by mutation in nuclear-encoded genes or in mitochondrial-encoded genes. There are no obvious genotype-phenotype correlations, and inference of the underlying basis from the clinical or biochemical presentation is difficult, if not impossible. However, the majority of cases are caused by mutations in nuclear-encoded genes.

https://www.ncbi.nlm.nih.gov/pubmed/10649489

+ Complex 1 deficiencies may be associated with clinical disorders, ranging from lethal neonatal disease to adult-onset neurodegenerative disorders. Phenotypes include macrocephaly with progressive leukodystrophy, nonspecific encephalopathy, hypertrophic cardiomyopathy, myopathy, liver disease, Leigh syndrome, Leber hereditary optic neuropathy, and some forms of Parkinson's disease.

https://www.ncbi.nlm.nih.gov/pubmed/9593934

+ Catalytic activity:
- NADH + ubiquinone + 5 H+(In) = NAD+ + ubiquinol + 4 H+(Out)
- NADH + acceptor = NAD+ + reduced acceptor

+ Molecular function:
- Electron carrier activity
- NADH dehydrogenase (ubiquinone) activity

- NADH dehydrogenase activity

+ Biological process:
  - Cellular metabolic process
  - Mitochondrial electron transport, NADH to ubiquinone
  - Negative regulation of cell growth
  - Negative regulation of intrinsic apoptotic signaling pathway
  - Reactive oxygen species metabolic process
  - Respiratory electron transport chain
  - Small molecule metabolic process
  - Substantia nigra development

+ Subcellular location:
  - Mitochondrial inner membrane

+ Cellular component:
  - Mitochondrial inner membrane
  - Mitochondrial membrane
  - Mitochondrial respiratory chain complex I
  - Mitochondrian
  - Myelin sheath
  - Nucleus

http://www.uniprot.org/uniprot/O75489

NDUFS7

+ **Overview for NDUFS7** *NADH dehydrogenase [ubiquinone] iron-sulfur protein 7, mitochondrial* (aka, NADH-ubiquinone oxidoreductase 20 kDa subunit), NDUFS7, rs1142530, rs11666067, rs2074895, rs2332496, rs7254913, rs7258846, rs809359, encode NADH dehydrogenase [ubiquinone] iron-sulfur protein 7, mitochondrial.

- The NDUFS7 protein is a subunit of NADH dehydrogenase (ubiquinone) that is located in the mitochondrial inner membrane and is the largest of the five complexes of the electron transport.

https://www.ncbi.nlm.nih.gov/pubmed/22484275

+ Catalytic activity:
  - NADH + ubiquinone + 5 H+(In) = NAD+ + ubiquinol + 4 H+(Out)
  - NADH + acceptor = NAD+ + reduced acceptor

+ Cofactor:
  - [4Fe-4S] cluster   Binds one [4Fe-4S] cluster

+ Molecular function:
- 4 iron, 4 sulfur cluster binding
- Metal ion binding
- NADH dehydrogenase (ubiquinone) activity
- Oxidoreductase activity, acting on NAD(P)H, quinone or similar compound as acceptor
- Quinone binding

+ Biological process:
- Cellular metabolic process
- Mitochondrial electron transport, NADH to ubiquinone
- Mitochondrial respiratory chain complex I assembly
- Respiratory electron transport chain
- Small molecule metabolic process

+ Subcellular location:
- Mitochondrial inner membrane

+ Cellular component:
- Mitochondrial inner membrane
- Mitochondrial respiratory chain complex I
- Neuronal cell body
- Neuron projection
- Synaptic membrane

http://www.uniprot.org/uniprot/O75251

+ Associated disease:
- Leigh syndrome - An early-onset progressive neurodegenerative disorder characterized by the presence of focal, bilateral lesions in one or more areas of the central nervous system, including the brainstem, thalamus, basal ganglia, cerebellum, and spinal cord. Clinical features depend on which areas of the central nervous system are involved and include subacute onset of psychomotor retardation, hypotonia, ataxia, weakness, vision loss, eye movement abnormalities, seizures, and dysphagia.

http://www.ncbi.nlm.nih.gov/pubmed/10360771

NDUFS8

+ **Overview for NDUFS8** *NADH dehydrogenase [ubiquinone] iron-sulfur protein 8, mitochondrial* (aka, NADH-ubiquinone oxidoreductase 23 kDa subunit), NDUFS8, rs1051806, rs1104739, rs1122731, rs2075626, rs3115546, rs4147776, rs999571, encodes NADH dehydrogenase [ubiquinone] iron-sulfur protein 8, mitochondrial.

- NDUFS8 encodes a subunit of mitochondrial NADH: ubiquinone oxidoreductase, or complex I, a multimeric enzyme of the respiratory chain responsible for NADH oxidation, ubiquinone reduction, and the ejection of protons from mitochondria.

https://en.wikipedia.org/wiki/NDUFS8

+ Molecular function:
- 4 iron, 4 sulfur cluster binding
- Metal ion binding

http://www.uniprot.org/uniprot/Q08E91

Section 4.2.2 – Mitochondria SNPs – Complex III

UQCRC2

+ **Overview for UQCRC2** *Cytochrome b-c1 complex subunit II, mitochondrial,* UQCRC2, rs11648723, rs12922362, rs2965803, rs4850, rs6497563, encodes Cytochrome b-c1 complex subunit II, mitochondrial.

- Its gene product is a subunit of the respiratory chain protein ubiquinol cytochrome c reductase (UQCR, Complex III or Cytochrome bc1 complex), which consists of the products of one mitochondrially-encoded gene, MTCYTB (mitochondrial cytochrome b) and ten nuclear genes.

https://en.wikipedia.org/wiki/UQCRC2

+ This is a component of the ubiquinol-cytochrome c reductase complex (complex III or cytochrome b-c1 complex), which is part of the mitochondrial respiratory chain. The core protein 2 is required for the assembly of the complex.

+ Molecular function:
- Metal ion binding
- Metalloendopeptidase activity

+ Biological process:
- Aerobic respiration
- Cellular metabolic process

- Oxidative phosphorylation
- Respiratory electron transport chain
- Small molecule metabolic process

+ Cellular component:
- Extracellular exosome
- Mitochondrial inner membrane
- Mitochondrial respiratory chain complex III
- Mitochondrian
- Myelin sheath

http://www.uniprot.org/uniprot/P22695

+ Associated disease:
- Mitochondrial complex III deficiency, nuclear 5 - A disorder of the mitochondrial respiratory chain resulting in a highly variable phenotype depending on which tissues are affected. Clinical features include, mitochondrial encephalopathy, psychomotor retardation, ataxia, severe failure to thrive, liver dysfunction, renal tubulopathy, muscle weakness, and exercise intolerance.

http://www.ncbi.nlm.nih.gov/pubmed/23281071

Section 4.2.3 – Mitochondria SNPs – Complex IV

COX5A

+ **Overview for COX5A** *Cytochrome c oxidase subunit 5a,* COX5A, rs8042694, encodes cytochrome *c* oxidase subunit 5a.
- Its gene product is a subunit of the cytochrome c oxidase complex, also known as complex IV, the last enzyme in the mitochondrial electron transport chain.
- This is the heme A-containing chain of cytochrome c oxidase, the terminal oxidase in mitochondrial electron transport.

+ During oxidative stress, Bcl-2 moderates mitochondrial respiration through cytochrome c oxidase (COX) activity to prevent an excessive buildup of reactive oxygen species (ROS) by-production from electron transport activities.

https://www.ncbi.nlm.nih.gov/pubmed/19834492

+ Molecular function:
- Cytochrome-c oxidase activity

- Electron carrier activity
- Metal ion binding

+ Biological process:

- Cellular metabolic process
- Gene expression
- Hydrogen ion transmembrane transport
- Respiratory electron transport chain
- Small molecule metabolic process
- Transcription initiation from RNA polymerase II promoter

+ Cellular component:

- Extracellular exosome
- Mitochondrial inner membrane
- Myelin sheath

http://www.uniprot.org/uniprot/P20674

COX6C

+ **Overview for COX6C** *Cytochrome c oxidase subunit 6c,* COX6C, rs1135382, rs12544943, rs4510829, rs4518636, rs4626565, rs7828241, rs7844439, encodes Cytochrome *c* oxidase subunit 5c.

- Cytochrome c oxidase (COX), the terminal enzyme of the mitochondrial respiratory chain, catalyzes the electron transfer from reduced cytochrome c to oxygen. It is a heteromeric complex consisting of 3 catalytic subunits encoded by mitochondrial genes and multiple structural subunits encoded by nuclear genes. The mitochondrially-encoded subunits function in electron transfer, and the nuclear-encoded subunits may be involved in the regulation and assembly of the complex. This nuclear gene encodes subunit VIc, which has seventy-seven percent amino acid sequence identity with mouse COX subunit VIc. This gene is up-regulated in prostate cancer cells. A pseudogene COX6CP1 has been found on chromosomes 16p12.

https://www.ncbi.nlm.nih.gov/pubmed/10072584

+ Lung epithelial cells resist influenza-A infection by inducing the expression of cytochrome c oxidase 6c, which is modulated by miRNA 4276.

https://www.ncbi.nlm.nih.gov/pubmed/25203353

+ Molecular function:

- Cytochrome-c oxidase activity

+ Biological process:

- Cellular metabolic process
- Gene expression
- Generation of precursor metabolites and energy
- Respiratory electron transport chain
- Small molecule metabolic process
- Transcription initiation from RNA polymerase II promoter

+ Subcellular location:
- Mitochondrial inner membrane

+ Cellular component:
- Integral component of membrane
- Mitochondrial inner membrane
- Mitochondrion

http://www.uniprot.org/uniprot/P09669

Section 4.2.4 – Mitochondria SNPs – Complex V

ATP5c1

+ **Overview for ATP5c1** *Mitochondrial ATP synthase,* ATP5c1, rs1244414, rs1244422, rs12770829, rs2778475, rs4655, encodes mitochondrial ATP synthase.

- Mitochondrial ATP synthase catalyzes adenosine triphosphate synthesis, utilizing an electrochemical gradient of protons across the inner mitochondrial membrane during oxidative phosphorylation.

https://www.ncbi.nlm.nih.gov/pubmed/8227057

> **Our Two Cents**: The importance of maintaining healthy membranes, both cell and mitochondrial, cannot be overstated. Phospholipids and healthy fats are good. Transfats are not.

+ Mitochondrial membrane ATP synthase (F1F0 ATP synthase or complex V) produces ATP from ADP in the presence of a proton gradient across the membrane which is generated by electron transport complexes of the respiratory chain. F-type ATPases consist of two structural domains, F1 - containing the extramembraneous catalytic core, and F0 - containing the membrane proton channel, linked together by a central stalk and a peripheral stalk. During catalysis, ATP synthesis in the catalytic domain of F1 is coupled via a rotary mechanism of the central stalk subunits to proton translocation. Part of the complex F1 domain and the central stalk that is part of the complex rotary element. The gamma subunit protrudes into the catalytic domain formed of alpha3beta3. Rotation of the central stalk against the surrounding alpha3beta3 subunits leads to hydrolysis of ATP in three separate catalytic sites on the beta subunits.

+ Molecular function:
- Poly (A) RNA binding
- Proton-transporting ATPase, rotational mechanism
- Proton-transporting ATP synthase, rotational mechanism
- Transmembrane transporter activity

+ Biological process:
- ATP biosynthetic process
- Cellular metabolic process
- Mitochondrial ATP synthesis coupled proton transport
- Oxidative phosphorylation
- Respiratory electron transport chain
- Small molecule metabolic process

+ Cellular component:
- Extracellular exosome
- Membrane
- Mitochondrial inner membrane
- Mitochondrial matrix
- Mitochondrial proton-transporting ATP synthase complex
- Mitochondrian
- Myelin sheath

http://www.uniprot.org/uniprot/P36542

ATP5g3

+ **Overview for ATP5g3** *ATP synthase lipid-binding protein, mitochondrial,* ATP5g3, rs185584, rs36089250, encodes ATP synthase lipid-binding protein, mitochondrial.
- Mitochondrial ATP synthase catalyzes adenosine triphosphate synthesis, utilizing an electrochemical gradient of protons across the inner mitochondrial membrane during oxidative phosphorylation.

https://www.ncbi.nlm.nih.gov/pubmed/8227057

+ Molecular function:
- Hydrogen ion transmembrane transporter activity
- Lipid bindingy

+ Biological process:

- ATP hydrolysis coupled proton transport
- ATP synthesis coupled proton transport

+ Cellular component:
- Integral component of membrane
- Proton-transporting ATP synthase complex, coupling factor F(o)

http://www.uniprot.org/uniprot/Q6LEU9

Chapter 5

My Favorite Books

You can order most of the books directly from Amazon, or get them on Audible for your Iphone. I do both for my favorites, and listen to Audible while driving and cooking.

For GI Issues:

- ✓ The Second Brain, by David Gershon (basics of GI health)
  http://www.amazon.com/Second-Brain-Groundbreaking-Understanding-Disorders/dp/0060930721/ref=sr_1_sc_1?ie=UTF8&qid=1440990509&sr=8-1-spell&keywords=Second+btrain

- ✓ The Bullet Proof Diet, by Dave Asprey
  http://www.amazon.com/Bulletproof-Diet-Reclaim-Energy-Upgrade/dp/162336518X/ref=sr_1_3?ie=UTF8&qid=1440990966&sr=8-3&keywords=Bullet+proof

- ✓ NOTE: As an aside, there was recently a Holistic Oral Health Summit organized by Jonathan Landsman. Most of us rarely consider oral hygiene and connections to disease, but the connection between oral health, GI function and overall health is unrefutable. Here is a link to ordering the 33 talks from experts in the field.
- ✓ http://holisticoralhealthsummit.com/order/

For Auto-immune Issues:

- ✓ Why Isn't My Brain Working?, by Datis http://www.amazon.com/Isnt-Brain-Working-Revolutionary-Understanding/dp/0985690437/ref=sr_1_2?ie=UTF8&qid=1440990605&sr=8-2&keywords=Datis

- ✓ Why Do I Still Have Thyroid Symptoms?, by Datis
  http://www.amazon.com/Still-Thyroid-Symptoms-Tests-Normal/dp/0985690402/ref=sr_1_1?ie=UTF8&qid=1440990605&sr=8-1&keywords=Datis

- ✓ I highly recommend ordering the Audible version, as you will want to listen and relisten. Besides being kind, Datis is brilliant so his books are full of well-reaserched info.

- ✓ The Autoimmune Solution, by Amy Meyers
  http://www.amazon.com/Autoimmune-Solution-Spectrum-Inflammatory-Symptoms/dp/0062347470/ref=sr_1_1?ie=UTF8&qid=1440990857&sr=8-1&keywords=Autoimmune

- ✓ The Bullet Proof Diet, by Dave Asprey
  http://www.amazon.com/Bulletproof-Diet-Reclaim-Energy-Upgrade/dp/162336518X/ref=sr_1_3?ie=UTF8&qid=1440990966&sr=8-3&keywords=Bullet+proof

For losing weight:

- ✓ The Belly Fat Effect, by Mike Mutzel (weight loss is the focus of the content, but really it's an excellent book about functional medicine application) http://www.amazon.com/Belly-Fat-Effect-Intestinal-Bacteria/dp/0991070313/ref=sr_1_1?ie=UTF8&qid=1440991018&sr=8-1&keywords=Mike+mutzel
- ✓ NOTE: Mike's wife, Deanna, is also publishing some great books and instagram postings on nutrition and recipes.

- ✓ The Bullet Proof Diet, by Dave Asprey
  http://www.amazon.com/Bulletproof-Diet-Reclaim-Energy-Upgrade/dp/162336518X/ref=sr_1_3?ie=UTF8&qid=1440990966&sr=8-3&keywords=Bullet+proof

- ✓ Snow Drop Herbals, The Healthy Mito (chondria) Cookbook, by Meggan Hurley for food recipes that address SNPs. Her next book is in the works.
  https://snowdropherbals.selz.com

- ✓ Sean Croxton's pod casts are another source of good info. His site is http://www.UndergroundWellness.com

Made in the USA
San Bernardino, CA
23 July 2019